**1991**
**YEAR BOOK OF**
**EMERGENCY MEDICINE**®

# The 1991 Year Book® Series

Year Book of Anesthesia®: Drs. Miller, Kirby, Ostheimer, Roizen, and Stoelting

Year Book of Cardiology®: Drs. Schlant, Collins, Engle, Frye, Kaplan, and O'Rourke

Year Book of Critical Care Medicine®: Drs. Rogers and Parrillo

Year Book of Dentistry®: Drs. Meskin, Currier, Kennedy, Leinfelder, Matukas, and Rovin

Year Book of Dermatology®: Drs. Sober and Fitzpatrick

Year Book of Diagnostic Radiology®: Drs. Reed, Hendee, Keats, Kirkpatrick, Miller, Osborn, and Thompson

Year Book of Digestive Diseases®: Drs. Greenberger and Moody

Year Book of Drug Therapy®: Drs. Lasagna and Weintraub

Year Book of Emergency Medicine®: Drs. Wagner, Burdick, Davidson, Roberts, and Spivey

Year Book of Endocrinology®: Drs. Bagdade, Braverman, Halter, Horton, Kannan, Molitch, Morley, Odell, Rogol, Ryan, and Sherwin

Year Book of Family Practice®: Drs. Berg, Bowman, Dietrich, Green, and Scherger

Year Book of Geriatrics and Gerontology®: Drs. Beck, Abrass, Burton, Cummings, Makinodan, and Small

Year Book of Hand Surgery®: Drs. Dobyns, Chase, and Amadio

Year Book of Health Care Management: Drs. Heyssel, King, and Steinberg, Ms. Avakian, and Messrs. Berman, Brock, Kues, and Rosenberg

Year Book of Hematology®: Drs. Spivak, Bell, Ness, Quesenberry, and Wiernik

Year Book of Infectious Diseases®: Drs. Wolff, Barza, Keusch, Klempner, and Snydman

Year Book of Infertility: Drs. Mishell, Paulsen, and Lobo

Year Book of Medicine®: Drs. Rogers, Des Prez, Cline, Braunwald, Greenberger, Utiger, Epstein, and Malawista

Year Book of Neonatal and Perinatal Medicine: Drs. Klaus and Fanaroff

Year Book of Neurology and Neurosurgery®: Drs. Currier and Crowell

Year Book of Nuclear Medicine®: Drs. Hoffer, Gore, Gottschalk, Sostman, Zaret, and Zubal

Year Book of Obstetrics and Gynecology®: Drs. Mishell, Kirschbaum, and Morrow

1991

# The Year Book of EMERGENCY MEDICINE ®

Editor

**David K. Wagner, M.D.**
*Professor and Chairman, Department of Emergency Medicine, The Medical College of Pennsylvania, Philadelphia, Pennsylvania*

Associate Editors

**William P. Burdick, M.D.**
*Associate Professor, Department of Emergency Medicine; Assistant Professor, Department of Internal Medicine; The Medical College of Pennsylvania, Philadelphia, Pennsylvania*

**Steven J. Davidson, M.D.**
*Professor, Department of Emergency Medicine, The Medical College of Pennsylvania, Philadelphia, Pennsylvania*

**James R. Robert, M.D.**
*Associate Professor of Emergency Medicine, The Medical College of Pennsylvania; Chairman, Department of Emergency Medicine, Mercy Catholic Medical Center, Philadelphia, Pennsylvania*

**William H. Spivey, M.D.**
*Assistant Professor, Department of Emergency Medicine, The Medical College of Pennsylvania, Philadelphia, Pennsylvania*

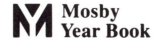

**Mosby Year Book**

St. Louis    Baltimore    Boston    Chicago    London    Philadelphia    Sydney    Toronto

Editor-in-Chief, Year Book Publishing: Nancy Gorham
Sponsoring Editors: Rebecca A. Ede
Senior Medical Information Specialist: Terri Strorigl
Assistant Director, Manuscript Services: Frances M. Perveiler
Associate Managing Editor, Year Book Editing Services: Elizabeth Fitch
Production Coordinator: Max F. Perez
Proofroom Supervisor: Barbara M. Kelly

Editorial Office:
Mosby–Year Book, Inc.
200 North LaSalle St.
Chicago, IL 60601

International Standard Serial Number: 0271-7964
International Standard Book Number:0-8151-9062-x

# Contributing Editors

**James T. Amsterdam, M.D., D.M.D.**
*Associate Professor of Emergency Medicine, Northeastern Ohio Universities College of Medicine, Chairman, Department of Emergency Medicine, Western Reserve Care System, Youngstown*

**Gail V. Anderson, M.D.**
*Professor and Chairman, Department of Emergency Medicine, University of Southern California School of Medicine, Los Angeles, California*

**David J. Cionni, M.D.**
*Instructor in Emergency Medicine, The Medical College of Pennsylvania, Philadelphia*

**Joseph E. Clinton, M.D.**
*Clinical Associate Professor of Emergency Medicine, Hennepin County Medical Center, Minneapolis*

**Frederick Henretig, M.D.**
*Associate Professor of Pediatrics, University of Pennsylvania School of Medicine, Children's Hospital of Philadelphia, Philadelphia*

**Jerome R. Hoffman, M.D.**
*Associate Professor of Medicine, Emergency Medicine Center, UCLA Medical Center, Los Angeles*

**William J. Koenig, M.D.**
*Assistant Director, Emergency Department, Long Beach Memorial Medical Center, Long Beach*

**Emily Jean Lucid, M.D.**
*Associate Professor, Division of Emergency Medicine, Medical College of Pennsylvania, Allegheny Campus, Allegheny General Hospital, Pittsburgh*

**Stephen Ludwig, M.D.**
*Professor of Pediatrics, University of Pennsylvania School of Medicine, Division Chief, General Pediatrics, Children's Hospital of Philadelphia, Philadelphia*

**Peter A. Maningus, M.D.**
*Executive Medical Director, Black Hills Institute for Prehospital Care, Rapid City*

**Robert M. McNamara, M.D.**
*Assistant Professor of Emergency Medicine, The Medical College of Pennsylvania, Philadelphia*

**Joyce M. Mitchell, M.D.**
*Assistant Professor and Associate Residency Director, Department of Emergency Medicine, East Carolina University School of Medicine, Pitt County Memorial Hospital, Greenville*

**James T. Niemann, M.D.**
*Director of Research, Department of Emergency Medicine, Los Angeles County-Harbor UCLA Medical Center, Torrance*

**Gary J. Ordog, M.D.**
*Assistant Professor of Emergency Medicine, University of California at Los Angeles, MLK/Drew Medical Center, Saugus*

**Harold H. Osborn, M.D.**
*Professor of Clinical Community and Preventive Medicine, New York Medical College, Our Lady of Mercy Medical Center, Bronx*

**Peter T. Pons, M.D.**
*Medical Director, Denver Paramedic Division, Department of Health and Hospitals, Denver General Hospital, Denver*

**Earl J. Reisdorff, M.D.**
*Assistant Clinical Professor and Assistant Residency Director—Education, Michigan State University, Emergency Medicine Residency, Ingham Medical Center, Lansing*

**Suzanne B. Repasky, D.O.**
*Assistant Professor of Emergency Medicine, The Medical College of Pennsylvania, Philadelphia*

**Ernest Ruiz, M.D.**
*Chief, Emergency Medicine, Department of Emergency Medicine, Hennepin County Medical Center, Minneapolis*

**Richard Rutstein, M.D.**
*Assistant Professor of Pediatrics and Medical Director, Special Immunology Service, Children's Hospital of Philadelphia, Philadelphia*

**Robert W. Schafermeyer, M.D.**
*Acting Chairman and Program Director, Department of Emergency Medicine, Carolinas Medical Center, Charlotte Memorial Hospital and Medical Center, Charlotte*

**John Schoffstall, M.D.**
*Assistant Professor of Emergency Medicine, The Medical College of Pennsylvania, Philadelphia*

**Kathy N. Shaw, M.D.**
*Attending Physician, Emergency Department, Children's Hospital of Philadelphia, Philadelphia*

**Thomas O. Stair, M.D.**
*Associate Professor of Emergency Medicine, Georgetown University School of Medicine, Washington, D.C.*

**Ellen H. Talafierro, M.D.**
*Associate Clinical Professor, Department of Surgery, Department of Emergency Services, San Francisco General Hospital, San Francisco*

**Henry D. Unger, M.D.**
*Assistant Professor of Emergency Medicine, The Medical College of Pennsylvania, Philadelphia*

**Suman Wason, M.D.**
*Associate Professor of Clinical Pediatrics and Emergency Medicine, University of Cincinnati, Toxicologist-in-Chief, Cincinnati Drug and Poison Information Center, Children's Hospital, Cincinnati*

# Table of Contents

The material in this volume represents literature reviewed up to April 1990.

# Journals Represented

Mosby–Year Book subscribes to and surveys nearly 850 U.S. and foreign medical and allied health journals. From these journals, the Editors select the articles to be abstracted. Journals represented in this YEAR BOOK are listed below.

Acta Dermato–Venereologica
Allergy
American Family Physician
American Heart Journal
American Journal of Cardiology
American Journal of Diseases of Children
American Journal of Emergency Medicine
American Journal of Medicine
American Journal of Obstetrics and Gynecology
American Journal of Public Health
American Journal of Roentgenology
American Journal of Sports Medicine
American Journal of Surgery
American Surgeon
Annales de Radiologie
Annals of Emergency Medicine
Annals of Internal Medicine
Annals of Surgery
Archives of Disease in Childhood
Archives of Emergency Medicine
Archives of Internal Medicine
Archives of Otolaryngology–Head and Neck Surgery
Archives of Surgery
British Journal of Radiology
British Medical Journal
Burns
Canadian Journal of Surgery
Chest
Circulation
Circulatory Shock
Clinical Chemistry
Clinical Imaging
Clinical Pediatrics
Clinical Pharmacology and Therapeutics
Clinical Radiology
Clinical and Laboratory Haematology
Critical Care Medicine
Ear, Nose, and Throat Journal
European Heart Journal
European Journal of Radiology
Foot and Ankle
Head and Neck
Human Toxicology
Injury
International Journal of Cardiology
Journal of Allergy and Clinical Immunology
Journal of Applied Physiology
Journal of Bone and Joint Surgery (American volume)

Journal of Bone and Joint Surgery (British volume)
Journal of Child Neurology
Journal of Clinical Investigation
Journal of Clinical Psychiatry
Journal of Clinical Ultrasound
Journal of Clinical and Experimental Neuropsychology
Journal of Emergency Medicine
Journal of Family Practice
Journal of Neurosurgery
Journal of Occupational Medicine
Journal of Oral and Maxillofacial Surgery
Journal of Orthopedic Trauma
Journal of Otolaryngology
Journal of Pediatric Surgery
Journal of Pediatrics
Journal of Thoracic and Cardiovascular Surgery
Journal of Trauma
Journal of Urology
Journal of Vascular Surgery
Journal of the American College of Cardiology
Journal of the American Geriatrics Society
Journal of the American Medical Association
Journal of the Royal College of Surgeons of Edinburgh
Lancet
Medical and Biological Engineering and Computing
Medicine and Science in Sports and Exercise
New England Journal of Medicine
New York State Journal of Medicine
Pediatric Emergency Care
Pediatric Infectious Disease Journal
Pediatric Radiology
Pediatrics
Physician and Sportsmedicine
Postgraduate Medical Journal
Postgraduate Medicine
Radiology
S.A.M.J./S.A.M.T.—South African Medical Journal
Southern Medical Journal
Stroke
Surgery
Urology
Western Journal of Medicine

---

### STANDARD ABBREVIATIONS

The following terms are abbreviated in this edition: acquired
immunodeficiency syndrome (AIDS), central nervous system (CNS),
cerebrospinal fluid (CSF), computed tomography (CT), electrocardiography
(ECG), and human immunodeficiency virus (HIV).

# Introduction

Clinical expertise in general emergency medicine continues to remain the dominant feature of the practicing emergency physician, but there appears to be an exponentially growing interest in the developing subspecialties of the discipline. As an example of that trend, the American Board of Emergency Medicine recently announced that it was in the early stages of considering credentialling criteria requirements in four such areas: pediatric emergency medicine, toxicology, prehospital care, and sports medicine. Further amplifying the trend toward subspecialization, the American College of Emergency Physicians has established, in addition to the aforementioned, an additional eight or ten sections, including observation medicine, occupational/industrial medicine, hyperbaric medicine, critical care medicine, and wilderness medicine. Such activities portend an expanded role of the emergency physician in the health care system wherever acute alteration of body form or function occurs.

In concert with this trend, your editor has identified leaders in emergency medicine who have particular expertise and interest in these developing subspecialties. These individuals have assumed the responsibility for the selection and oversight of material pertinent to their specific body of knowledge. These Associate Editors are Steven J. Davidson, M.D., who has assumed responsibility for prehospital care and EMS material; James R. Roberts, M.D., for toxicology; William H. Spivey, M.D., for basic research; and William P. Burdick, M.D., for critical care medicine. Each, in turn, will further identify contributing editors whose expertise can be expected to best represent current and contemporary thoughts and comments in the field.

The overall purpose of the YEAR BOOK OF EMERGENCY MEDICINE, namely, to be clinically focused and provide comments pertinent to the day-to-day practice of emergency medicine, continues. Rapid, accurate bedside diagnosis and treatment remain the hallmarks of exemplary emergency physician behavior. The YEAR BOOK is committed to enhance such a response.

Again, more than anyone else, one individual maintains the role of supervising manager of the manuscript. She is well known to all of us for her pleasant, yet persuasive means of keeping us relatively on time and always well organized. Thanks, again, from all of us to you, Rose! That's Rose G. Schulberger.

David K. Wagner, M.D.

# 1 Acute Systems Pathophysiology

## Cardiopulmonary, Cerebral Resuscitation

**Effect of Epinephrine on End-Tidal Carbon Dioxide Monitoring During CPR**
Martin GB, Gentile NT, Paradis NA, Moeggenberg J, Appleton TJ, Nowak RM
(Henry Ford Hosp, Detroit)
*Ann Emerg Med* 19:396–398, 1990                                     1–1

Coronary perfusion pressure (CPP) has been shown to correlate with survival in both animals and human beings. Recent studies have shown that end-tidal carbon dioxide ($ETCO_2$) is correlated with CPP during cardiopulmonary resuscitation (CPR). Monitoring of $ETCO_2$ during CPR therefore could be a useful noninvasive check of CPR efficacy. To measure the change in CPP and $ETCO_2$ after epinephrine administration during CPR, ventricular fibrillation was induced with a transthoracic electric shock in 6 dogs. At the end of 5 minutes of ventricular fibrillation without therapy, CPR was initiated. After 5 minutes of CPR, epinephrine was given intravenously in a dose of .045 mg/kg. The CPP and $ETCO_2$ were compared immediately before and 2 minutes after epinephrine administration.

The correlation between CPP and $ETCO_2$ before epinephrine administration was significant. Epinephrine caused a significant increase in CPP and a significant decrease in $ETCO_2$. However, the correlation between $ETCO_2$ and CPP after epinephrine administration was decreased.

That $ETCO_2$ is a good indicator of CPP during CPR was confirmed. However, the increases in CPP induced by intravenous administration of epinephrine were not reflected in the $ETCO_2$. Caution therefore must be taken when $ETCO_2$ is used to evaluate the efficacy of CPR after therapeutic administration of epinephrine.

▶ This paper raises a very important point, which is that $ETCO_2$ is significantly affected by circulating levels of epinephrine. As demonstrated in a previous paper by Kern et al. (see Abstract 1–8), there is wide variation in catecholamine levels in animals in cardiac arrest. This has also been shown to be true in a clinical series of patients undergoing resuscitation. It brings into question whether or not patients with high circulating epinephrine levels who are probably more likely to be resuscitated could, in fact, have a lower $ETCO_2$ than patients with lower catecholamine levels. Although the reverse of this has been shown in both animal and clinical studies, this paper does raise the theoretical concern that higher doses of both endogenous and exogenous epinephrine may alter the data that we get from an $ETCO_2$ monitor.—W.H. Spivey, M.D.

### Effects of Epinephrine and Norepinephrine on Cerebral Oxygen Delivery and Consumption During Open-Chest CPR

Lindner KH, Ahnefeld FW, Pfenninger EG, Schuermann W, Bowdler IM (Universität Ulm, Germany)
*Ann Emerg Med* 19:249–254, 1990                                            1–2

The duration of a cardiac arrest and the oxygenation of the cerebrum during subsequent cardiopulmonary resuscitation (CPR) both determine neurologic outcome. Epinephrine improves regional cerebral blood flow under these conditions. Recent experiments showed that resumption of spontaneous circulation after electrically induced ventricular fibrillation took significantly less time after administration of norepinephrine than after epinephrine administration. The effects of epinephrine and norepinephrine on cerebral oxygen delivery and consumption after 5 minutes of cardiopulmonary arrest and 3 minutes of open-chest CPR were compared.

Twenty-one anesthetized pigs in whom ventricular fibrillation was electrically induced were used. The animals were randomly divided into 3 groups of 7 animals each. After 3 minutes of open-chest CPR, 7 pigs were given saline solution, 7 were given 45 μg of epinephrine/kg and 7 were given 45 μg of norepinephrine/kg administered over 30 seconds.

Norepinephrine and epinephrine injections given after a 5-minute cardiac arrest and 3 minutes of CPR resulted in identical increases in cerebral oxygen delivery. Cerebral perfusion pressure with either drug was significantly higher than that with saline solution. Both drugs enhanced cerebral oxygen delivery more than cerebral oxygen consumption, and oxygen extraction decreased with both drugs under these conditions. There was no significant difference between the effects of epinephrine and norepinephrine on the cerebral delivery and consumption of oxygen and glucose. Because of its positive effect on cerebral oxygenation, the use of norepinephrine as an alternative to epinephrine for restoring spontaneous circulation after cardiac arrest should be further investigated.

▶ Although not stated by the investigators, I think this study was based on the premise or hypothesis that cerebral blood vessels would respond to exogenous catecholamines in the setting of cardiac arrest. Although cerebral vessels have adrenergic receptors, it is unclear what role they play in regulating brain blood flow under any physiologic circumstances, since cerebral flow is strictly and locally autoregulated.

The animals used in this study were young swine; it is well known that adrenergic receptor density changes with age in this animal model. Only a single dose of epinephrine and norepinephrine was evaluated. The number of animals in each study group is most likely to have been too small to detect a difference in study variables (β error). Prearrest control values of cerebral flow for drug-treated animals were not measured. Cerebral blood flow was measured with radiolabeled microspheres, but the technique and values reported by investigators are substantially different from those reported from other laboratories with experience in this technique.

This study does not support the use of one agent over another. Although differences might exist, study design deficiencies preclude any meaningful conclusion.—J. Niemann, M.D.

---

**Effects of Cardiac Configuration, Paddle Placement and Paddle Size on Defibrillation Current Distribution: A Finite-Element Model**
Ramirez IF, Eisenberg SR, Lehr JL, Schoen FJ (Boston Univ; Brigham and Women's Hosp, Boston)
*Med Biol Eng Comput* 27:587–594, 1989                                          1–3

---

Clinical experiences have led to empirically based strategies for the selection of paddle size and paddle position when defibrillating patients with ventricular arrhythmias. The technique is the same for different paddle positions and anatomic chest configurations. The effects of paddle size and paddle position on the distribution of myocardial current during defibrillation were assessed, and a method was developed for quantitatively assessing the potential of a defibrillating shock to cause myocardial damage.

A moderately detailed 2-dimensional finite-element model of the conductive anatomy of the human thorax was constructed. Five paddle positions, 2 paddle sizes, and 3 variations of thoracic anatomy were examined in a model of an average man. Some of the electrode pairings examined roughly corresponded to paddle placements used clinically.

Variations in paddle placement significantly affected myocardial-current distributions, whereas variations in paddle size had only small effects. Paddle positions close to the heart with bony structures interposed between the heart and electrode produced focal regions of much greater than average myocardial current magnitudes. Myocytes in those areas that were exposed to the greater current intensity dissipated 49 times the energy dissipated by myocytes exposed to threshold current magnitudes, potentially causing focal myocardial damage. Variations in cardiac configuration had essentially no effect on myocardial current distributions. An alternative paddle position significantly improved myocardial current distribution. Maximum energy dissipation was reduced to 4.8 times threshold energy while defibrillation efficiency was reduced by less than 7%. Use of this alternative paddle position would reduce the risk of myocardial damage significantly.

Paddle position plays a dominant role in determining myocardial current distributions. The paddle placements currently in clinical use may cause current density distributions that expose focal regions of the heart to significantly larger current magnitudes than are required to attain myocyte inactivation, thus increasing the likelihood of myocardial damage.

▶ This is a well-performed study using a computer-based, 2-dimensional, finite element model of the human heart and thorax (including electrical resistance) to determine optimums for transthoracic defibrillation. To my knowledge, this is the first application of finite element modeling relevant to emergency medical care and a common clinical problem. The findings of this study suggest that currently recommended paddle placement may be incorrect in that defibrillation produces greater myocyte injury. This has obvious clinical implications related to postresuscitation outcome as well as success of defibrillation.—J. Niemann, M.D.

---

**Postresuscitation Electrolyte Changes: Role of Arrhythmia and Resuscitation Efforts in Their Genesis**
Salerno DM, Murakami MM, Winston MD, Elsperger KJ (Univ of Minnesota)
*Crit Care Med* 17:1181–1186, 1989                                                    1–4

---

Hypokalemia frequently occurs after ventricular fibrillation (VF) resuscitation. The causal roles of VF and resuscitation in electrolyte changes after resuscitation were studied in 6 groups of dogs. Of the dogs, 9 had cardiopulmonary resuscitation (CPR) and electrical cardioversion, 9 had no intervention, 5 had CPR without arrhythmia, 5 had electrical cardioversion without arrhythmia, 5 had CPR and cardioversion without arrhythmia, and 5 had rapid right ventricular pacing. Blood was obtained before and sequentially for 3 hours after the intervention to analyze potassium, calcium, magnesium and glucose levels. A maximum change of .3 mEq/L in magnesium was recorded in the VF group 7 minutes after resuscitation; there were no changes in magnesium levels in the other groups. A maximum change of 79 mg/dL occurred in glucose content in the VF group 7 minutes after resuscitation, and calcium levels decreased by a maximum of .4 mg/dL 15 minutes after resuscitation. There were no changes in calcium or glucose levels in the other groups. Potassium decreased by a maximum of .8 mEq/L in the VF group 60 minutes after resuscitation, but by lesser amounts in the other groups.

Basic CPR, including chest massage, electrical cardioversion, and tachycardia with moderate hypotension does not produce the metabolic changes noted after VF resuscitation. These alterations seem to be caused by the severe hypotension associated with VF.

▶ This is a very well-designed study that in some ways raises more questions than it answers. It does clearly show that animals subjected to brief VF with its ensuing hypotension and hypoxia have brief electrolyte abnormalities that are rapidly corrected. The changes in magnesium and calcium are not surprising when one looks at the common response of these electrolytes to stress. Routinely, they show a decrease in patients undergoing stress. For instance, asthmatics who are acutely hypoxic often have low magnesium levels.

Several important questions are raised: First, what is the significance of this drop in potassium and magnesium? A more important question is: What are the effects of long-term arrest on electrolytes, and what, if any, permanent damage may these changes produce? Finally, would early replacement of these electrolytes have any beneficial effect on outcome?—W.H. Spivey, M.D.

## pH-Dependent Effects of Lidocaine on Defibrillation Energy Requirements in Dogs

Echt DS, Cato EL, Coxe DR (Vanderbilt Univ)
*Circulation* 80:1003–1009, 1989                1–5

Lidocaine suppresses cardiac arrhythmias and increases the energy required for ventricular defibrillation in dogs. To investigate whether the mechanism by which lidocaine affects defibrillation energy requirements (ED) is determined by its action on the fast inward sodium channel current, the effect of acidosis and alkalosis on defibrillation ED in the presence of lidocaine was studied in 28 dogs.

Hydrochloric acid infusion was used to produce acidosis. The arterial pH was reduced from approximately 7.4 to 7.2, without significantly affecting the defibrillation ED. Therapeutic lidocaine infusion at normal pH, increased the ED. Acidosis exacerbated the effect of lidocaine on defibrillation energy. Respirator hyperventilation was used to induce alkalosis, increasing arterial pH from approximately 7.4 to 7.6, which decreased the ED. Alkalosis reversed the effect of lidocaine on ED.

In dogs, lidocaine increases the defibrillation ED. This effect is enhanced by acidosis and reversed by alkalosis. Lidocaine exhibited pH-dependent effects on defibrillation ED consistent with its sodium channel–blocking properties.

▶ Antiarrhythmic drugs are used to treat those patients at greatest risk for developing life-threatening rhythm disturbances. Lidocaine is commonly used in emergency care, particularly in patients with suspected, acute myocardial infarction either as a prophylactic agent or to treat significant ventricular ectopy in the setting of acute myocardial ischemia. However, patients treated with lidocaine can still develop primary ventricular fibrillation. This study suggests that therapy used to prevent VF may affect therapy (countershock), should VF occur (i.e., increase ED for successful defibrillation).

This study used a common animal model for studies of defibrillation: a canine anesthetized with pentobarbital, an epicardial patch electrode system for defibrillation, and a short period of VF (10 seconds) before defibrillation attempts and determination of "threshold" energy levels. Acidosis was produced by an acute infusion of hydrochloric acid, and alkalosis was induced by mechanical hyperventilation. Multiple studies were performed in all animals.

Although the methods used by the authors are technically well founded and accepted or used by other investigators, I find it difficult to relate this study to clinical emergency medicine practice. Changes in ED induced by lidocaine were statistically significant (3–10 J) in this study model. In the patient population, transthoracic countershock "doses" are administered in increments of 100 J or more in the management of VF. Although lidocaine had statistically significant effects on defibrillation ED in this animal model, there is no evidence that such an effect would be clinically significant.—J. Niemann, M.D.

### The Effect of an Unsuccessful Subthreshold Shock on the Energy Requirement for the Subsequent Defibrillation

Murakawa Y, Gliner BE, Shankar B, Thakor NV (Johns Hopkins School of Medicine)
Am Heart J 117:1065–1069, 1989                    1–6

Does an unsuccessful low-energy defibrillating shock influence the success of subsequent attempts? This question was examined in 10 anesthetized dogs, in which defibrillation was attempted using a spring catheter electrode in the superior vena cava and a patch electrode on the anteroapical wall of the left ventricle. Success rates of defibrillation 20 seconds from the onset of ventricular fibrillation were compared at 3 different energy levels with and without a preceding subthreshold shock.

A total of 637 episodes of fibrillation-defibrillation were analyzed. Without subthreshold shocks, the predicted energy levels for successful defibrillation rates of 50% and 80% were .0303 and .0367 J/g, respectively. With an unsuccessful subthreshold shock, the respective values were .0325 and .0380 J/g; the differences were not significant.

An unsuccessful subthreshold shock appears not to alter significantly the energy requirement for subsequent defibrillation using an implantable defibrillator. It therefore makes sense to deliver shocks relatively near the defibrillation threshold at the outset.

▶ In this study, the investigators found that a subthreshold countershock delivered via an epicardial patch electrode system after a brief period of ventricular fibrillation (10–20 seconds) did not alter the energy requirement for subsequent, successful defibrillation in canines.

Does this finding have any clinical relevance to the emergency department management of ventricular fibrillation? I suspect not. One of the major determinants of successful closed-chest defibrillation of VF is transthoracic resistance, which is most closely related to thoracic dimensions and varies widely. It has been shown that transthoracic resistance declines only slightly with a second shock at the same energy level and that more substantial reductions in resistance and increases in current flow can be achieved by using large paddles and applying firm paddle contact (1). To my knowledge, there are no studies that indicate that a "subthreshold" or unsuccessful transthoracic defibrillation attempt alters the defibrillation energy threshold requirement. In the clinical setting, there is ample evidence to indicate that adjusting energy dose based on transthoracic resistance is more likely to result in a favorable outcome (2, 3).— J. Niemann, M.D.

*References*

1. Kerber RE, et al: *Circulation* 63:676, 1981.
2. Kerber RE, et al: *Circulation* 71:136, 1985.
3. Kerber RE, et al: *Circulation* 77:1038, 1988.

**The Effect of Applied Chest Compression Force on Systemic Arterial Pressure and End-Tidal Carbon Dioxide Concentration During CPR in Human Beings**
Ornato JP, Levine RL, Young DS, Racht EM, Garnett AR, Gonzalez ER (Med College of Virginia, Richmond)
*Ann Emerg Med* 18:732–737, 1989                                    1–7

To determine how applied chest compression force relates to blood pressure and end-tidal carbon dioxide during closed-chest cardiopulmonary resuscitation in humans beings, 12 adults with cardiac arrest were studied as they received cardiopulmonary resuscitation (CPR) by computerized Thumper. When the decision was made to cease resuscitative effort, applied force was lowered in 20-lb force ($lb_f$) increments at 30-second intervals as the radial artery pressure and end-tidal carbon dioxide were monitored.

Arterial systolic pressure was linearly related to applied chest compression force, whereas diastolic pressure did not change significantly with the applied force. End-tidal carbon dioxide also related linearly to applied force. An applied piston compression force of greater than 100 $lb_f$ led to significantly higher systolic pressure and end-tidal carbon dioxide values than the standard 60–80 $lb_f$ recommended by the American Heart Association (AHA).

A 3-in. displacement stop on the Thumper piston allows better arterial pressure and flow without producing obvious thoracic injury. A thoracic vest device encircling the chest might maximize intrathoracic and intravascular pressures while minimizing chest displacement at any given point.

▶ The physiologic effects of "high-impulse" chest compression, when compared with conventional CPR, were reported by Maier et al. in 1984 (1). What "high impulse" really means remains uncertain, but any physiologic benefit from this CPR method appears to be related to chest compression rate during cardiac arrest. The physiologic effects of a more rapid chest compression rate played a major role in the 1986 AHA revisions of advanced cardiac life support guidelines.

In this study, the investigators used a fixed rate of chest compression at an increasing force (depth of sternal depression). In my opinion, this combination does not really represent high-impulse CPR. The application of the critical study variable (i.e., varying compression force) was studied in a nonrandomized manner in what appears to be a convenience population sample. Figures 1 and 2 in the original article do not represent regression plots. The reported *r* values are weak but attain statistical significance. No data are provided to indicate that increasing compression force significantly increased either CPR systolic arterial pressure or end-tidal carbon dioxide.

The major measurements in this study were CPR systolic arterial pressure and end-tidal carbon dioxide. Cardiopulmonary resuscitation systolic arterial pressure has not been shown to be a determinate of cardiac resuscitation outcome. Cardiopulmonary resuscitation diastolic arterial pressure is a major determinant of myocardial perfusion during cardiac arrest and CPR but was not effected by compression force in this study. Similarly, a relation between systemic perfusion during CPR, end-tidal carbon dioxide, and cardiac resuscitation outcome is supported by a growing body of literature. In this study, end-tidal carbon dioxide does not appear to have been effected by chest compression force.

This study neither supports nor refutes the value of high-impulse CPR and does not support any single proposed mechanism for blood flow during closed-chest CPR. Clearly, additional studies are needed in the clinical population.—J. Niemann, M.D.

*Reference*

1. Maier GW, et al: *Circulation* 70:86, 1984.

---

**Plasma Catecholamines and Resuscitation From Prolonged Cardiac Arrest**
Kern KB, Elchisak MA, Sanders AB, Badylak SF, Tacker WA, Ewy GA (Univ of Arizona; VA Med Ctr, Tucson, Ariz; Univ Med Ctr, Tucson; Purdue Univ)
*Crit Care Med* 17:786–791, 1989                                    1–8

---

Extraordinarily high levels of endogenous epinephrine (EPI) and norepinephrine (NE) levels have been reported during cardiac arrest and attempted cardiopulmonary resuscitation (CPR). The significance of these high catecholamine plasma levels was assessed in 9 mongrel dogs. Plasma EPI and NE levels were obtained before cardiac arrest and after 8 and 14 minutes of cardiac arrest and CPR. Epinephrine was administered intravenously 1 minute before the last plasma level was drawn.

Plasma catecholamine levels increased markedly during cardiac arrest and attempted resuscitation. Plasma EPI levels increased significantly from 15.9 pmol/mL at baseline to 396.0 pmol/L after 8 minutes of cardiac arrest. Similarly, NE levels increased significantly from 4.4 to 66.5 pmol/mL. Neither the absolute catecholamine plasma concentration nor the response to cardiac arrest of the endogenous catecholamine concentration differed significantly between successfully resuscitated animals and those not resuscitated. However, catecholamine response to exogenous EPI administration correlated with resuscitation outcome. Despite extraordinarily high levels of endogenous plasma catecholamines, animals successfully resuscitated had a 53-fold increase in plasma EPI concentrations compared with a 23-fold increase in animals not resuscitated. Resuscitated animals also had increased NE levels after exogenous EPI, whereas unsuccessfully resuscitated animals had either no change or a decrease in NE levels. A significant increase in coronary perfusion pressure was found after EPI administration in animals eventually resuscitated compared with those who were not resuscitated.

Despite markedly elevated endogenous catecholamine levels during resuscitative efforts for cardiac arrest, exogenous EPI administration appears beneficial during prolonged CPR.

▶ The authors in this paper make the point that animals with higher plasma EPI levels have an improved resuscitation rate when compared with those animals with lower plasma EPI levels. We have observed a very similar finding in our own laboratory and can often tell in the first 5–10 minutes which animals will be resuscitated and which ones will not be resuscitated. It seems that animals that start with a high circulating catecholamine level and are supplemented with exogenous EPI do much better than those that start with lower EPI levels and lower blood pressure. Interestingly, animals that require 2 or 3 electrical shocks to produce ventricular fibrillation seem to have a better survival rate. This probably reflects stress that increases circulating catecholamines just before arrest.

I have often wondered if patients who suddenly go into cardiac arrest are less likely to be resuscitated with CPR than those that experience increased stress before the arrest such as hypoxia or severe anxiety. It may be that a short period of stress immediately before cardiac arrest does have a beneficial effect for those patients who undergo subsequent CPR.—W.H. Spivey, M.D.

---

**Metabolic and Hemodynamic Consequences of Sodium Bicarbonate Administration in Patients With Heart Disease**
Bersin RM, Chatterjee K, Arieff AI (Univ of California, San Francisco; VA Med Ctr, San Francisco)
*Am J Med* 87:7–14, 1989                                         1–9

---

The use of sodium bicarbonate ($NaHCO_3$) in patients with cardiopulmonary arrest has been questioned. The increase in intracellular carbon dioxide from $NaHCO_3$ infusion can exacerbate the intracellular acidosis already present in hypoxic states and cardiopulmonary arrest. Because the clinical circumstances of patients with heart failure are similar to patients in cardiopulmonary arrest, although not as severe, the effects of $NaHCO_3$ in patients with congestive heart failure were studied prospectively. Ten patients with stable congestive heart failure received $NaHCO_3$ and control infusions of equimolar sodium chloride ($NaCl$), and the metabolic and hemodynamic consequences of these infusions were evaluated.

Arterial oxygen tension decreased by an average of 10 mm Hg after $NaHCO_3$ administration, whereas it increased with $NaCl$ infusion. After $NaHCO_3$ administration, myocardial oxygen consumption decreased by 17% as a result of reduced myocardial oxygen extraction. Systemic oxygen consumption also decreased by a mean 21% because of a significant reduction of systemic oxygen extraction. Red blood cell 2,3-diphosphoglyceric acid levels, which were elevated at baseline, did not change with $NaHCO_3$ administration. The arterial and mixed venous carbon dioxide tensions increased with $NaHCO_3$, but decreased significantly with $NaCl$ administration. Administration of $NaHCO_3$ reduced the oxygen pressure at 50% hemoglobin saturation significantly and shifted the oxygen-hemoglobin binding curve toward normal (Bohr effect). Arterial lactate concentration increased with $NaHCO_3$ infusion. Net myocardial lactate generation developed in 3 patients during $NaHCO_3$ administration;

symptoms of angina developed in 2 of these patients. Blood glucose concentration decreased significantly with $NaHCO_3$ administration. Coronary blood flow did not change with $NaHCO_3$ infusion, but increased with NaCl. Four patients had transient reductions of cardiac output, and 2 patients had transient pump failure during $NaHCO_3$ administration.

Administration of $NaHCO_3$ to patients with congestive heart failure impairs arterial oxygenation and reduces systemic and myocardial oxygen consumption. The reduction in oxygen utilization is associated with anaerobic metabolism, enhanced glycolysis, and elevation of blood lactate levels, which may lead to transient myocardial ischemia in some patients. Thus, the use of $NaHCO_3$ in these patients may have potentially deleterious consequences and warrants reevaluation.

▶ This article adds to the growing body of evidence that clearly shows that $NaHCO_3$ has adverse effects in cardiac arrest and congestive heart failure. This paper has impressively demonstrated that $NaHCO_3$ has an adverse effect on arterial oxygen tension.

One particularly strong aspect of this paper is the patient population studied. It is virtually impossible to conduct a study like this in patients in cardiac arrest, so the authors used the next best patient population—those in congestive heart failure. Although there are always dangers in extrapolating findings of studies such as this to patients in cardiac arrest, I think that because the patient population is so similar to those in cardiac arrest, the findings here are applicable. One major question yet to be answered, however, is whether or not there is a beneficial effect of $NaHCO_3$ when patients are acidotic. Is there a point at which the change in arterial oxygen tension is outweighed by the adverse effects of a very low blood pH?—W.H. Spivey, M.D.

## Four Case Studies: High-Dose Epinephrine in Cardiac Arrest
Martin D, Werman HA, Brown CG (Ohio State Univ)
*Ann Emerg Med* 19:322–326, 1990                                    1–10

Results of hemodynamic studies in animals and human beings suggest that epinephrine at doses higher than currently recommended may improve resuscitation rates after prolonged cardiac arrest.

Four cardiac arrest victims failed to respond after 20–45 minutes of cardiopulmonary resuscitation and standard 1.0-mg doses of epinephrine. Thereafter, larger doses of epinephrine, .12–.22 mg/kg, were administered by peripheral intravenous bolus injection. Within 5 minutes, perfusing rhythms developed in all 4 patients, with maximum systolic blood pressures ranging from 134 to 222 mm Hg. Cardiac dysrhythmias and metabolic alterations did not occur after these high doses. Cardiac enzyme levels were increased in all patients, but only 1 had pathologic evidence of acute myocardial infarction, which, historically, appeared before the administration of high-dose epinephrine. All patients sustained severe brain injury and died. This was probably because of prolonged cardiopulmonary arrest and global brain ischemia.

Clinical trials are warranted to establish the role of high-dose epinephrine as the initial pharmacologic intervention in selected patients during prehospital resuscitation.

▶ This series of case reports adds to a growing body of evidence that higher than currently recommended doses of epinephrine do have the beneficial effect in resuscitating the heart. I would caution, however, that there has yet to be a published, controlled study that has demonstrated that high doses of epinephrine are beneficial in cardiac arrest. Although I personally believe very strongly that increased doses of epinephrine probably do have a beneficial effect, I also believe a lot of questions need to be answered before we all begin to empty our code carts of epinephrine every time there is a cardiac arrest. This brings to mind the experience we had 7 or 8 years ago when it appeared that calcium-bound blockers had a beneficial effect in preventing brain injury. Resuscitated patients quickly got a dose of verapamil regardless of whether they needed it. Consequently, we sent a lot of patients to the intensive care unit (ICU) in complete heartblock and never did anything for their brain. As has been demonstrated by the Brain Resuscitation Clinical Trial Group and numerous animal studies, calcium-bound blockers have no beneficial effect in patients who have suffered cerebral anoxia.

Currently in the United States several trials are underway to examine standard vs. various high doses of epinephrine. I would urge readers to pay very close attention to these trials, not just the number of patients who are resuscitated but, more important, the number of patients who leave the hospital alive. One major concern I have about high-dose epinephrine is that we will start more hearts, but we may be doing it in patients who are brain dead. It doesn't do anyone any good to bring back a patient who will never leave the ICU.—W.H. Spivey, M.D.

## Shock

### Hypertonic Saline Resuscitation in a Porcine Model of Severe Hemorrhagic Shock

Stanford GG, Patterson CR, Payne L, Fabian TC (Univ of Tennessee)
*Arch Surg* 124:733–736, 1989                                         1–11

Reportedly, administration of small volumes of hypertonic saline solution (HTS) rapidly restores tissue perfusion and corrects the hemodynamic deficits of hemorrhagic shock. However, these effects appear to be transient. The efficacy of a resuscitation regimen for hemorrhagic shock that incorporates an initial infusion of HTS solution with the standard regimen of lactated Ringer's solution (LR) was assessed in a porcine model.

Twenty-two young pigs were bled to 50% of their total blood volume in a 30-minute period. Each animal was then kept in shock for 60 minutes by maintaining its mean arterial pressure at 40–60 mm Hg by reinfusing shed blood or withdrawing more blood. Eight animals did not survive the hemorrhage. Seven surviving animals were treated with LR, 20 mL/kg, for 10 minutes and 7 animals were treated with HTS, 10 mL/kg for 10 minutes. All animals then received LR at a dose of 2 mL/kg/min until the mean arterial pressure reached 80 mm Hg.

Two of 7 pigs treated with only LR did not survive the 2-hour resuscitation period; the other 5 were resuscitated successfully. Two of 5 surviving animals achieved adequate urine output. None of the HTS-treated pigs died. All 7 HTS-treated animals rapidly achieved a rise in mean arterial pressure during the first 10 minutes of resuscitation. The increase in the cardiac index was significantly greater in HTS-treated animals than in LR-treated animals during the early resuscitation period. All HTS-treated pigs regained adequate urine output. Thus, HTS may offer a superior alternative for the initial resuscitation of patients in hemorrhagic shock.

▶ This is the first in a series of articles that investigates HTSs for the treatment of hemorrhagic shock. Having been one of the original investigators of this new resuscitation solution, I am gratified to see the area the subject of intense scientific scrutiny.

The use of HTS for the treatment of hemorrhagic shock arose out of both a civilian and military need. In the present era of "scoop and run" policies for urban trauma, a need exists for a more effective solution in the small volumes delivered during the short transport times encountered in urban emergency medical service. During military conflicts, it is logistically impossible for the field medic to carry out sufficient quantities of crystalloid or blood to treat significant numbers of combat casualties. Therefore, small-volume resuscitation with HTS offers a unique solution to both clinical problems.—P.A. Maningas, M.D.

---

**Effects of Bicarbonate Therapy on Tissue Oxygenation During Resuscitation of Hemorrhagic Shock**
Mäkisalo HJ, Soini HO, Nordin AJ, Höckerstedt KAV (Helsinki Univ, Finland)
*Crit Care Med* 17:1170–1174, 1989                                    1–12

---

Transfusion of colloids assists hemodynamic recovery in hypovolemic shock. Hydroxyethyl starch (hetastarch) is effective in the treatment of hypovolemic shock of pigs, although acidosis resolves slowly. The effects of a 7.5% dose of bicarbonate on tissue oxygenation during treatment of hypovolemic shock with hetastarch was investigated in 12 piglets.

Both the 6 animals receiving colloid alone and the 6 receiving colloid plus bicarbonate recovered hemodynamically. However, tissue oxygen measurements recovered more slowly in the bicarbonate group. Pulmonary artery wedge pressure and arterial bicarbonate concentration were greater in the bicarbonate group during early resuscitation than in the control group. Arterial plasma lactate levels were greater in the bicarbonate group at the end of the 40-minute follow-up period.

Bicarbonate adjunct therapy for hypovolemic shock has no beneficial effect on hemodynamics. Addition of bicarbonate may be harmful to tissue oxygenation when resuscitation involves hetastarch.

▶ Bicarbonate therapy continues to fall into disfavor for the treatment of several disease processes. In cardiac arrest, bicarbonate therapy does not facilitate defibrillation or improve outcome. In diabetic ketoacidosis, bicarbonate therapy offers no therapeutic advantage when the pH is greater than 7.1. This article demonstrates delayed tissue oxygenation when bicarbonate therapy is used for the treatment of hemorrhagic shock, presumably from the shift of the oxyhemoglobin curve to the left. In all of these disease processes, it appears that the key to successful management is the reversal of the primary pathophysiology process that has produced the acidosis rather than an attempt to manipulate the pH with bicarbonate.— P.A. Maningas, M.D.

---

### Effect of Hemorrhage and Resuscitation on Subcutaneous, Conjunctival, and Transcutaneous Oxygen Tension in Relation to Hemodynamic Variables

Gottrup F, Gellett S, Kirkegaard L, Hansen ES, Johansen G (Univ of Aarhüs, Denmark)
*Crit Care Med* 17:904–907, 1989                                    1–13

---

Tissue oxygen measurements, using subcutaneous ($PsCO_2$), conjunctival ($PcJO_2$), or transcutaneous ($PtCO_2$) polarographic oxygen monitors, have been considered as potential indices of perfusion. These 3 methods were compared in 8 anesthetized dogs during controlled hemorrhage and reperfusion. Intravascular pressure, hemodynamic variables, and oxygen transport variables were also measured.

During the controlled hemorrhage phase, $PsCO_2$ was the first tissue oxygen measurement to change significantly from baseline. During continuous bleeding, $PsCO_2$ and $PcJO_2$ declined significantly more than $PtCO_2$. After reinfusion, $PsCO_2$ was the last tissue oxygen measurement to return to baseline. $PvO_2$ decreased significantly during hemorrhage and returned to baseline during resuscitation, whereas arterial oxygen pressure remained constant. Unheated instruments were reliable for indicating peripheral perfusion.

Transcutaneous polarographic oxygen monitor was the first tissue oxygen measurement to be perturbed by hemorrhage and the last to recover to baseline after resuscitation. Therefore $PsCO_2$ was the most sensitive index of blood loss. It was more sensitive than the standard cardiopulmonary variables, and it may be a clinically useful index of perfusion.

▶ Transcutaneous and $PcJO_2$ measurements of oxygen tension have been studied since the early 1980s, primarily as indicators of tissue perfusion in shock states. The $PtCO_2$ method has inherent problems because of the need for a heated sensor. The $PsCO_2$ technique is a relatively new method for measuring tissue oxygen (an indicator of systemic perfusion), and the $PsCO_2$ and $PcJO_2$ methods do not require a heated sensor. In this study, both the $PsCO_2$ and $PcJO_2$ oxygen measurements were sensitive, noninvasive indicators of hypoperfusion in a canine model of hemorrhagic shock. They were also useful in assessing adequacy of resuscitation following reinfusion of shed blood.

The technology to measure tissue oxygen tensions has been available for nearly 1 decade. It is my impression that such technology has not been "embraced" by the medical community, probably because published studies are limited and usually address hemorrhagic shock, few investigations have studied human subjects, and the method offers no clear advantage over invasive monitoring conventionally used in the management of patients in shock not caused by blood loss.—J. Niemann, M.D.

---

**Effect of Crystalloid Infusion on Hematocrit in Nonbleeding Patients, With Applications to Clinical Traumatology**
Stamler KD (Torrance Mem Med Ctr, Torrance, Calif)
*Ann Emerg Med* 18:747–749, 1989                                                  1–14

Slow or delayed intra-abdominal bleeding often is difficult to identify in patients who have sustained blunt abdominal injury. A decrease in the hematocrit value on serial determinations, frequently used as an indicator of intraperitoneal bleeding, may be related to intravenous infusion of crystalloid solution. The change in hematocrit value produced by such infusions was evaluated in 20 nonbleeding individuals tested under a simulated trauma treatment protocol.

Eight healthy volunteers and 12 patients with renal colic were pooled into a single study group. All were tested at baseline and after an initial infusion of 20 mL of normal saline/kg over 45 minutes. Ten (group A) had a third hematocrit determination after infusion of an additional 15 mL/kg over 1 hour; in 10 (group B), the final hematocrit test was made after infusion of an additional 15 mL/kg over 3 hours.

One half of the 20 study participants had decreases in hematocrit value of more than 5 points after the initial infusion. In group A, the mean decrease in hematocrit value after the initial infusion was 4.4; after the second infusion, the mean hematocrit value increased by .6. The corresponding values in group B were a decrease of 4.0 and an increase of 0.6 after the second infusion.

A dilutional effect clearly occurs in nonbleeding patients during crystalloid infusion, although only the initial infusion of 1,500 mL lowers the hematocrit value. This decrease, however, may be as great as 6 points. Thus, patients who have sustained blunt abdominal trauma may exhibit significant drops in hematocrit value even though they are not bleeding.

▶ This article gives yet another reason that following changes in hematocrit values in the setting of trauma is an unnecessary waste of resources. First, the hemodilution and subsequent drop in hematocrit value that does occur following hemorrhage because of the translocation of fluid into the intravascular space does not occur until hours after injury (false negative response). Second, as demonstrated in this article, a drop in hematocrit value may occur in nonbleeding patients as a consequence of fluid infusion (false positive response).

In the setting of blunt abdominal injury, further credence is given to peritoneal lavage as the diagnostic procedure to rule out intraperitoneal hemorrhage.— P.A. Maningas, M.D.

### Treatment of Uncontrolled Hemorrhagic Shock by Hypertonic Saline and External Counterpressure

Landau EH, Gross D, Assalia A, Krausz MM (Hadassah Univ Hosp, Jerusalem)
*Ann Emerg Med* 18:1039–1043, 1989                                1–15

The combined use of hypertonic saline and external counterpressure was examined in rats with "uncontrolled" hemorrhagic shock induced by incising branches of the ileocolic artery. Groups of animals were observed for 3 hours after receiving either physiologic or 7.5% saline solution, 5 mL/kg, either alone or in conjunction with inflation of a binder to 50 mm Hg.

Hypertonic saline alone was associated with many deaths compared with the use of normal saline. Combined use of hypertonic saline and compression was followed by a rise in arterial pressure, which was sustained (Fig 1–1). All of these animals survived.

The combination of hypertonic saline and external counterpressure is worth trying in patients with multiple injuries and severe hemorrhagic shock. Hypertonic saline infusion may lower the risk of impaired oxygen perfusion and its attendant complications when the military antishock trousers are inflated.

▶ There has been considerable discussion concerning the value of aggressive prehospital fluid resuscitation with either standard crystalloids or hypertonic saline. An increasing number of clinicians believe that a sudden elevation of blood

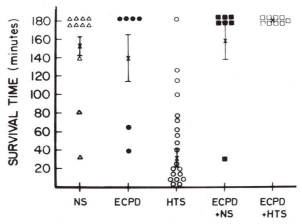

**Fig 1–1.**—Survival time of animals in "uncontrolled" hemorrhagic shock treated by normal saline (NS), hypertonic saline (HTS), and external counterpressure (ECPD). (Courtesy of Landau EH, Gross D, Assalia A, et al: *Ann Emerg Med* 18:1039–1043, 1989.)

pressure in a traumatized individual before surgical hemostasis has achieved results in the dislodging of a thrombus surrounding the injured vessel and could actually hasten bleeding. Bickell and co-workers (1) demonstrated that the rapid administration of lactated Ringer's solution in an aortotomy model in swine resulted in an increase in the volume of hemorrhage and, more important, resulted in the death of all treated animals compared with no mortality in untreated controls. This information has led to a study in Houston that is evaluating the value of fluid vs. no fluids in the hypotensive trauma patient before surgery.— P.A. Maningas, M.D.

*Reference*

1. Bickell WH, et al: *Ann Emerg Med* 19:476, 1989.

---

### The Hemodynamic and Cardiovascular Effects of Near-Drowning in Hypotonic, Isotonic, or Hypertonic Solutions
Orlowski JP, Abulleil MM, Phillips JM (Cleveland Clinic Found)
*Ann Emerg Med* 18:1044–1049, 1989                                    1–16

---

It has been proposed that near-drowning in fresh water can cause hemodilution and hypervolemia, whereas near-drowning in seawater produces hypovolemic shock secondary to its hypertonicity. Solutions of varying tonicity were instilled into the lungs of anesthetized dogs in a volume of 20 mL/kg. Control animals were made anoxic for 5 minutes. The solutions compared were sterile water, .225% sodium chloride, .45% sodium chloride, normal saline, 2% sodium chloride, and 3% sodium chloride.

The hemodynamic effects of hypotonic, isotonic, and hypertonic solutions did not differ from the changes seen in anoxic control dogs. Cardiac output fell immediately as pulmonary capillary wedge pressure rose. Dynamic compliance of the lungs fell markedly in all groups. Wedge pressure and central venous pressure peaked at 10 minutes and then fell gradually over 4 hours. Cardiac output and lung compliance remained depressed throughout the study, and pulmonary vascular resistance gradually deteriorated.

It appears that the cardiovascular sequelae of near-drowning do not depend on the tonicity of the aspirated fluid but result directly from anoxia. Because anoxia also causes cerebral dysfunction and some degree of respiratory compromise in this setting, hypoxia must be rapidly corrected.

▶ The majority of near-drowning patients do not aspirate a sufficient quantity of fluid (22 mL/kg) to cause clinically significant electrolyte abnormalities. Moreover, 15% of drowning patients are "dry" drownings where little, if any, fluid has been aspirated. Hypoxia results from laryngospasm in response to the cold water stimulus or the mechanical irritation of swallowed water.— P.A. Maningas, M.D.

### Resuscitation of Conscious Pigs Following Hemorrhage: Comparative Efficacy of Small-Volume Resuscitation

Wade CE, Hannon JP, Bossone CA, Hunt MM, Loveday JA, Coppes R, Gildengorin VL (Letterman Army Inst of Research, Presidio of San Francisco, Calif)

*Circ Shock* 29:193–204, 1989                                        1–17

Infusion of small volumes of hypertonic or hyperoncotic solutions, or both, effectively improves cardiovascular function after hemorrhage. To assess their efficacy in improving survival, the functional consequences of small volume resuscitation (4 mL/kg) with isotonic saline (NS, .9% sodium chloride), hypertonic saline (HS, 7.5% sodium chloride), hyperoncotic colloid (D, dextran), or a combination hypertonic-hyperoncotic solution (HSD, 7.5% sodium chloride in 6% dextran 70) were

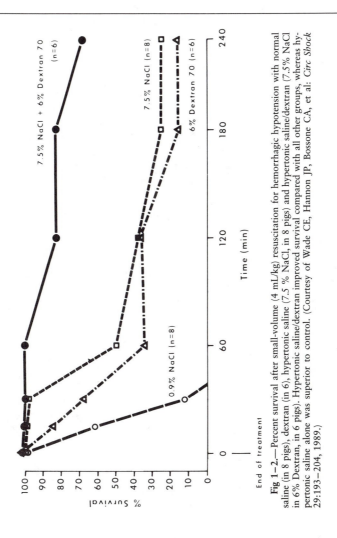

**Fig 1–2.**—Percent survival after small-volume (4 mL/kg) resuscitation for hemorrhagic hypotension with normal saline (in 8 pigs), dextran (in 6), hypertonic saline (7.5 % NaCl, in 6) and hypertonic saline/dextran (7.5% NaCl in 6% Dextran, in 6 pigs). Hypertonic saline/dextran improved survival compared with all other groups, whereas hypertonic saline alone was superior to control. (Courtesy of Wade CE, Hannon JP, Bossone CA, et al: *Circ Shock* 29:193–204, 1989.)

compared in 28 conscious immature swines bled 37.5 mL/kg over 60 minutes.

Four-hour survival after administration of HSD (67%) was significantly greater than after HS (25%), D (17%), or NS (0%) (Fig 1–2). Survival also was improved after HS injection, only when compared with NS. The improved resuscitation after injection of HSD, and to a lesser extent after HS infusion, was associated with rapid volume expansion, improved cardiac index and stroke volume, and decreased heart rate. The acute increases in cardiac index and stroke volume with HSD persisted throughout the 4 hours of recovery. Also found was a transient increase in mean arterial pressure with HSD. Plasma sodium concentration and osmolality were increased to a similar extent with HSD and HS injection, whereas plasma potassium levels were initially decreased, returning to control levels within 60 minutes.

Small-volume resuscitation with 4 mL of HSD solution/kg improved short-term survival after hemorrhagic hypovolemia in conscious swines. The HSD solution increases cardiac output, the latter effect being largely attributed to increased stroke volume index.

▶ Contrary to the previous article by Stanford et al. (Abstract 1–11), a number of articles have shown the hemodynamic response to HS alone is rather transient, because sodium is rapidly lost out of the intravascular compartment. This has led to the investigation of HSD. This article demonstrates even greater improvement in hemodynamic response and survival with HSD compared with HS, D, or NS. Initially, the hypertonicity of HS draws fluid out of the extracellular space into the intravascular space. The dextran component of the solution, by its oncotic properties, retains that redistributed fluid in the vascular compartment. (See also Abstract 1–18.)—P.A. Maningas, M.D.

## Intravenous Fluid Therapy in the Prehospital Management of Hemorrhagic Shock: Improved Outcome With Hypertonic Saline/6% Dextran 70 in a Swine Model

Chudnofsky CR, Dronen SC, Syverud SA, Zink BJ, Hedges JR (Univ of Cincinnati)
*Am J Emerg Med* 7:357–363, 1989                    1–18

The benefits of intravenous fluid resuscitation therapy in the field treatment of patients with hemorrhagic shock are unproved. Administration of small volumes of hypertonic saline (HTS) rapidly improves hemodynamics and significantly increases survival in animal shock models. To determine whether HTS administration would be useful in the prehospital management of hypotensive trauma patients, a lightly anesthetized, splenectomized porcine continuous hemorrhage model was used in a simulated prehospital resuscitation setting.

Twenty-eight immature swine were divided into 2 groups. Hemorrhage was initiated at time 0 at a rate of 1.25 mL/kg/minute in all animals. After 20 minutes of hemorrhage, 14 animals were treated with normal saline solution and 12 received 7.5% HTS in 6% dextran 70 (HTS/DEX) at 1 mL/kg/min for 22.5 minutes, simulating the time required for completion of prehospital patient evaluation, treatment, loading, and transport to the hospital. At 42.5 minutes, simulating hospital arrival, the infusion rate in the normal saline group was increased to 3 mL/kg/minute. In the HTS/DEX group, infusions were changed to normal saline at 3 mL/kg/min. At 45 minutes, after a total infusion of 30 mL/kg of crystalloid, the resuscitation fluid was changed to equal proportions of normal saline and shed blood at 3 mL/kg/min. Hemorrhage was discontinued at 65 minutes or at 25 minutes after simulated hospital arrival. Hemodynamic parameters were recorded at baseline and at 15-minute intervals for 120 minutes or until death of the animal.

All 12 HTS/DEX-treated animals but only 8 of 14 normal saline–treated animals survived. The cardiac index, mean arterial pressure, oxygen delivery, and central venous pressure all were significantly higher in the HTS/DEX-treated group compared with the normal saline–treated group. Values obtained at each period after hemorrhage also were greater in the HTS/DEX group than in the normal saline group. These findings are encouraging and warrant clinical investigation.

▶ This article evaluates the efficacy of HSD in an animal model simulating the prehospital management of hemorrhagic shock. The success of HSD in the animal laboratory has led to preliminary studies in human beings. A study in Houston (1) demonstrated the feasibility of prehospital infusion of HSD by paramedics. There were no complications related to the infusion of HSD, and there were trends in improvement in blood pressure and survival. Recently, a large multicenter clinical trial has been completed, and the results are forthcoming.— P.A. Maningas, M.D.

*Reference*

1. Maningas PA, et al: *Am J Surg* 157:528, 1989.

---

**Assessing Acid–Base Status in Circulatory Failure: Differences Between Arterial and Central Venous Blood**
Adrogué HJ, Rashad MN, Gorin AB, Yacoub J, Madias NE (Baylor College of Medicine, Houston; Tufts Univ)
*N Engl J Med* 320:1312–1316, 1989                                   1–19

Arteriovenous differences in acid-base status were studied by measuring pH and carbon dioxide tension ($PCO_2$) in blood taken simultaneously from the arterial and central venous circulations of 26 patients with normal cardiac output, 36 with moderate circulatory failure, and 5 with severe failure. Thirty-eight patients in cardiac or cardiorespiratory arrest also were evaluated.

The acid-base composition of central venous and mixed venous blood was similar in patients with normal function and those with moderate

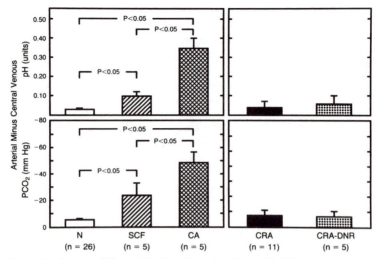

Fig 1–3.—Arteriovenous differences in pH and $P_{CO_2}$ in patients with different hemodynamic conditions. *N*, normal hemodynamic status (group I); *SCF*, severe circulatory failure (group III); *CA*, cardiac arrest (group IV A); *CRA*, cardiorespiratory arrest (group V A), and *CRA-DNR*, cardiorespiratory arrest in nonresuscitated patients (group VI B). Means ± SEM are shown. To convert values for $P_{CO_2}$ to kilopascals, multiply by .1333. (Courtesy of Adrogué HJ, Rashad MN, Gorin AB, et al: *N Engl J Med* 320:1312–1315, 1989.)

failure. In patients with normal function, venous pH was lower by .03 unit and venous $P_{CO_2}$ was higher by .8 kPa. In hypotensive patients with severe circulatory failure, significant differences existed between mean arterial and central venous pH values and $P_{CO_2}$ values (Fig 1–3). Large arteriovenous differences also were found during cardiac arrest when ventilation was mechanically supported, whether or not sodium bicarbonate was given. In contrast, large arteriovenous differences occurred in patients to whom only bicarbonate was given.

In patients who are severely compromised hemodynamically, both arterial and central venous samples are needed to assess acid-base status. If severe hypoperfusion is present, tissue acidemia and hypercapnia are best reflected in central venous blood.

▶ An arteriovenous difference in $P_{CO_2}$ and pH is known to occur during cardiac arrest and closed-chest cardiopulmonary resuscitation, as well as during vigorous exercise. This study demonstrates that a similar rise in venous $P_{CO_2}$ and fall in pH (when compared with arterial blood values) occurs during severe circulatory failure. This phenomenon is most probably the result of tissue anoxia, lactic acidosis, increased generation of carbon dioxide, and decreased pulmonary blood flow. Carbon dioxide is freely diffuseable across cell membranes and can worsen intracellular acidosis.

The findings of this study raise another issue, namely, should sodium bicarbonate be used to treat the lactic acidosis that accompanies circulatory shock. Administering sodium bicarbonate raises central venous $P_{CO_2}$ and could worsen intracellular acidosis and cellular function. I am unaware of a single study that demonstrates in a scientific manner any benefit of sodium bicarbonate therapy in the management of lactic acidosis. There are studies that indicate that sodium bicarbonate use in lactic acidosis is, in fact, detrimental (1).—J. Niemann, M.D.

*Reference*

1. Graf H, et al: *Science* 227:754, 1985.

## Neurorespiratory Dysfunction

**The Bone Marrow as a Source of Laboratory Studies**
Orlowski JP, Porembka DT, Gallagher JM, Van Lente F (Cleveland Clinic Found)
*Ann Emerg Med* 18:1348–1351, 1989                                                    1–20

The intraosseous route is an emergency alternative for the administration of drugs and fluids when intravenous access cannot be achieved. One drawback of using the intraosseous route is that blood samples for blood gases, laboratory tests, and blood cultures still need to be obtained. To determine whether bone marrow samples could be used instead of venous and arterial blood samples for performing essential laboratory tests, bone marrow samples and venous and arterial blood samples were obtained simultaneously from 10 anesthetized healthy dogs. The samples were used for measuring blood electrolytes, blood chemistries, blood gases, and hemoglobin levels. In addition, bone marrow samples from 16 children and 8 adults with hematologic malignancies were cultured. All patients required bone marrow aspiration to assess oncologic status and to identify the source of sepsis.

The only tests that gave marginally significantly different values were blood glucose, alkaline phosphatase, and lactate dehydrogenase. Venous and bone marrow glucose levels were identical, but each was less than the arterial glucose level. Alkaline phosphatase and lactate dehydrogenase levels were elevated in bone marrow but were identical in arterial and venous blood samples. The measured hemoglobin levels from all 3 sites were identical. Blood gases were significantly different among the 3 sites, with bone marrow values falling between those measured in arterial and venous blood samples. The 15 patients who had blood cultures that were positive for bacteria or fungus had bone marrow samples that were positive for the same organisms.

These preliminary findings suggest that bone marrow samples obtained via the intraosseous route are not only useful in an emergency setting but also may serve as a viable alternative for obtaining initial diagnostic laboratory studies when intravenous access is unobtainable.

► Several years ago, we conducted a very similar study in which we compared blood chemistries obtained from venous and marrow cavity blood. We found essentially the same results as the authors (i.e., electrolytes and other blood chemistries are not significantly different when drawn from a venous vs. intraosseous site). One problem that we did have with the technique, however, was obtaining a complete blood cell (CBC) count. In virtually every tube of blood that was drawn from the intraosseous route through an 18-gauge spinal needle, the blood clotted. In fact, we were unable to get any data about the CBC count because of difficulty with the blood clotting so rapidly. We postulated at that time that it may be caused by the platelet precursors or small, bony spicules that induced clotting. Nevertheless, there is no reason as indicated by this study and our previous work that the intraosseous route should not be used for blood chemistries. Furthermore, it may be used for blood cultures. If you're going to place a needle for fluid or drug administration, you may as well use this stick to get as much information as possible.—W.H. Spivey, M.D.

---

**Comparison of Serum Phenobarbital Levels After Single Versus Multiple Attempts at Intraosseous Infusion**
Brickman K, Rega P, Choo M, Guinness M (St Vincent Med Ctr–The Toledo Hosp, Toledo, Ohio)
*Ann Emerg Med* 19:31–33, 1990                                                  1–21

---

Intraosseous infusion is being used increasingly to rapidly obtain vascular access in pediatric emergencies. It is possible, however, that inexperienced persons could make multiple attempts and thereby produce significant extravasation from intramedullary entrance sites. Serum drug levels were compared in dogs given phenobarbital when multiple intraosseous attempts were made and when a single intraosseous attempt was made in nontraumatized bone. In the former cases, 3 punctures were made 1 cm apart into the intramedullary space of the proximal tibia.

None of the animals had hemodynamic instability. Extravasation of the drug in normal saline was evident in all multiple-puncture cases but not in single-puncture attempts. Consistently, higher phenobarbital levels were found in the single-attempt group. Peak drug levels occurred at 1 minute in both groups.

If an initial attempt at intramedullary placement fails, a totally different site should be chosen. Regular practice is necessary to succeed consistently at intraosseous drug infusion.

▶ Emergency physicians can be credited with the reinterest in interosseous infusion, particularly with reference to resuscitation. This study confirms the suspicion that defects occurring with multiple attempts to obtain medullary access will delay central circulation of the pharmacologic agent. In addition to the recommended operator training, a good "first puncture" needle must be made available. In the authors' model, 3 " successful" punctures were made in the multiple puncture animal. In the failed clinical situation, one might postulate that unsuccessful marrow entry had occurred, possibly limiting the extraosseous loss. (See also Abstract 5–13.)—D.K. Wagner, M.D.

**Hyperbaric Oxygen Increases Survival Following Carotid Ligation in Gerbils**
Reitan JA, Kien ND, Thorup S, Corkill G (Univ of California, Davis)
*Stroke* 21:119–123, 1990                                                                                     1–22

A major criticism of studies on the use of hyperbaric oxygen (HBO) therapy is the lack of controlled prospective analysis. The efficacy of graded exposure to HBO (1,875 mm Hg) for the treatment of evolving stroke was studied prospectively in an animal model. After unilateral carotid artery interruption, gerbils were assigned at random to a specific therapeutic regimen, including pentobarbital alone, superoxide dismutase alone, 2 and 4 hours of HBO alone, and each agent combined with HBO, to investigate possible mechanisms of protection from cerebral ischemia. Because excessive oxygen has toxic pulmonary effects, a pilot mortality study was performed. The $LD_{50}$ was 7.26 hours, and none of the gerbils died during 4 hours of HBO exposure. Survival rates and neurologic deficit scores over 5 days were compared between treatment groups and controls.

Compared with control animals, survival rates at 5 days were significantly higher in animals treated with 2 and 4 hours of HBO and those treated with pentobarbital. Although there was a dose-dependent relation between survival and increasing HBO exposure, the combination of pentobarbital or superoxide dismutase with HBO offered no apparent additive protection. There were no significant differences in neurologic deficit scores at 5 days between groups.

Graded doses of HBO increases survival in a gerbil model of stroke. Because it is noninvasive and relatively safe, HBO treatment remains an attractive treatment for stroke and other neuroischemic conditions.

▶ The authors of this article state that the effect of hyperbaric oxygen on these animals is paradoxical. On one hand, it causes marked tissue damage and toxicity, while on the other hand, it provides apparent treatment for neuronal ischemia. Hyperbaric oxygen does seem to provide a beneficial role in animal models of stroke, but no one seems to know why. This makes skeptics of hyperbaric oxygen very uneasy about the entire field. To complicate things, there are very few good, controlled clinical trials using hyperbaric oxygen. This is especially true for stroke. This is a field where there definitely needs to be good, controlled clinical trials, addressing the effect of hyperbaric oxygen on both focal and general cerebral ischemia.—W.H. Spivey, M.D.

# 2 Trauma Emergencies

## General Trauma Evaluation

### Outcome of Trauma Patients Who Present to the Operating Room With Hypotension

Wiencek RG Jr, Wilson RF, Demaeo P (Wayne State Univ, Detroit)
Am Surg 55:338–342, 1989                                                  2–1

Despite attempts at restoring intravascular volume and tissue perfusion, some trauma patients will be hypotensive when arriving in the operating room. Of 101 such patients who needed emergency surgery with systolic blood pressures less than 90 mm Hg, blood pressures were not obtainable for 35.

Overall mortality was 48% in this series. Mortality was 6% for those with systolic pressures of 70–89 mm Hg; 79% for those with 50–69 mm Hg; and 86% for patients with nonobtainable pressures. Mortality was much higher when the duration of shock in the emergency department and operating room exceeded 30 minutes. Nineteen of 42 patients responded favorably to prelaparotomy thoracotomy with cross-clamping of the thoracic aorta, and 42% of them survived. None of the 23 unresponsive patients survived surgery. Among 12 patients with systolic blood pressures less than 70 mm Hg who did not have prelaparotomy aortic cross-clamping, only 1, who had an aortic compressor applied, survived.

Early aortic cross-clamping will limit blood loss from and promote survival of patients who are in severe shock after trauma, especially when shock lasts longer than 30 minutes. It is increasingly clear that patients who fail to respond to aortic cross-clamping usually do not respond to prolonged surgery and large amounts of blood and blood products.

▶ There is a plethora of data and comparisons presented in this study. Expectedly, the paper points out that the degree of hypotension, duration of shock, and number of units of blood transfused is directly related to eventual mortality. All efforts to aggressively treat hypotension should be made, and, in particular, this study addresses the usefulness of aortic cross-clamping in attaining this goal. Although it clearly decreased the amount of transfused blood products required, its overall effect on mortality was limited. Of the 42 patients who underwent aortic cross-clamping, 19 displayed at least a transient increase in blood pressure, but only 8 of these victims survived. The remaining 23 patients who were cross-clamped, did not increase their blood pressure, and none of this group survived. It is the authors' contention that, based on their data, if the hypotensive trauma patient does not respond to aortic clamping, laparotomy may not be warranted since their survival was zero. It would be difficult for most surgeons to refrain from exploratory surgery in these patients since identifiable, repairable lesions may be found. Rapid movement to the operating room would limit blood loss and duration of shock, and this may have a greater bearing on outcome. (See also Abstracts 1–1, 1–14, and 1–15.)—H. Unger, M.D.

---

**Physician Exposure to Ionizing Radiation During Trauma Resuscitation: A Prospective Clinical Study**
Weiss EL, Singer CM, Benedict SH, Baraff LJ (Univ of California, Los Angeles)
*Ann Emerg Med* 19:134–138, 1990                                                            2–2

---

Care of the critical trauma patient often requires continuous resuscitative efforts during radiographic procedures. A 3-month prospective study was conducted to determine whole-body and extremity exposure to ionizing radiation of emergency physicians during trauma patient resuscitation. A total of 150 patients with major trauma requiring 481 radiographic studies were treated.

During radiographic examinations of these patients, the trauma team wore leaded aprons with permanently attached radiation film badges and thermoluminescent dosimeter finger rings. One emergency medicine resident monitored the airway and, when necessary, stabilized the neck during cervical spine radiography (A-CS resident). Another resident supervised trauma care and wore a separate set of dosimeters. Additional garment shieldings were not worn.

Mean monthly cumulative whole-body exposures were 136.7 mrem for the A-CS resident and 103.3 mrem for the supervising resident. Mean weekly hand exposures were 523 mrem for the A-CS resident and 48 mrem for the supervising resident. Assuming the 2 residents worked 200 12-hour shifts per year, their respective mean monthly cumulative whole-body exposure values were 9.2% and 6.8% of the upper occupational exposure limits established by the National Council of Radiation Protection (NCRP) in the United States. The respective mean weekly cumulative extremity values were 15.2% and 1.4% of the recommended limits. Assuming they work 200 12-hour shifts per year, the A-CS and supervising residents have to treat 9.2 and 11.9 trauma patients per shift to exceed the whole-body annual limit of the NCRP, and 5.9 and 67.8 patients, respectively, to exceed the extremity limit of the NCRP.

During radiographic evaluation of trauma victims, physicians are at risk of significant whole-body and extremity radiation exposure. The level of risk is a function of trauma volume and trauma management technique. The risk is increased in activities that require close patient proximity and use of unshielded hands to restrain the patient. Appropriate shielding devices should be used by physicians during radiographic evaluation of trauma patients.

▶ This is an alarming study. Although the radiation exposure of the physicians caring for trauma patients appeared to be within the safe limits set by the

NCRP in the United States, many questions are raised. Why does the Health and Safety Executive (HSE) in England set the safety levels at 10% of the NCRP? In England, the physician would exceed the safe radiation level after having cared for only 2 trauma patients. What about hospitals such as the King/Drew Medical Center where we see more than 40 trauma patients every day?

What is a safe level of radiation exposure? The only safe level is none. Some geneticists suggest that the protective mechanisms of the body may be able to deal with only 100 mREM above background before irreparable mutagenic DNA changes occur. This is the exposure received by the physician holding the cervical spine for only 2 patients.

Every emergency physician should read and seriously consider this study, including possible methods of reducing radiation exposure. One final note: Even the NCRP standards indicate that a health professional stabilizing only 1 cervical spine per day will double his or her work-related death rate.—G. Ordog, M.D.

---

**Epidemiology and Pathology of Traumatic Deaths Occurring at a Level I Trauma Center in a Regionalized System: The Importance of Secondary Brain Injury**
Shackford SR, Mackersie RC, Davis JW, Wolf PL, Hoyt DB (Univ of California, San Diego)
*J Trauma* 29:1392–1397, 1989                                          2–3

---

To determine if the epidemiology of traumatic death can be affected by developments in regionalized system of trauma care, the hospital records and autopsy data of all deaths occurring at a level I trauma center during a 1-year interval were reviewed.

Of the 1,581 adult major trauma victims seen, 104 (6.6%) died. The incidence of gunshot wounds and pedestrians struck by vehicles was significantly higher in nonsurvivors (NS). Compared with survivors (S), NS were significantly older, had a lower trauma score, higher injury severity scores, and lower probability of survival; the scene time and transport time did not differ between NS and S. Of the NS, 91.4% died within 7 days, and 8.6% after 7 days. The leading cause of death was injury to the CNS (48.1%), followed by hemorrhage (36.8%), and cardiovascular disease (5.7%). Sepsis was the cause of death in 5.5%. Autopsy showed evidence of secondary brain injury, such as diffuse cerebral edema, tonsillar or uncal herniation, or frank necrosis, in 66% of patients dying of CNS injury. Patients dying of head injury had significantly heavier lungs than other patients dying of all other causes except sepsis. No deaths were assessed as frankly preventable, and only 4 (3.8%) were judged potentially preventable.

Compared with Baker's classic study on the epidemiology of traumatic death, there is a significant reduction in the incidence of late deaths and in the percentage of deaths caused by sepsis in the present study. This could be because of improvements in treatment associated with regionalization of trauma care. Despite rapid transport and evacuation of mass lesions, secondary brain injury occurs in a significant number of patients dying of CNS injury. These changes are caused by reduction in oxygen delivery to the brain because of either hypoxia or decrease in cerebral perfusion pressure caused by hypotension with a normal or elevated intracranial pressure. In addition, these patients have a type of "secondary injury" that extends to the lungs; edematous lungs may contribute further to secondary brain injury by causing hypoxia. These data suggest that secondary brain injury may play an important role in the pathophysiology of head trauma.

▶ The fact that the majority of patients with head trauma had indirect sequelae throughout the brain, in addition to the primary injury, is not surprising. Since the majority (40 of 50) of patients with fatal CNS injury had brain contusion diagnosed at autopsy, I don't see a "window" for salvaging these patients. The authors don't report how many had isolated intracranial hematoma without significant contusion, a group where initial intervention might have prevented secondary brain injury. If, however, cerebral edema, necrosis, or hematoma were reported in any of the patients without significant head injury, I would worry about anoxic injury in the interval before hemodynamic resuscitation. It is not clear how closely this was studied.—W.P. Burdick, M.D.

---

## A Comparison of the Trauma Score, the Revised Trauma Score, and the Pediatric Trauma Score

Eichelberger MR, Gotschall CS, Sacco WJ, Bowman LM, Mangubat EA, Lowenstein AD (Children's Natl Med Ctr, Washington, DC; Tri-Analytics, Inc, Bel Air, Md)
*Ann Emerg Med* 18:1053–1058, 1989                                          2–4

---

Triage criteria for use in pediatric populations have not been well studied. Previous studies have shown that the trauma score (TS) and the Revised Trauma Score (RTS) can be used for predicting survival in injured children, but their usefulness as triage tools has not been evaluated. The Pediatric Trauma Score (PTS), designed specifically for field triage of children, has not yet been tested in a triage setting. The abilities of the TS, RTS, and PTS were compared to retrospectively identify severely injured children who needed triage to a pediatric trauma center.

The study population consisted of 1,334 children, aged 14 years or younger, who had been admitted to a primary pediatric trauma center with blunt or penetrating injuries. Complete index data and Injury Severity Score (ISS) values were available for all children. The ISS values of more than 15 and 20 or higher were used as criteria of severe injury and the need for triage to a pediatric trauma center. The RTS was modified to accommodate the higher respirations of children aged younger than 3 years (RTSC). The TS, RTSC, and PTS were computed from admission data.

Forty children (3%) died and 1,294 children (97%) survived. The median ISS value was 5, and the mean ISS value was 8.5. A total of 183 children (14%) had ISS values of 16 or greater, and 115 (8.6%) had ISS values of 20 or greater. A TS of less than 15, a RTSC of less than 12, and a PTS of less than 9 proved to be the most efficient threshold values for triage to a pediatric trauma center. There was no significant difference in the sensitivity, specificity, and positive and negative predictive values of the 3 scales. All 3 scales produced a relatively large number of false positive results, but the precise level of overtriage was not determined. Because of the equivalence of the 3 triage scoring systems, other factors, such as reliability ease of use, and quality assurance should be considered in the selection of a pediatric triage tool.

▶ This study shows no significant difference between the TS and the PTS in identifying severely injured children. When the RTS was adjusted to the higher respiratory rate of children, all 3 performed similarly. We would hope that all of these instruments can be combined into one that is easy to use and is also reliable.—G.V. Anderson, M.D.

---

**Seizure Disorders and Trauma**
Fallon WF Jr, Robertson LM, Alexander RH (Univ of Florida Health Science Ctr, Jacksonville)
*South Med J* 82:1093–1095, 1989                                          2–5

---

Seizures may increase a person's risk for injury by adversely influencing his or her performance in a particular situation. To determine the relationship between seizure disorder and the frequency and severity of injury, data on 30 patients with injury-related seizures and admitted to a trauma service during a 3-year period were evaluated. The 16 male and 14 female patients represented 1.6% of all admissions for that period. Their mean age was 34.8 years.

Twenty-eight patients (93%) had histories of seizure immediately before injury. The mean duration of seizure activity was 16.5 years (range 3–40 years). The mechanism of injury was exclusively blunt trauma, the most frequent causes being falls (50%), motor vehicular accidents (40%), and burns (10%). Injury severity was low. Nine patients (30%) required surgery, mostly for repair of skeletal injuries. Both seizure diagnosis and etiology were multifactorial. Multiple drug therapy predominated, the most common drug being phenytoin. Overall compliance was poor among 16 patients (53%), and 7 (23%) had breakthrough seizure activity despite anticonvulsant therapy. Six patients (20%) had alcohol in their blood.

Patients with a history of seizure who are noncompliant, have breakthrough seizures, or have the metabolism of their drug altered by alcohol or other drugs are likely to be at increased risk for injury. These patients should be identified and counseled to prevent potentially serious injury.

▶ We all are familiar with the seizure patient we repeatedly see in our department who sustained some degree of trauma because of a seizure and in whom we find that blood levels of their medications are extremely low because of noncompliance. This is a very difficult problem because we cannot force a patient to take his or her medication. The article emphasizes that all physicians caring for these patients must take the time to educate the patient regarding the hazards of not taking the medication. This is alien to the adolescent diabetic who refuses to be compliant with diet and insulin.

Although we should not be the primary physicians of these patients, anyone working in an inner-city hospital emergency department knows that we frequently serve that role and must do our part to educate these patients.—E.J. Lucid, M.D.

---

**The Use of an Emergency Department Observation Unit in the Management of Abdominal Trauma**
Henneman PL, Marx JA, Cantrill SC, Mitchell M (Denver Gen Hosp; Harbor-UCLA Med Ctr, Torrance, Calif)
*Ann Emerg Med* 18:647–650, 1989                                                    2–6

---

Diagnostic peritoneal lavage (DPL) is an accurate predictor of the need for laparotomy in patients with blunt and penetrating abdominal trauma. However, DPL lacks sensitivity for certain organ injuries and does not provide evaluation of the retroperitoneum where a pathologic lesion may not show signs for hours. Postinjury monitoring is therefore required. The safety and efficacy of monitoring trauma patients with a normal DPL for 12 hours in an ED observation unit was retrospectively evaluated.

During a 29-month study period, 984 patients with blunt or penetrating abdominal trauma underwent DPL in the ED. All patients with a negative DPL and no other indication for hospital admission were sent to the ED observation unit where they were observed for 12 hours. Blunt trauma accounted for 66% of the injuries and penetrating trauma for 34%. The incidence of laparotomy was 17% for blunt trauma and 32% for penetrating trauma.

Of the 984 patients, 729 had a normal DPL, including 485 who were directly hospitalized for associated injuries and 14 who were transferred from the ED. The remaining 230 patients, 35 women and 195 men with a mean age of 30.3 years, were admitted to the observation unit. Of these 230 patients, 188 were discharged home from the unit after 12 hours of observation, 37 were admitted to the hospital, 3 signed out against medical advice, and 2 were transferred to another hospital. Five of the hospital admissions were to the intensive care unit. Four patients transferred from the ED observation unit required laparotomy, 3 of whom had hollow viscera injuries and 1 had a renal injury. There were no deaths. None of the 230 patients with trauma showed instability or sustained complications related to their stay in the ED observation unit. The potential savings realized by the use of an ED observation unit came to $51,329.

Admitting selected patients with significant blunt or penetrating abdominal trauma and a normal DPL to an ED observation unit for 12 hours of observation is a safe and cost-effective policy.

▶ Establishment of an ED observation unit should not be taken lightly. Space and personnel requirements are cost effective in consistently full hospitals. Hospitals with empty, but staffed, beds have fixed costs needing to be met by filling the beds, not an observation unit. The long-term benefits of bed reduction to the point of needing an observation unit are debatable. The evil of ED overcrowding must be balanced with the real benefit of an observation unit.

The authors described an observation unit that seems to be functioning effectively.

This busy urban hospital makes optimum use of the observation unit as a buffer on the demand for its limited inpatient capacity. (See also Abstract 3–23.)—J.E. Clinton, M.D.

---

**Prophylactic Antibiotics in Trauma: The Hazards of Underdosing**
Ericsson CD, Fischer RP, Rowlands BJ, Hunt C, Miller-Crotchett P, Reed L II
(Univ of Texas, Houston; Queen's Univ, Belfast)
*J Trauma* 29:1356–1361, 1989                                              2–7

---

The optimal regimen of antibiotics in trauma patients who require laparotomy remains controversial. Because prophylactic antibiotic regimens in trauma patients may be significantly altered by large fluid shifts and hyperdynamic physiologic responses, the effects of duration of coverage, dosing interval, and dose of prophylactic amikacin and clindamycin were assessed in 150 patients with abdominal trauma who required laparotomy. After intravenous administration of clindamycin (1,200 mg) and amikacin (7.5 mg/kg) in the emergency room, additional doses of clindamycin and amikacin were randomly administered 12 hours later (24-hour therapy): clindamycin and amikacin every 12 hours for 5 doses (72-hour therapy) or clindamycin (600 mg) every 6 hours for 11 doses and amikacin (7.5 mg/kg) for 5 doses (72-hour therapy). The patients were followed up for 30 postoperative days for the development of wound or intra-abdominal infections.

Rates of infection did not differ significantly between the 24- and 72-hour (21% vs. 19%) antibiotic coverage. Clindamycin dosed at 1,200 mg every 12 hours achieved acceptable serum concentrations, but infection rates with this regimen were not significantly higher than those seen with 600 mg every 6 hours (21% vs. 12%). In some patients who received amikacin, 6.7–7.5 mg/kg, the observed peak concentrations of amikacin were lower than generally accepted peak values, correlating with higher volumes of distribution, and the half-life of amikacin was shorter than expected. Increasing the amikacin dose to 11 mg/kg significantly decreased the infection rate in patients with high blood loss and high Injury Severity Scores and in patients without colon penetration. In trauma patients who require laparotomy, high doses of antibiotics are more effective than long courses of antibiotics in reducing the incidence of infection.

▶ Previous studies have already demonstrated that cefoxitin is as effective as clindamycin plus an aminoglycoside in preventing infection in penetrating abdominal trauma (1). The cost for clindamycin plus gentamicin was 15% higher than cefoxitin in that study. In the present study, the authors chose amikacin, which, at $46/day, is about 10 times the cost of gentamicin. Underdosing of aminoglycosides has been studied in septic patients and has been shown to be caused by an increase in the volume of distribution in the drug in sepsis. It is easy to explain the difficulty these authors had in achieving therapeutic levels. If determining the dosage of aminoglycosides is so difficult and the costs are so much higher, why bother using or, for that matter, studying this drug combination at all when cefoxitin works just as well? Perhaps the makers of Cleocin (clindamycin) who supported this research can explain.—W.P. Burdick, M.D.

*Reference*

1. Nichols RL, et al: *N Engl J Med* 311:1065, 1984.

## Cranial, Neck, and Laryngeal Vertebral Trauma

**Cervical Spine Injury and Radiography in Alert, High-Risk Patients**
McNamara RM, Heine E, Esposito B (Med College of Pennsylvania; Frankford Hosp, Philadelphia)
*J Emerg Med* 8:177–182, 1990                                   2–8

There is much controversy over the indications for routine cervical spine radiography (CSR) in blunt trauma patients who are at high risk for cervical spine injury but who have no cervical signs or symptoms. It is generally accepted that intoxicated patients or those with altered mental status must undergo CSR after sustaining injuries with the potential for cervical spine injury. However, because the need for CSR in alert, asymptomatic, nonintoxicated blunt trauma victims is less clear, medical charts were reviewed retrospectively to further examine the need for routine CSR.

During a 14-month period, 751 alert, nonintoxicated victims of blunt trauma were admitted to a level II trauma center, 401 of whom were at high risk for cervical spine injury by virtue of the mechanism of injury. Of these 401 patients, 115 subsequently were excluded from analysis because neck pain or tenderness were either absent or not recorded (Fig 2–1). None of the 115 excluded patients later were found to have sustained

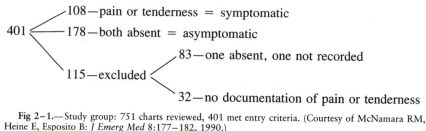

Fig 2–1.—Study group: 751 charts reviewed, 401 met entry criteria. (Courtesy of McNamara RM, Heine E, Esposito B: *J Emerg Med* 8:177–182, 1990.)

cervical spine fracture or ligament disruption. Of the remaining 286 patients, 178 were asymptomatic and 108 were symptomatic. Five patients had proved cervical spine fracture or ligament disruption, but all 5 were symptomatic at arrival in the ED.

None of the asymptomatic patients had fractures or ligament disruptions of the cervical spine. Not performing mandatory CSR in this group would have resulted in a significant cost saving and would likely have allowed for a more time-effective evaluation of these patients.

Routine CSR in alert, nonintoxicated, asymptomatic victims of blunt trauma is a costly practice that should be investigated further in a larger prospective trial.

▶ Very relevant. These patients frequently are admitted to the ED. The addition of routine CSR is costly in time, money, and possible accumulative radiation exposure to the ED staff. This article concludes that these x-ray studies can be safely eliminated in the clinically alert and asymptomatic patient. (See also Abstracts 2–9 and 4–55.)—E.H. Taliaferro, M.D.

---

**Unsuspected Upper Cervical Spine Fractures Associated With Significant Head Trauma: Role of CT**
Kirshenbaum KJ, Nadimpalli SR, Fantus R, Cavallino RP (Illinois Masonic Med Ctr, Chicago)
*J Emerg Med* 8:183–198, 1990                                                             2–9

---

Early and accurate diagnosis of cervical spine injuries is essential for patients with acute head and neck trauma because of a high risk of neurologic damage in such patients. Several recent studies have shown that CT is far more sensitive than traditional plain radiography for evaluating cervical spine fractures and spinal cord pathology. Despite these reports, cervical CT scanning in most institutions is limited to follow-up examinations of those patients with equivocal or suspicious findings on initial plain films that are suggestive of cervical spine injury.

Recently, 3 patients with significant head and neck trauma were evaluated with both CT and standard plain radiography of their cervical spines. Computed tomography showed significant C1–C2 fractures, whereas plain films were completely normal in all 3 cases. In a prospective study of the next 50 patients admitted with significant head trauma through an ED, CT evaluation of the upper cervical spine showed significant C1–C2 fractures in 4 patients that could not be detected with plain radiographic studies. Thus, at 1 institution alone, a total of 7 upper cervical spine fractures were detected with CT after plain films were found to be normal. All 7 patients had significant intracranial hemorrhage, and 4 of them had sustained significant skull fractures.

It is suggested that accepted trauma protocols be changed to include CT in the initial evaluation of patients with significant head trauma who may also have occult cervical spinal fracture, because plain films cannot be relied on to exclude fracture of the upper cervical spine.

▶ ,Right on. This is a significant contribution to the emergency medical literature.

For all practical purposes, skull films have been eliminated at our trauma center. It is tempting to eliminate cervical spine x-ray studies also.

This article suggests that cervical spine radiographs can be eliminated in favor of CT scan when cervical fractures of the upper spine are detected. It does not address lower cervical spine fractures. More research is in order before we throw away those x-ray requisition forms.— E.H. Taliaferro, M.D.

---

**Early Fresh Frozen Plasma Prophylaxis of Abnormal Coagulation Parameters in the Severely Head-Injured Patient is Not Effective**
Winter JP, Plummer D, Bottini A, Rockswold GR, Ray D (Hennepin County Med Ctr, Minneapolis)
*Ann Emerg Med* 18:553–555, 1989                                                2–10

---

Recently, early prophylactic treatment with fresh frozen plasma (FFP) has been recommended in severely head-injured patients to prevent the development of abnormal coagulopathy, but the efficacy of this approach has not been studied. In a retrospective study, data on 149 head-injured patients with a Glasgow Coma Scale of 9 or less were studied to evaluate the effect of early FFP in these patients. Of these, 106 patients received FFP in the absence of coagulopathy. Based on the time of administration of FFP, group 1 received FFP within an assigned time from injury ("early") and group 2 received FFP after time ("later") or not at all.

There were no differences in the posttreatment coagulation parameters (e.g., prothrombin time, partial thromboplastin time, and platelet concentration), between patients given FFP at an "early" time or those given FFP "later" or not at all.

The time of FFP administration is not critical for effective prophylaxis against coagulopathy in severely head-injured patients. Because of the accompanying risks of transfusions, a prospective study is warranted to evaluate the early use of FFP in severely head-injured patients.

▶ This study casts doubt on the efficacy of FFP to prevent coagulopathies in head-injured patients. The weight of the literature reflects that FFP should be reserved for those conditions in which a coagulopathy is either present or impending (a rapidly declining fibrinogen level). Early and aggressive use of FFP or other blood component therapy is advocated at first signs of coagulopathy in the head-injured patients.— E.J. Reisdorff, M.D.

---

**Relationship Between Admission Hyperglycemia and Neurologic Outcome of Severely Brain-Injured Patients**
Young B, Ott L, Dempsey R, Haack D, Tibbs P (Univ of Kentucky)
*Ann Surg* 210:466–473, 1989                                                2–11

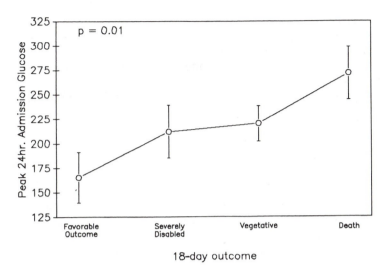

**Fig 2–2.**—Peak 24-hour admission serum level of glucose versus Glasgow Outcome Scale score 18 days after injury in 59 severely head-injured patients. All values are mean ± standard error of mean. (Courtesy of Young B, Ott L, Dempsey R, et al: *Ann Surg* 210:466–473, 1989.)

The possibility of a relationship between hyperglycemia and the severity of brain injury was examined in 59 consecutive patients who had a mean peak Glasgow Coma Scale score of 6.9 during the first 24 hours after hospital admission.

Forty-eight percent of patients had a peak admission blood level of glucose of greater than 200 mg/dL and less than 7% had a peak serum level of glucose of less than 120 mg/dL. A lower mean 24-hour admission peak blood level of glucose correlated with a better outcome at 18 days (Fig 2–2). Patients with a peak 24-hour level of glucose of greater than 200 mg/dL had a 2-unit increase in Glasgow Coma Scale scores during the 18-day study period, and those with lesser values had a 4-unit increase. The findings were the same after adjusting for the amount of glucose given within 24 hours after injury, the administration of steroid or insulin, and the presence of diabetes or multiple injuries.

Hyperglycemia at admission for head injury is frequent and is a useful indicator of the severity of injury. It also significantly predicts the outcome. A randomized study will be needed to determine whether prevention of hyperglycemia after head injury will improve the outcome.

▶ This article somewhat raises the chicken or the egg issue regarding poor neurologic outcomes in the setting of hyperglycemia. The authors' conclusion is that given a group of patients with head injury, those with higher-peak 24-hour glucose levels will have a less favorable outcome. The unanswered question is whether the poorer outcome is the result of more severe injury with greater stress response and higher glucose levels or is secondary to the hyperglycemia itself. Numerous studies utilizing anoxic ischemia cerebral injury models implicate the hyperglycemia itself with resultant greater brain lactate levels as the culprit. The take-home point for emergency physicians is not to be cavalier with the administration of D50 or other glucose preparations in the patient with such a potential cerebral insult. Every ED and prehospital team should strongly consider rapid serum glucose testing before routine dextrose administration in comatose patients.

An excellent review of this issue is available (1).—R.M. McNamara, M.D.

*Reference*

1. Browning DG, et al: *Ann Emerg Med* 19:683, 1990.

---

**The Tooth as a Foreign Body in Soft Tissue After Head and Neck Trauma**
Houck JR, Klingensmith MR (Pennsylvania State Univ, Hershey; Geisinger Med Ctr, Danville, Pa)
*Head and Neck* 11:545–549, 1989                                                2–12

Examination of the teeth should be an integral part of the evaluation of head and neck trauma. Aspiration or swallowing of avulsed or fractured teeth can lead to serious complications. Two cases of dental injury in which the tooth lodged as a foreign body in the soft tissues of the head and neck are evaluated.

Both patients had a missing tooth after a motor vehicle accident. In the first patient, a superficial examination and x-ray films failed to show the missing tooth. Chest radiographs showed possible foreign body, but flexible bronchoscopy failed to show the missing tooth. Reevaluation of the facial films showed the missing tooth displaced superiorly into the soft tissues, near the anterior nasal spine. In the second patient, cervical spine films showed the tooth embedded in the soft tissue of the left side of the neck, as well as a small fragment of bone in the retropharyngeal space at the level of C3, and extensive subcutaneous emphysema. These findings were confirmed by CT. The tooth was removed.

All missing teeth should be accounted for after head and neck trauma. Rarely, avulsed teeth can be propelled as foreign body into the soft tissues of the head and neck, which can lead to diagnostic confusion.

▶ As physicians, we receive very little emphasis on dental subjects in our training. Because of this fact, although it makes perfect sense that a tooth can be a troublesome foreign body, we frequently have a very low index of suspicion about the potential for such a problem. When this is coupled with the fact that our attentions are more appropriately directed to the initial resuscitation parameters such as airway control, we tend to overlook "the missing tooth." This article should certainly make us think about the problem more than we usually do. Of course, the prolonged search for the missing tooth is probably not going to be undertaken by the emergency physicians but by the trauma surgeon or other specialist such as the oral and maxillofacial surgeon or otolaryngologist.—E.J. Lucid, M.D.

## Laryngeal Paralysis as the Presenting Sign of Aortic Trauma
Woodson GE, Kendrick B (Univ of California, San Diego; Baylor College of Medicine, Houston)
*Arch Otolaryngol Head Neck Surg* 115:1100–1102, 1989                    2–13

Thoracic aorta disruption is usually fatal without prompt surgical intervention. Left recurrent laryngeal nerve paralysis has been reported in 10% of patients who survived long enough for a pseudoaneurysm to occur, but the time of onset has not been established. The incidence of laryngeal paralysis as the presenting sign in 50 patients with aortic pseudoaneurysms was compared with 50 patients with atherosclerotic aneurysms matched for location.

The group with traumatic aortic arch aneurysm had an average age of 42 years and a male/female ratio of 4:1. Injuries suggesting internal thoracic damage in the trauma group included rib fractures in 15 patients, clavicle or scapula fracture in 4, and soft-tissue injury in 8; 23 had no apparent injury. Hoarseness caused by the aneurysm developed in 6 patients with atherosclerotic vascular disease. The hoarseness came on slowly over several days to a few months; 4 patients in the trauma group were hoarse, 3 of whom had immediate onset.

Hoarseness may be the only indication of mediastinal trauma. Prompt radiologic examination of the mediastinum in patients with laryngeal paralysis after trauma will allow earlier diagnosis and treatment of thoracic aorta disruption.

▶ Isolated laryngeal paralysis, manifested as a change in voice (hoarseness), should prompt careful evaluation and reevaluation of the mediastinum in patients with major trauma (particularly thoracic deceleration injuries). (See also Abstracts 2–14, 2–15, and 2–16.)—J.R. Hoffman, M.D.

## Diagnosis and Management of Acute Laryngeal Trauma
Ganzel TM, Mumford LA (Univ of Louisville)
*Am Surg* 55:303–306, 1989                    2–14

Laryngeal fractures are unusual and may go unrecognized because patients with such fractures often have incurred multiple serious injuries in motor vehicle accidents. However, a missed or delayed diagnosis may result in laryngeal stenosis and the need for prolonged tracheostomy and multiple reconstructive procedures. Over a 4-year period, 13 patients with acute laryngeal injury were admitted to 1 hospital's trauma service.

Twelve of the 13 were men; 9 were involved in motor vehicle accidents. Three gunshot victims had penetrating injuries to the larynx. One patient had a sports injury. Hoarseness, stridor, and airway distress were the primary clinical indications of laryngeal trauma. Direct or indirect laryngoscopy was used to determine the location and extent of injury. The most common site of fracture was the thyroid cartilage.

Ten patients underwent tracheostomy; 4 had this procedure during initial resuscitation. Three patients recovered with bed rest, humidity, and short-term steroid therapy. All patients were treated successfully, although 1 continued to have hoarseness at follow-up.

Laryngeal fractures most often result when the neck strikes the steering wheel or dashboard. In addition to gunshot and knife wounds, "clothesline" injuries, such as those sustained when a motorcyclist hits an outstretched wire, account for a number of penetrating wounds. A blunt trauma may have no obvious external signs of injury. Computed tomography is helpful when fractures cannot be confirmed by clinical signs. Endoscopy is the definitive diagnostic procedure, although emergency tracheostomy should precede endoscopy when airway compromise is severe.

▶ Laryngeal fracture is a challenging problem for the emergency physician. Patients can precipitously decline, and establishing an adequate airway can be difficult. Indirect laryngoscopy and CT are the most useful adjuncts for evaluation. Fiberoptic nasopharyngoscopy is also helpful. Four patients in this study underwent tracheostomy in the ED. Tracheostomy is probably not appropriate for the emergency physician and should be reserved for the trauma surgeon or otolaryngologist. Percutaneous translaryngeal or transtracheal ventilation is the preferred technique for the emergency physician if gentle, directly visualized intubation is not possible. By performing percutaneous transtracheal ventilation first, tracheostomy can be performed in a more controlled environment and with a better-oxygenated patient. Other conditions can mimic laryngeal fracture such as soft tissue edema associated with cervical spine injury.—E.J. Reisdorff, M.D.

---

**Blunt Laryngeal Trauma: Classification and Management Protocol**
Fuhrman GM, Stieg FH III, Buerk CA (Orlando Regional Med Ctr, Fla)
*J Trauma* 30:87–92, 1990                                                                 2–15

---

Experience with 10 patients seen in an 18-month period with diagnoses of blunt laryngotracheal trauma was reviewed. The patients represented fewer than 1% of all blunt trauma victims seen in this period. Six patients were unrestrained occupants of motor vehicles. Two sustained direct blows, 1 was struck by a car, and 1 had a "clothesline" injury when riding a motorcycle.

Eight patients needed tracheotomy. All patients received antibiotics, which were continued if open repair was necessary. The most reliable clinical findings were hoarseness, tenderness, and subcutaneous emphysema; only 4 patients had externally evident injury of the anterior neck. Three of 6 CT scans showed laryngeal injury. Eight patients had a total of 12 operations. None of the patients died, and 6 of 8 patients have been decannulated to date. Six of the 10 patients had good voice quality, and 4 had fair voice quality when last assessed.

Both Gussack and Schaefer (Fig 2–3) have proposed protocols for

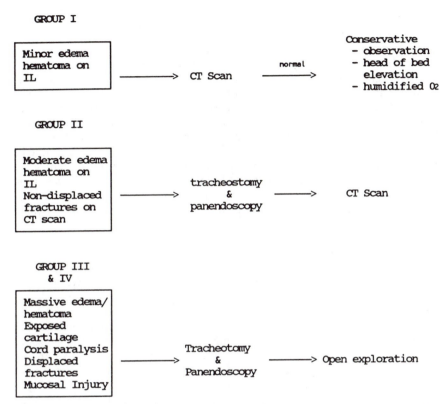

GROUP I

| Minor edema hematoma on IL | ———→ | CT Scan | —normal—→ | Conservative<br>- observation<br>- head of bed elevation<br>- humidified O₂ |

GROUP II

| Moderate edema hematoma on IL Non-displaced fractures on CT scan | ———→ | tracheostomy & panendoscopy | ———→ | CT Scan |

GROUP III & IV

| Massive edema/ hematoma Exposed cartilage Cord paralysis Displaced fractures Mucosal Injury | ———→ | Tracheotomy & Panendoscopy | ———→ | Open exploration |

Fig 2–3.—Summary of Schaefer's protocol. (Courtesy of Fuhrman GM, Stieg FH III, Buerk CA: *J Trauma* 30:87–92, 1990.)

managing laryngotracheal injuries. Both recommend indirect laryngoscopy as the initial diagnostic study. Early operation is appropriate for blunt laryngotracheal trauma.

▶ Luckily, laryngeal trauma is rare, occurring in less than 1% of all blunt traumas seen in this level I trauma center. Common presenting symptoms include hoarseness, shortness of breath, inability to tolerate the supine position, and pain. Usually the involved region will be tender to palpation and may have evidence of subcutaneous air. In the patient without an adequate airway or one unable to tolerate the supine position, the authors suggest emergent intervention. Because their operative experience revealed that separation of the proximal and distal segments of a completely transected larynx can approach 8 cm, they believe that oral intubation is dangerous and unlikely to be successful. Cricothyroidotomy must be performed. In the patient with a stable airway, initial ED evaluation should include visualization of the larynx. Rapid and unexpected compromise of the airway should always be of concern. Use of a fiberoptic nasopharyngoscope is desirable. It should be a basic tool in all EDs.— H. Unger, M.D.

### Evaluation and Treatment of Acute Laryngeal Fractures

Schild JA, Denneny EC (Univ of Illinois, Chicago)
Head Neck 11:491–496, 1989                                    2–16

Treatment of laryngeal fractures has advanced in recent years, and the airway can now be restored without aspiration or stenosis in most patients. Because the best treatment of vocal chord dysfunction from trauma remains controversial, data on 12 patients with blunt, neck trauma and 3 with penetrating laryngeal trauma were reviewed in reference to symptoms, type of injury, and treatment to determine the value of CT and photographic documentation. Photographs of each patient were taken during direct laryngoscopy. All patients had normal cervical spine radiographs. Axial CT scans were obtained and compared with clinical findings. Treatment results were evaluated for speech and for adequate airway patency.

The patients were aged 16–67 years; 11 were male. Symptoms ranged from mild neck discomfort to dyspnea and hoarseness; 5 patients had respiratory distress and stridor, 6 had dysphagia or odynophagia, and 3 had hemoptysis. Treatment varied according to severity of injury; 7 patients were observed only and 8 required surgery. Endoscopic photographs were valuable in assessing the patients' progress, particularly in those with more severe injuries. Computed tomography was reliable for defining the extent of soft-tissue injury and for diagnosing the presence and displacement of fractures. At completion of treatment, all 15 patients had satisfactory airways for normal activity and normal deglutition. All patients returned to preinjury activities without dyspnea. Of the 12 patients with voice abnormalities, 3 had permanent voice changes, but none required amplification devices.

In all patients, CT was extremely valuable for accurate evaluation of soft-tissue trauma and fractures; it also enabled better visualization of the cricoarytenoid area, where severe abnormalities produced later vocal cord dysmotility than did plain films. Patients with minor injuries were accurately evaluated by CT for conservative management, whereas severely injured patients had better surgical treatment planning.

▶ Although no formal evaluation was done, the authors of this clinical series believed that CT was helpful in stable patients to determine the scope of laryngotracheal injury and especially to help avoid surgery, when appropriate.—J.R. Hoffman, M.D.

---

### Penetrating Neck Injuries: Recommendations for Selective Management

Wood J, Fabian TC, Mangiante EC (Univ of Tennessee, Memphis; Presley Mem Trauma Ctr, Memphis)
J Trauma 29:602–605, 1989                                    2–17

---

Ever since a 1956 study demonstrated that mandatory neck exploration decreased morbidity and mortality from penetrating neck injuries, this approach has been standard policy. However, normal findings of exploration in as high as 76% of patients have been reported. To determine the relative accuracy and safety of traditional and more selective concepts in the management of penetrating neck trauma, data were reviewed on 225 patients admitted with penetrating neck injuries over a 4-year period.

Patients were divided into 5 groups, based on clinical presentation, site of injury, and method of management. The first group (31 patients) included 29 with shock or active hemorrhage, or both, and 2 with respiratory distress. All 31 had immediate exploration. The second group (76 patients) was clinically stable but had anterior wounds and equivocal physical findings, with or without normal results on contrast studies. All had mandatory exploration.

The third group (17 patients) and the fourth group (80 patients) were clinically similar to those in the second group. However, the third group had abnormal findings on contrast studies and underwent exploration; the fourth had normal results on contrast studies and was kept under observation for 24 hours. The last group (21 patients) had wounds in the posterior triangle or minimal physical findings.

There were no missed injuries in the fourth or fifth group. Two esophageal injuries were missed in the second group, and a carotid injury was missed in the third group.

The findings were used as the basis for the following new guidelines for selective management of penetrating neck injuries. Immediate exploration should be performed in patients with major blood loss or respiratory distress; stable patients can be managed according to information obtained by arteriography and diagnostic esophageal studies; patients sustaining wounds with low probability of serious injury because of lateral or posterior location or prolonged time from injury can be observed; and all patients with reasonable likelihood of esophageal injury, regardless of surgical exploration, should have barium esophagram or esophagoscopy, or both.

▶ The issue of mandatory neck exploration for penetrating injuries is once again studied. Abnormal x-ray studies or the presence of severe patient compromise increased the percentage of explorations with abnormal findings. Based on this study, the authors recommend that even though immediate exploration is indicated in those patients with hemodynamic or respiratory compromise, stable patients could be managed according to the presence or absence of abnormal arteriography or diagnostic esophageal studies.

Meyer et al. (1) studied 120 patients with zone 2 penetrating neck wounds. In all but 7 (who required immediate surgery), extensive radiographic evaluation preceded neck exploration. The results of 24% of explorations were abnormal (significant injuries). Five patients with normal preoperative examinations and x-ray studies had significant injuries at exploration. There have been several studies done that have either advocated mandatory exploration or recommended selective management. An argument can be made to individualize decision making according to the institution, the clinician, and the clinical status of the patient. The ready availability of quality radiographic studies as well as laryngoscopy and esophagoscopy will be required if one chooses the selective management approach. The clinician must decide whether he or she is willing to perform a substantial number of neck explorations.—J.M. Mitchell, M.D.

*Reference*

1. Meyer JP, et al: *Arch Surg* 122:592, 1987.

---

**Incidence and Diagnosis of C7-T1 Fractures and Subluxations in Multiple-Trauma Patients: Evaluation of the Advanced Trauma Life Support Guidelines**
Gisbert VL, Hollerman JJ, Ney AL, Rockswold GL, Ruiz E, Jacobs DM, Bubrick MP (Hennepin County Med Ctr, Minneapolis)
*Surgery* 106:702–709, 1989                                    2–18

The consequences of a delayed diagnosis of traumatic fracture or subluxation of the cervical spine can be devastating. The Committee on Trauma of the American College of Surgeons recommends that all 7 cervical vertebrae be identified on radiographs for all patients who sustain multiple trauma. To determine whether C7–T1 injuries occur often enough to warrant cervical spine radiologic examination of all trauma patients, the records of 201 patients with cervical spine fracture or fracture-dislocation injuries seen during a 5-year period were reviewed retrospectively.

Of the 201 patients, 22 had fracture or subluxation at C7 or C7–T1. Fourteen of these 22 were injured in motor vehicle accidents, 6 were injured in falls, and 2 sustained direct blows to the neck. Nineteen patients had neck pain, tenderness, or neurologic findings on initial examination, but the other 3 were awake and asymptomatic.

Diagnoses could be made in only 3 patients from the initial lateral cervical spine radiograph. For the remaining 19 patients, diagnoses were confirmed by swimmer's view, oblique views, flexion-extension views, or CT scans. Diagnoses were not made in 2 patients until 24 hours later. Follow-up radiographs were abnormal in 3 of 22 cervical spine films, 10 of 14 swimmer's views, 2 of 3 oblique views, and 2 of 3 flexion-extension views. Fourteen of 20 follow-up CT scans were abnormal.

These findings support the recommendation for the liberal use of cervical spine radiography in trauma patients. However, the lateral cervical spine film as a single screening view is inadequate because of its inability to visualize the C7 vertebral body in most patients. The inclusion of a swimmer's view to visualize C7 and the C7–T1 intervertebral space is recommended. Strong consideration should be given to the routine use of a 5-view trauma series.

▶ It is standard practice at our facility that the C7–T1 junction be visualized radiographically in the multiple trauma patient during the initial screening examinations done in the ED. Like the authors' experience, the swimmer's view is often required to accomplish this because of the inability to view this area adequately on most lateral spine films. Because of injury severity, many patients do not have complete cervical spine series performed initially but are appropriately immobilized until the study is completed.

Liberal use of cervical spine films is advocated, even in the alert patient without neck pain, since 3 of their 22 patients with cervical fractures were asymptomatic. All 3 had stable injuries. One is cautioned that severe, painful injuries elsewhere can divert the patient's and physician's attention away from the cervical spine.—J.M. Mitchell, M.D.

---

## Early Mobilisation and Outcome in Acute Sprains of the Neck

McKinney LA (Royal Victoria Hosp, Belfast)
*BMJ* 299:1006–1008, 1989                                   2–19

---

Acute sprains of the neck have usually been treated by rest, analgesia, and the wearing of collars. Many patients with acute neck sprains continue to have symptoms 2 years after the injury. Early mobilization appears to be an effective treatment, but its long-term value has not been reported. This prospective study compared recovery in 167 patients randomized to receive 1 of 3 treatments.

Patients had sustained their injuries in traffic accidents. Treatment consisted of rest for 10 to 14 days, physiotherapy, or self-mobilization. Those receiving physiotherapy were treated for 6 weeks with hot and cold applications, hydrotherapy, traction, and active and passive repetitive movements. The self-mobilization program consisted of a 30-minute advice session on posture, movement, and analgesia. These patients were advised to avoid excessive reliance on a collar.

After 2 years, patients completed a questionnaire on duration and severity of pain. Those who were given advice on mobilization exercises to do at home did significantly better than the other 2 patient groups. Nearly one half of those treated with rest (46%) or physiotherapy (44%) still had symptoms compared with 23% of the early mobilization group. Sixty percent of the 104 patients who recovered within the follow-up period had done so within 3 months of their injury; only 10% recovered later than 6 months. Those with persistent symptoms had used a collar for significantly longer periods. Initial severity of neck pain (but not original range of cervical movement) was associated with lack of recovery.

Early mobilization significantly reduces long-term outcome and is a more effective treatment than rest or physiotherapy. Before this trial was completed, all patients were given instruction about effective mobilization, and the rest protocol was discontinued.

▶ This is another in a series of British studies (this one from Ireland) suggesting that early mobilization is optimal treatment, in the long-term as well as the short, for a variety of musculoskeletal injuries. Although I suspect the author's conclusions are very likely to be correct, major limitations in the study design (a single unblinded author/investigator who both instructed all the patients, followed them up himself, and decided how well they were doing, using apparently only a yes/no test regarding "continuing symptoms" he himself administered) make it impossible to support as definitively early mobilization for "whiplash" as for ankle sprains, or muscular low-back pain, for example.—J.R. Hoffman, M.D.

---

**Comparison of Five-View and Three-View Cervical Spine Series in the Evaluation of Patients With Cervical Trauma**
Freemyer B, Knopp R, Piche J, Wales L, Williams J (Valley Med Ctr, Fresno, Calif)
*Ann Emerg Med* 18:818–821, 1989                                    2–20

---

Trauma patients with suspected cervical spine injury have traditionally been evaluated with a 3-view trauma series consisting of cross-table lateral, anteroposterior, and open-mouth odontoid views. Because of an ongoing controversy over the need for additional views in the initial screening, a prospective study was conducted to determine whether the addition of supine oblique views would improve the diagnostic sensitivity of plain radiography in the diagnosis of cervical spine injury.

During a 2-year period, trauma patients were prospectively selected to have the standard 3-view series and supine oblique views. Only patients with a neurologic deficit, neck pain, or decreased ability to perceive pain from an altered mental status were included in the study. The 58 high-risk patients also underwent conventional thin-section tomography of the cervical spine, which served as the gold standard. Radiographic findings were classified as abnormal, suspicious, or normal.

Of the 58 patients, 25 had normal tomographic scans and 33 had 68 abnormal tomographic findings. The diagnoses were correct in 30 of the 33 patients who had the standard 3-view series. The addition of supine oblique views did not identify any additional patients. Although the supine oblique views did not identify any fractures or subluxations missed on the 3-view series, the addition of these views did allow a more specific diagnosis in some patients. The routine use of supine oblique views when screening trauma patients for suspected cervical spine injuries does not appear warranted.

▶ This study suggests that the experienced emergency physician is not likely to miss cervical fractures or dislocations using the standard 3-view series. Supine obliques may make for more accurate diagnosis in certain specific injuries such as unilateral-locked facets, articular mass fractures, pedicle fractures, lamina fractures, and subluxation from posterior ligamentous sprain.—G.V. Anderson, M.D.

---

**Cervical Injuries: Perils of the Swimmer's View: Case Report**
Davis JW (Univ of California, San Diego)
*J Trauma* 29:891–893, 1989                                    2–21

Occasionally, a swimmer's view, with 1 arm elevated above the head and the other by the patient's side, is required to visualize adequately the C7–T1 junction in a patient with cervical injury. This procedure is generally believed to be without risk if performed with adequate head and neck immobilization. A subluxation of an unstable cervical spine injury occurred during swimmer's positioning.

Man, 21, presented with tenderness at C5 and complete quadriplegia below that level after a major trauma. Cervical spine radiographs showed posterior element fractures at C5 but failed to show C7–T1. A swimmer's view was obtained and showed a subtotal subluxation of C5 on C6 not shown on the previous film. A repeated lateral radiograph, with the patient returned to the neutral position, showed complete reduction at C5–C6.

A swimmer's positioning may cause movement in the unstable spine, which caused subluxation of the cervical spine in this patient. It is recommended that the initial radiographs should be obtained and reviewed without traction or swimmer's positioning. If the patient has clinical or radiographic evidence of injury, bilateral oblique views, plain lateral tomography, or CT may be necessary to evaluate the C7–T1 junction.

▶ Past cineradiographic studies have demonstrated that even with inline traction, any manipulation of the airway will cause movement within the cervical spine. This article now reports a very interesting finding of cervical movement with a swimmer's view. Of course, one does not know what other movement may have occurred when this view was obtained. Once the standard lateral radiograph has demonstrated cervical injury, especially in the symptomatic patient, great care must be taken with any further movement of the patient until the cervical spine has been well stabilized. A study would be nice to determine the amount of cervical displacement that occurs with simply pulling on the patient's arms with no traction on the head; such a technique is, perhaps, the most commonly used in trying to view C7–T1.—J.T. Amsterdam, M.D.

**Management Strategy for Penetrating Oropharyngeal Injury**
Singer JI (Wright State Univ, Dayton, Ohio)
*Pediatr Emerg Care* 5:250–252, 1989                    2–22

Children who fall while holding an object in their mouth typically have transient oral bleeding and intraoral pain. Even a benign-appearing peritonsillar injury in a child with few symptoms can lead to devastating consequences.
The most frequent injury is a V-shaped tear at the junction of the hard and soft palates. Impalement of the hard palate, laceration of the labial or buccal mucosa or tongue, and penetration of the sublingual, retropharyngeal, or precervical space are less frequent injuries. A pencil point can produce a life-threatening vascular injury, tissue emphysema, or infected wound. Penetration of the retromolar region can lead to delayed injury of

the internal carotid artery. Endogenous organisms can become pathogens after a penetrating or crush injury of the oral cavity. Adequate lighting is important for an accurate oral examination. A short-acting barbiturate or benzodiazepine can facilitate the examination.

Intraoral injuries should not be sutured because the gingiva and palate have great potential for spontaneous healing. Antibiotics should be considered for lacerations longer than 1 cm. A patient with a laceration in the parapharyngeal region may receive salicylate for 4–5 days as an anticoagulant. If the patient has an impalement injury of the lateral soft palate or tonsillar region, vascular injury should be assumed, and the patient should be admitted for at least 24 hours. Retropharyngeal involvement also calls for inpatient observation for 1 day.

▶ Three cases do not settle the issues, but the authors provide some guidelines for managing kids who fall with a pencil in the mouth. Palatal lacerations may require antibiotics but not suturing. Lateral parapharyngeal injuries may damage carotid arteries, but aspirin may be sufficient antithrombotic prophylaxis. Retropharyngeal injuries can communicate with the mediastinum and should also be closely observed.—T. Stair, M.D.

---

**Stab Wounds to the Neck: Role of Angiography**
Hartling RP, McGahan JP, Lindfors KK, Blaisdell FW (Univ of California, Davis, Sacramento)
*Radiology* 172:79–82, 1980                                              2–23

The role of angiography in penetrating neck trauma remains controversial. Angiographic findings in 61 stab wounds in 45 patients were correlated with physical findings. Wounds were classified into 3 anatomic zones: zone 1, below the cricoid cartilage; zone 2, cricoid cartilage to mandibular angle; and zone 3, mandibular angle to skull base.

Eighteen stab wounds involved major physical findings, including pulse deficit, active bleeding or expanding hematoma, bruit or murmur, neurologic deficit, or hypotension. Only 2 of these wounds involved significant vascular injuries; both occurred in patients with zone 1 trauma. The remaining 43 wounds involved minor physical findings, and the only indications for angiography were nonexpanding hematoma or proximity of trauma to major vessels. None of these resulted in significant vascular trauma. On the basis of angiographic results, there were 2 true positive, 16 false positive, 43 true negative, and no false negative physical examinations for significant arterial injury.

Angiography is indicated in zone 2 and zone 3 stab wounds associated with major physical findings because of possibile underlying vascular trauma. Angiography also is recommended in zone 1 stab wounds, regardless of physical findings, because of possible clinically occult vascular trauma. Angiography may not be warranted in patients with zone 2 and

3 stab wounds with minor physical findings, because occult vascular injury is unlikely.

▶ According to this study, stab wounds in the neck below the cricoid cartilage (zone 1) should receive angiography regardless of findings because of the probability of occult vascular damage. However, minor stab wounds of the neck area between the cricoid cartilage and the angle of the mandible (zone 2) or between the angle of the mandible and base of the skull (zone 3) are much less likely to have occult vascular injury. These general guidelines for the evaluation of the wounds of the neck may seem to be helpful, but each case has to be individualized. There are few absolutes in medicine!—G.V. Anderson, M.D.

## Chest and Cardiac Trauma

**Traumatic Asphyxia: Report of a Case**
Ghali GE, Ellis E III (Univ of Texas, Dallas)
*J Oral Maxillofac Surg* 47:867–870, 1989                    2–24

The clinical syndrome of traumatic asphyxia appears indistinguishable from the clinical signs of maxillofacial trauma. A patient was seen with classic traumatic asphyxia.

Man, 35, who was a construction worker, was pinned down with a large metal beam on his chest. Examination revealed bilateral periorbital ecchymosis, bilateral subconjunctival hemorrhage, generalized facial erythema, and ecchymosis over the upper thorax. The left clavicle was fractured. Maxillofacial injuries were not observed clinically or radiographically. Results of an ophthalmologic examination were normal.

Traumatic asphyxia is a rare condition, usually resulting from a force applied in an anteroposterior direction to the victim's abdomen, chest, or both. It appears that a concurrent chest compression and closure of the airway after deep inspiration may play an integral role in the pathogenesis of traumatic asphyxia. The clinical syndrome of traumatic asphyxia includes subconjunctival and periorbital hemorrhage, facial edema, and cyanosis, combined with ecchymotic hemorrhages of the upper part of the chest and face. Associated injuries are common. Long-term sequelae are uncommon, although visual impairments have been reported.

▶ This is an outstanding example of the often-used phrase "a picture is worth a thousand words." These are excellent facial and upper chest, colored photographs of a 35-year-old construction worker who was pinned down for several minutes with a large, heavy steel beam on his chest. The gross appearance of the face, conjunctiva, and upper part of the chest suggest major maxillofacial trauma. Somehow the term "traumatic asphyxia" doesn't provide the necessary imagery for the reader to "grasp the picture."—G.V. Anderson, M.D.

### A Triage System for Stab Wounds to the Chest

Wormald PJ, Knottenbelt JD, Linegar AG (Groote Schuur Hosp, Cape Town, South Africa)
*S Afr Med* 76:211–212, 1989                              2–25

Ideally, all patients with chest wounds should have chest radiography, but radiographic facilities may not be available on a 24-hour basis in many parts of the world. To determine whether clinical signs could be used as a guide for effective triage of patients with chest wounds, 5 clinical parameters, including pulse rate (>100/min), blood pressure (<100 mm Hg systolic), respiratory rate (>20/min), auscultation (reduced breath sounds on affected side), and hemoglobin value (<13 g/dL), were evaluated in 200 patients with chest wounds before chest radiography or thoracostomy were undertaken.

Chest radiographs were abnormal in 131 patients. Respiratory rate and chest auscultation were the most sensitive indicators for chest lesions, but all signs were valuable. The sensitivity of 1 or more positive signs was 99.2%, specificity was 61%, positive predictive value was 95%, and negative predictive value was 98%. The sensitivity of 2 or more positive signs was 86% and the specificity was 99%. The positive predictive value was 99%, and the negative predictive value was 78%.

This simple system could be valuable in areas without a 24-hour radiographic facility. Patients with no signs initially should be monitored closely for delayed hemothorax or pneumothorax.

▶ This paper is interesting because it makes one realize that despite all the sophistication of medicine in the United States, there are many places worldwide where access to radiography is not readily available. To me, the important message in this paper is that not only can the physical examination be used initially to triage patients but that continued, frequent observation and reassessment of these patients must occur during the early phase of their management. This dictum should apply even in sophisticated systems where technology is available. We must take care not to let technology take the place of clinical judgment.—E.J. Lucid, M.D.

### Pneumothorax: Appearance on Lateral Chest Radiographs

Glazer HS, Anderson DJ, Wilson BS, Molina PL, Sagel SS (Washington Univ, St Louis)
*Radiology* 173:707–711, 1989                          2–26

Because pneumothorax usually is obvious on the erect posteroanterior projection, little attention has been paid to the findings on the erect lateral projection. Lateral chest radiographs were reviewed for 100 patients with pneumothorax who had a total of 122 examinations. Their mean age was 55 years.

Pneumothorax was identified on the posteroanterior projection in 97% of studies and on the lateral view in 89%. For 19 lateral films findings were subtle. The lateral view was considered helpful in 14% of examinations. A displaced pleural line was seen most often anteriorly or posteriorly and less often at the lung apex or at a subpulmonic site. In 11 cases an air-fluid level was the only sign of pneumothorax on the lateral projection. The lung base was the most frequent site of an air-fluid level.

Confirmatory signs of pneumothorax usually are discernible on lateral chest radiographs, and in nearly 15% of cases, this projection can provide helpful additional information.

▶ Occasionally, pneumothorax is a subtle finding on chest radiographs, and I'll take all of the help I can get in reading them. This study reminded me of what to look for on the lateral view, but I am not going to start ordering posteroanterior and lateral views to rule out pneumothorax. An expiratory posteroanterior view will still be my choice if the routine posteroanterior view is not diagnostic.— E. Ruiz, M.D.

---

**Traumatic Pneumothorax: A Scheme for Rapid Patient Turnover**
Knottenbelt JD, van der Spuy JW (Groote Schuur Hosp; Research Council, Cape Town, South Africa)
*Injury* 21:77–80, 1990                                          2–27

---

A protocol developed for managing traumatic pneumothorax by tube thoracostomy for a minimal time was based on early mobilization and drain removal. Removing a drain within 24 hours usually was possible with minimal morbidity and an excellent outcome. Patients were encouraged to move about the ward and to exercise vigorously, taking their drain bottles where necessary. Enough analgesia was provided for patients to breathe deeply and cough without undue pain. Drains were removed during sustained Valsalva's maneuver when lungs had reexpanded and bubbles were absent from drain bottles. Removal was delayed 12 hours if a continual air leak had been present.

Of 690 patients with penetrating injuries and 114 with blunt chest trauma, 333 initially had conservative management. Thirty-three of them eventually needed drainage for enlarging pneumothoraces, and 4 of these patients should have had drainage at the outset. One of 471 patients having tube thoracostomy before admission to a ward needed early thoracotomy for massive air leakage. One fifth of all patients having drainage needed suction for air leakage. Six patients underwent operative pleurodesis. Ten patients needed repeat drainage because air reaccumulated.

This protocol is effective and safe and allows a high turnover of patients with traumatic pneumothorax. Patients must be followed up after discharge. Whether this approach is feasible for patients with missile injuries of the chest is not clear.

▶ The authors present a prospective study of 804 patients with a pneumothorax caused by chest injury of any kind. Patients treated with closed thoracostomy were actively exercised, once expansion occurred, to see if an air leak could be precipitated. In the absence of a demonstrated leak, the tube was removed. "Leakers" were placed on high-volume suction, and the test was repeated after 12 hours. According to a rather elaborate decision-making protocol, approximately 42% of the patients were initially treated without thoracostomy. Ten percent of these subsequently required closed thoracostomy. Chest x-ray films were taken at 2-hour intervals throughout the evaluation of all patients. Many would question whether this was a sensible utilization of resources (see also Abstract 3–13 for a more aggressive treatment protocol for a less serious [i.e., nontraumatic] pneumothorax).—D.K. Wagner, M.D.

---

**Five Thousand Seven Hundred Sixty Cardiovascular Injuries in 4459 Patients: Epidemiologic Evolution 1958 to 1987**
Mattox KL, Feliciano DV, Burch J, Beall AC Jr, Jordan GL Jr, DeBakey ME (Baylor College of Medicine, Houston; Ben Taub Gen Hosp, Houston)
*Ann Surg* 209:698–705, 1989                                    2–28

---

Like many major American cities, Houston is in the throes of an epidemic of cardiovascular injuries that has continued since the mid-1970s. A total of 4,459 patients were treated for 5,760 such injuries at a single civilian trauma center in the past 3 decades. All but 14% of the patients were male; the average age was 30 years.

Penetrating injuries accounted for a majority of cases. Presently stab wounds outnumber gunshot wounds, but for the entire review period, more than half of all injuries were caused by gunshot wounds. Two thirds of all treated injuries involved the trunk (including the neck). Another fifth were lower extremity injuries. One third of the injuries involved the abdominal vasculature. Virtually all named major vessels in the body were injured. Thoracic and upper limb injuries have continued to increase in the most recent years of the survey period.

The rise in vascular trauma in Houston is out of proportion to the population growth in the past 30 years. Penetrating wounds of the trunk have predominated in the past 15 years, as in other series. The present data do not indicate that gunshot wounds are being produced by increasingly larger-caliber and higher-velocity missiles.

▶ This retrospective record review is of interest to the emergency physician as an illustration of the penetrating injury.—J.E. Clinton, M.D.

---

**Cardiac Injuries: A Clinical and Autopsy Profile**
Kulshrestha P, Das B, Iyer KS, Sampath KA, Sharma ML, Rao IM, Venugopal P (All India Inst of Med Sciences, New Delhi)
*J Trauma* 30:203–207, 1990                                    2–29

---

The number of cardiac injuries seen in urban hospitals is increasing, the most frequent of which are pericardial tamponade and excessive bleeding. Of 102 cardiac injuries seen in a 4-year period, 45 were blunt,

36 were stab, and 21 were gunshot injuries. A ventricle was involved in a majority of cases. One third of the patients died at the scene, and 57% died during transportation. Only 11 patients reached the hospital alive; 10 of them survived thoracotomy with repair of the injury. Blunt cardiac trauma was associated with the worst prognosis. Patients with atrial or pulmonary artery injuries had better chances of surviving than those with ventricular injuries. Right ventricular trauma was less lethal than injury to the left ventricle. Surviving patients were doing well up to 4 years after operative treatment.

Rapid transportation of cardiac injury victims and aggressive surgical management hold the most hope of improving the outcome of these injuries.

▶ This paper fails to answer one of the most important questions concerning cardiac trauma: What is the best strategy for handling the patient with a penetrating cardiac injury who arrives at the hospital without vital signs? Although it is clear that the salvage rate for patients with blunt chest trauma and no vital signs approaches 0%, most trauma centers will still attempt resuscitation in patients without vitals who have evidence of penetrating chest trauma. This is true especially if there were vital signs at the scene. This paper would seem to suggest that at the All India Institute of Medical Sciences, no resuscitative efforts will be made on this group of patients. Of the 91 patients entered in the study who fit this criteria, the only procedure performed was an autopsy.—H. Unger, M.D.

---

**Blunt Cardiac Injury: Is This Diagnosis Necessary?**
Healey MA, Brown R, Fleiszer D (McGill Univ, Montreal)
*J Trauma* 30:137–146, 1990                                2–30

---

Blunt cardiac injury in multiply injured patients remains problematic because there is substantial confusion and disagreement over its diagnosis, incidence, implications, and treatment. Cardiac selective creatine kinase (CK-MB) assays and ECGs often correlate poorly with diagnoses made on clinical grounds or by other laboratory methods. Because of this lack of consensus, the records of all patients treated for blunt trauma during a 6-year period were retrospectively studied.

Of 342 patients admitted to the intensive care unit with blunt trauma, cardiac contusion on clinical grounds was diagnosed in 44 patients (13%). There were 31 men and 13 women with an average age of 40 years. The mean injury severity score was 35. Fifteen patients (34%) arrived at the ED in shock.

Twenty-seven patients (61%) subsequently had abnormalities of cardiac function, 13 (30%) of whom required treatment. Ectopy and aberrant conduction usually resolved spontaneously without treatment. Twenty-two patients underwent surgical procedures, 8 of whom had intraoperative cardiac-related complications. There were no intraoperative deaths, but 4 patients died shortly after operation. The overall mortality was 27%.

Neither findings on the chest radiograph nor physical examination correlated with subsequent cardiac complications. Admission ECG abnormalities did correlate with the subsequent development of cardiac abnormalities. Many patients had normal CK-MB levels at admission despite a clinical diagnosis of blunt cardiac injury. However, there was a strong correlation between CK-MB elevation and the development of cardiac complications. Very high CK-MB levels of greater than 200 μ/L were associated with a 100% incidence of cardiac complications. The combination of abnormal ECG findings plus elevated CK-MB levels predicted cardiac complications in all cases.

Blunt cardiac injury is an important source of morbidity and mortality in blunt trauma victims. However, as there is as yet no definitive method of diagnosing all blunt cardiac injuries, the traditional high index of suspicion and clinical impression derived from the patient's history, physical examination, and chest radiograph should be used to identify those patients who are at high risk for cardiac injury. It is then more important to determine which of these patients will have clinically significant complications than it is to confirm whether there is blunt heart injury.

▶ The weight of evidence shows that myocardial contusion contributes to mortality in patients with other serious injuries but can be innocuous in isolation. We should prepare for infarction, arrhythmias, and failure in patients with significant chest trauma but seldom need to make this diagnosis. (See also Abstract 4–66.)—T. Stair, M.D.

---

**A Plea for Sensible Management of Myocardial Contusion**
Baxter BT, Moore EE, Moore FA, McCroskey BL, Ammons LA (Denver Gen Hosp; Univ of Colorado)
*Am J Surg* 158:557–562, 1989                                    2–31

---

Cardiac evaluation of blunt myocardial injury in patients with nonpenetrating chest trauma from motor vehicle accidents commonly consists of the same diagnostic procedures as used in the evaluation of patients with atherosclerotic coronary artery disease. However, unlike acute myocardial infarction, cardiac muscle ischemia from blunt chest trauma causes only a transient decrease in ventricular function after which coronary perfusion is rapidly normalized. The clinical course in patients with nonpenetrating cardiac trauma was evaluated prospectively to delineate a safe but more cost-effective policy.

During a 3-year study, 280 patients with a mean age of 39 years were evaluated to exclude myocardial contusion after they had sustained blunt chest trauma. During the initial 48 hours after trauma, serial determinations of creatinine phosphokinase (CPK) and lactate dehydrogenase (LDH) and their isoenzymes were determined at baseline and at 8-hour intervals thereafter. All patients underwent continuous cardiac monitoring for 24 hours.

Myocardial contusion was diagnosed in 35 (13%) of the 280 patients. The diagnosis was based on ECG abnormalities in 30 patients, an increase in CPK isoenzymes in 9 patients, and on both in 4 patients. The increase in CPK isoenzyme levels always occurred within the first 24 hours after admission; the levels remained abnormal for more than 24 hours in only 2 patients. Total LDH levels were elevated in only 2 patients, and the elevation appeared to be a false positive finding in 1 of those patients. Two patients died of refractory cardiogenic shock 4 and 12 hours after injury. Seven patients required treatment of arrhythmias or myocardial failure. None of the remaining 271 patients had cardiac symptoms.

Patients who sustain blunt chest trauma in motor vehicle accidents are at low risk for myocardial contusion. The clinical diagnosis of myocardial contusion can be safely excluded when a normal ECG and normal cardiac enzyme levels are present during the initial 24-hour observation.

▶ This prospective study of patients considered at risk for blunt cardiac injury attempted to define the therapeutic complications of suspected or confirmed diagnosis of myocardial contusion. This is an important consideration in terms of health care economics and often overburdened trauma facilities and critical care units. From their study, the authors suggest that if the patient is initially hemodynamically stable, without arrhythmias or a history of coronary artery disease, complications of myocardial contusion usually occur within the first 12 hours. They also suggest that these complications are transient conduction disburbance arrhythmias, easily managed in a monitored but not necessarily critical care setting. They attempted to define relative risk factors for cardiac contusion based on other injuries. Their patient population was typically small; of 280 patients studied at risk, only 35 were confirmed to have myocardial contusion, and of these, only 9 had CPK isoenzyme elevation. This raises the never-ending question of what criteria really make the diagnosis of myocardial contusion. With their small numbers, none of their statistical evaluations could be significant. The authors should be commended for raising the question of more sensible management of myocardial contusion.— J.M. Mitchell, M.D.

---

**Complications Following Blunt and Penetrating Injuries in 216 Victims of Chest Trauma Requiring Tube Thoracostomy**

Helling TS, Gyles NR III, Eisenstein CL, Soracco CA (St Luke's Hosp and Truman Med Ctr, Kansas City, Mo; Univ of Missouri, Kansas City)
*J Trauma* 29:1367–1370, 1989                                    2–32

---

Many advances in the treatment of blunt and penetrating injuries to the chest occurred during military practice. Tube thoracostomy (TT) and thoracotomy came into widespread use during the Vietnam conflict and resulted in a sharp decline in the incidence of empyema. This more aggressive approach is now used in civilian trauma cases. Two hundred six-

Complications of Chest Trauma and Location
of Tube Thoracostomy

| Complications | ED | OR & ICU |
|---|---|---|
| Empyema | 3 | 3 |
| Recurrent pneumothorax | 38 | 13 |
| Residual hemothorax | 16 | 23 |
| requiring decortication | 6 | 1 |
| Air leak | 5 | 2 |
| Total patients | 52/140 (37%) | 26/76 (34%) |

Note: P = nonsignificant.
(Courtesy of Helling TS, Gyles NR III, Eisenstein CL, et al: *J Trauma* 29:1367–1370, 1989.)

teen patients treated with 324 chest tubes were reviewed to assess the risks and benefits of TT and to determine whether the procedure is less effective in blunt than in penetrating trauma.

The mean age of the patient group was 33 years; 180 were men. Blunt trauma was responsible for 94 of the cases; 122 patients received injuries from penetrating trauma. None of the 18 deaths was directly attributed to TT. Complications occurred more frequently in patients with blunt trauma (44%) than in those with penetrating trauma (30%). In addition, those with blunt trauma had a significantly longer intensive care unit (ICU) stay, duration of TT, and need for mechanical ventilation. Complications were not related to the place (ED, operating room, ICU, or ward) of TT insertion (table).

Empyema occurred in 6 (3%) patients, residual hemothorax in 39 (18%), and recurrent pneumothorax in 51 (24%). Seven patients with residual hemothorax required decortication. Of those with empyema or requiring decortication, only 7 of 13 had blunt trauma. Overall, the early use of TT to expand lung, obliterate pleural space, and evacuate blood is as effective in blunt chest trauma as in penetrating injuries. The procedure carries no increased risk for infection in patients with blunt trauma.

▶ This vaguely focused retrospective study confirms 2 facts. The first is that patients with blunt lung injuries who require chest tubes take longer to heal and have more air leaks than patients with penetrating lung injury. The other fact is that despite possibly more expedient chest tube insertion in the ED, the rate of complications was the same.—W.P. Burdick, M.D.

---

**Blunt Rupture of the Diaphragm: Mechanism, Diagnosis, and Treatment**
Kearney PA, Rouhana SW, Burney RE (Univ of Kentucky; Gen Motors Research Labs, Warren, Mich; Univ of Michigan)
*Ann Emerg Med* 18:1326–1330, 1989                    2–33

Diaphragmatic rupture after blunt trauma from motor vehicle accidents in the presence of massive visceral herniation or strangulation can be rapidly fatal. However, in the absence of respiratory distress and massive visceral herniation, the diagnosis of diaphragmatic rupture in multiply injured patients can be difficult. The exact mechanism of diaphragmatic injury after blunt trauma has not been defined, but it is known that victims of lateral impact motor vehicle collisions are more likely to sustain rupture of the diaphragm than victims of frontal collisions. The role of impact direction as a causal factor in blunt diaphragmatic rupture was investigated in 83 patients who were in motor vehicle accidents.

Impact direction was lateral in 45 patients, frontal in 28, and unknown in 10. Sixty patients had left hemidiaphragmatic ruptures, 13 had right hemidiaphragmatic ruptures, and 3 had bilateral ruptures; the side of rupture was unknown in 7. Mortality rates were 42% after lateral impact, 57% after frontal impact, and 70% after impact of unknown direction.

Accident victims with diaphragmatic disruption after right lateral impact collisions and rollover crashes were more severely injured and had a higher mortality rate than those involved in frontal or left-sided collisions. Of those with diaphragmatic rupture after a right-sided collision, 50% had injury to the left hemidiaphragm, 90% of whom had severe hepatic injuries. This finding suggests that the liver affords protection to the right hemidiaphragm. The side of diaphragmatic rupture correlated well with the direction of impact. The right hemidiaphragm appears to be more resistant to rupture than the left hemidiaphragm because a more severe collision was required to disrupt the right hemidiaphragm.

Knowledge of the mechanisms that produced the injury, an accident victim's seat position, and the impact direction should lead to a high index of clinical suspicion for diaphragmatic rupture. Because these ruptures do not heal spontaneously, operation is always indicated after a diagnosis of diaphragmatic disruption has been confirmed.

▶ Diagnosis of diaphragmatic rupture is difficult, and this article points out that a mechanism with lateral impact should heighten one's suspicion for this. Left-sided ruptures are, by far, more common than right-sided impacts. In this study, 60% of the diaphragm ruptures were on the right.—R.M. McNamara, M.D.

---

### Computed Tomography in Traumatic Defects of the Diaphragm
Demos TC, Solomon C, Posniak HV, Flisak MJ (Loyola Univ Med Ctr, Maywood, Ill)
*Clin Imaging* 13:62–67, 1989                                                    2–34

---

Abdominal viscera may herniate into the chest after blunt or penetrating trauma or through a congenital diaphragmatic defect. The resultant symptoms often are overlooked or may not develop for some time after injury, and conventional radiographic studies may be normal or nonspecific. Two such cases were diagnosed with CT.

*Case 1.*—Woman, 25, pregnant, and with severe epigastric pain, had had similar symptoms in 2 past pregnancies; CT showed bowel and omental fat in the left hemithorax and a diaphragmatic defect. At surgery her transverse colon and splenic flexure were herniated through a left hemidiaphragmatic defect.

*Case 2.*—Woman, 22, with a stab wound in the neck had bowel in her right hemithorax. Computed tomography showed a diaphragmatic defect that was confirmed operatively.

If herniation of abdominal viscera into the chest is missed, symptoms mimicking a variety of disorders including peptic ulcer, heart disease, and cholecystitis may develop. Bowel obstruction or strangulation can occur at any time after injury. Computed tomography allows direct visualization of parts of the diaphragm and adjacent structures. Herniated omental fat may be identified. If no constriction exists or if herniation is intermittent, the actual diaphragmatic defect may be visible on a CT scan. Defects should be sought on CT scans of patients with chronic or recurrent chest or abdominal symptoms, especially if patients have histories of penetrating or severe blunt abdominal trauma.

▶ Although the diagnosis of traumatic injury to the diaphragm remains difficult, especially in that subset where the rent is initially small and not incarcerating any intra-abdominal viscera. The classic example is the patient with a stab wound to the left posterolateral aspect of the chest in which a hemothorax without pneumothorax occurs. Such a patient may initially receive treatment with closed thoracostomy and spontaneous resolution of symptoms, only to return some months later when the diaphragmatic injury has enlarged and entrapped intra-abdominal viscera, most commonly the splenic flexure of the large bowel. No specific diagnostic maneuver short of direct visual inspection of the diaphragm will currently totally exclude diaphragmatic injury. However, as the authors point out in this article, selected areas of the diaphragm are generally more easily evaluated by a CT scan. Fortunately, this includes the posterolateral and posteromedial aspects on the left side, that area most likely injured by a penetrating event at or below the nipple line. Emergency physicians may do well to remind their diagnostic imaging colleagues to scrutinize the diaphragm carefully in situations where a subtle injury may be suspect.—D.K. Wagner, M.D.

## Abdominal Trauma

### Intra-Abdominal Seatbelt Injury
Asbun HJ, Irani H, Roe EJ, Bloch JH (Kern Med Ctr, Bakersfield, Calif)
J Trauma 30:189–193, 1990                                          2–35

Motor vehicle accidents still are a leading cause of death among persons aged less than 40 years. Although restraint definitely is indicated, a new group of injuries has emerged as seat restraints have come into wide use. Of more than 1,400 restrained occupants involved in motor vehicle

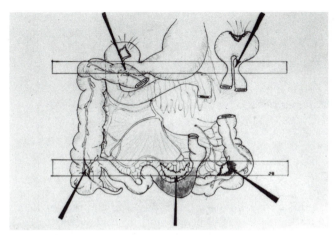

**Fig 2–4.**—Intestinal and mesenteric injuries seen in restrained victims of motor vehicle accidents. *Clockwise:* duodenal rupture ("fixed point"), closed loop perforation, mesenteric tears at sigmoid colon and small bowel areas with ischemic intestinal loops, seromuscular tear with intact mucosa. (Courtesy of Asbun HJ, Irani H, Roe EJ, et al: *J Trauma* 30:189–193, 1990.)

accidents in a recent 28-month period, 8 sustained intra-abdominal injuries associated with use of a seat belt.

Six of the 8 patients were wearing shoulder-lap restraints, and 2, who were rear seat passengers, wore lap belts. Two patients had false negative results of abdominal CT scans. One of 4 diagnostic peritoneal lavages (DPLs) was false negative. Seven patients had shearing injuries of 1 or more intestinal loops and mesenteric tears resulting in bowel ischemia. Three patients for whom surgery was delayed had ischemic necrosis and perforation by the time they were operated on. All 8 patients were discharged in stable condition.

Mechanisms proposed for seat belt–related bowel and mesenteric injuries (Fig 2–4) include compression of the abdominal wall and viscera between the belt and the spine, a sudden rise in intraluminal pressure, shearing and deceleration forces acting against fixed intestinal points, and "submarining" of the body. The most dangerous injury is a devascularized bowel loop from which mesentery is avulsed. Use of seat belts unquestionably should be continued, but better restraining devices might lower the rate of restraint-related injuries.

▶ It seems unlikely that an exploratory laparotomy would be performed on a patient based solely on the presence of a seat belt sign. This paper points out that some authors suggested this plan even if the patient appears relatively uninjured and has a normal DPL. In this study of 8 patients, all of whom suffered intraperitoneal injuries secondary to a seat belt lap restraint system, all but 1 victim had evidence of abdominal bruising from the belt. Two patients had CT scans and 1 a DPL, which was false negative. Based on these findings, it would seem prudent to closely observe a patient with a seat belt sign despite normal or inconclusive diagnostic studies. If the surgeons are not convinced, a prolonged observation stay in the ED might be the best alternative. The physician should also keep in mind the potential for associated lumbar spine fractures with this mechanism of injury. (See also Abstract 2–36.)—H. Unger, M.D.

---

**Intestinal Injuries Missed by Computed Tomography**
Sherck JP, Oakes DD (Stanford Univ; Santa Clara Valley Med Ctr, San Jose, Calif)
*J Trauma* 30:1–7, 1990                                                                 2–36

Isolated intestinal injuries from blunt trauma often are difficult to diagnose with physical examination and routine laboratory studies only, but delayed diagnosis may increase morbidity and the risk of death. Ten recently seen patients had small bowel injuries that were missed by CT examination. A total of 36 patients with small bowel injury were seen in the 8-year review period.

The 10 patients (table) averaged 31 years of age. All were injured in motor vehicle accidents, 4 while wearing seat belts. All had physical findings suggesting possible abdominal trauma, but in no case was the plain abdominal radiograph abnormal. All of the patients were observed but eventually had laparotomies, 7 within 24 hours of admission. All had intestinal injuries that needed surgical treatment; 9 patients had free perforation. One patient died.

Three CT studies were suboptimal. Two scans were diagnostic of perforation on review, and careful review of the remaining scans demonstrated other abnormalities. Five patients had free intraperitoneal fluid not explained by liver or spleen abnormality.

Patients having abdominal CT should be stable enough to receive sedation, if required, to limit motion. Gastric contrast always should be used, but in dilute solution. Proper diagnosis and management of bowel injuries still rely on serial evaluation by an experienced surgeon.

▶ Recent studies comparing the accuracy of different imaging modalities (i.e., CT and ultrasonography vs. diagnostic peritoneal lavage) in the assessment of abdominal trauma all have hinged on the skills of the interpreting radiologist. Although it is not clearly stated in the paper, it is implied that many of the abdominal radiographs in this study were initially interpreted by second-year radiology residents. This might account for the fact that 4 of the 6 "normal" CAT scans revealed significant pathologic conditions on review. Since subsequent patient care is dependent on accurate interpretation of these radiologic studies, immediate review by experienced radiologists should be mandatory. Trauma foundations have established guidelines to improve patient care and have dramatically altered hospital staffing patterns. It seems appropriate that policies addressing radiology support should be established as well.

It is noteworthy that the most sensitive test employed in this paper was serial abdominal examinations and prolonged observation. The emergency physician should have a high index of suspicion in abdominal trauma and should con-

Ten Patients With CT and Intestinal Injuries

| Patient No. | Initial Findings | Retrospective Review Findings | | | Operative Findings | |
|---|---|---|---|---|---|---|
| | | Fluid | SBT* | Other | Fluid | Other |
| 1 | Normal | – | – | Possible retroperitoneal air | + | Duodenal crush |
| 2 | Normal | – | – | Ileus pattern | – | Necrotic ileum |
| 3 | Normal | – | – | Small bowel dilated | + | Perforated ileum |
| 4 | Fluid | + | + | – | + | Perforated jejunum |
| 5 | Fluid | + | + | – | + | Perforated jejunum |
| 6 | Fluid | + | – | Hematoma, mass | + | Perforated ileum |
| 7 | Normal | + | + | – | + | Perforated ileum |
| 8 | Normal | – | – | Free air | + | Perforated ileum |
| 9 | Normal | + | – | Free air and contrast | + | Perforated jejunum |
| 10 | Fluid | + | – | – | + | Perforated cecum |

*SBT, small bowel thickening.
(Courtesy of Sherck JP, Oakes DD: *J Trauma* 30:1–7, 1990.)

sider the use of ED observationin the high-risk patient even when the initial CT scan is read as normal.—H. Unger, M.D.

## Is Diagnostic Peritoneal Lavage for Blunt Trauma Obsolete?
Hawkins ML, Bailey RL Jr, Carraway RP (Med College of Georgia, Augusta; Carraway Methodist Med Ctr, Birmingham, Ala)
*Am Surg* 56:96–99, 1990                                                              2–37

Since diagnostic peritoneal lavage (DPL) was first introduced in 1965, it has been a mainstay in the evaluation of severely injured patients. Recent studies have shown that CT is highly accurate in detecting intra-abdominal injuries after blunt trauma. This study was done to determine whether the continued use of DPL is justified.

During a 5-year study period, 414 trauma patients underwent 415 DPLs. One patient had a repeat study several hours after admission. Diagnostic peritoneal lavage was considered grossly abnormal if 10 mL of gross blood was aspirated and microscopically abnormal if greater than 100,000 red blood cells/mm$^3$, greater than 500 white blood cells/mm$^3$, elevated amylase or bilirubin levels, or bacteria or vegetable fibers were found in the effluent.

None of the patients had elevated bilirubin levels, elevated amylase levels, or bacteria in the effluent. Of the 415 DPLs, 117 (28%) were true positive, 286 (69%) were true negative, 7 (2%) were false positive, and 5 (1%) were false negative, yielding a 97% accuracy rate. Rare vegetable fibers found in 4 cases were false positives. Three of the 5 patients with false negative lavages had a ruptured diaphragm as the only intra-abdominal injury. The only complication in this study population was an inadvertently penetrated urinary bladder, which was successfully treated with Foley catheter drainage.

The hospital charge for peritoneal lavage is $94.50 compared with $350 for abdominal CT scanning, not including the radiologist's charges. Because DPL is accurate, rapid, and safe, avoids the disruption of patient care that results in the radiology suite, and is much less expensive than CT, DPL remains the procedure of choice for evaluating blunt abdominal trauma in the adult patient at this institution.

▶ The answer is "no." Although abdominal CT (and even ultrasound) may obviate DPL, few centers have this level of imaging support for trauma. Diagnostic peritoneal lavage remains the quickest way to find the hemoperitoneum in an unstable, multiple trauma victim. Don't believe vegetable fibers.—T. Stair, M.D.

## Bowel and Mesenteric Injury Following Blunt Abdominal Trauma: Evaluation With CT
Rizzo MJ, Federle MP, Griffiths BG (Univ of California, San Francisco)
*Radiology* 173:143–148, 1989                                                          2–38

Blunt abdominal trauma is a frequently reported injury in a mechanized society and is associated with small bowel or mesenteric injury in a small but significant percentage of patients with this trauma.

Computed tomographic scans were carried out in 51 patients (39 males and 12 females, aged 3–18 years) with suspected bowel or mesenteric injury resulting from blunt abdominal trauma. Data on 24 of these patients have been reported previously. Thirty-seven of the 51 patients were injured in motor vehicle-related accidents. Assaults, falls from heights, and jogging-related falls were also involved.

In 19 patients treated nonoperatively, CT scans suggested a bowel or mesenteric injury. One patient with massive internal injuries, hemoperitoneum, and hypotension died after CT but before indicated and intended surgery. Scans of 16 patients revealed suspected bowel wall hematomas shown as focal bowel wall thickening or luminal narrowing, and scans of 5 patients demonstrated mesenteric hematomas. Scans of 4 of the patients revealed small-to-moderate hemoperitoneum related to bowel or mesenteric hematoma. Except for the 1 death, all other patients who were treated nonoperatively were discharged in stable condition, suggesting correct CT diagnoses.

In 32 patients who underwent laparotomy, 28 preoperative CT scans (88%) revealed hemoperitoneum or other free peritoneal fluid. Twenty-seven scans (84%) demonstrated diffuse or focal mesenteric infiltration suggestive of mesenteric edema or hematoma. In 41% of the operative reports, a hematoma in the specified mesenteric area was confirmed; the other operative reports noted only retroperitoneal hematoma, free peritoneal blood, or associated mesenteric laceration. Sixteen of 20 patients who had single or multiple areas of bowel thickening on CT scans had bowel injuries consisting of transmural perforation, serosal laceration, or mural hematoma verified at laparotomy. In contrast to the nonoperated patients 50% of the 32 patients who underwent laparotomy had associated abdominal injuries, including 9 pancreatic contusions, 4 liver and 2 spleen lacerations, 2 gallbladder injuries, and 1 rectus muscle tear with ventral hernia. The CT scans revealed all injuries except 1 splenic and 1 gallbladder laceration obscured by other injuries necessitating surgery.

Computed tomography is both sensitive and accurate in revealing bowel and mesenteric injuries and in confirming the severity of associated solid visceral injury in this area. Furthermore, CT scans may have advantages over other diagnostic procedures in distinguishing operative from nonoperative cases, thus reducing the incidence of nontherapeutic laparotomy and accompanying postoperative complications without sacrificing significant sensitivity.

▶ This retrospective survey makes a strong case for the routine use of CT scanning in stable patients with blunt abdominal trauma. The authors report that CT scanning (administered with intravenous contrast) was highly sensitive in detecting intra-abdominal injuries and helpful in deciding which patients needed surgery. Abnormal CT findings included bowel wall thickening greater than 3 mm, hemoperitoneum or other free abdominal fluid, pneumoperitoneum, extravasated contrast, mesenteric thickening or hematoma, and associated abdominal findings. Significantly, the authors fail to tell us who reads the CT scans.

The authors state that all patients in the nonoperated group were discharged in good condition, thus claiming essentially perfect sensitivity for CT scanning. However, they later report that the CT scans of 2 patients in the operated group were misinterpreted as revealing no significant injury. Thus, the sensitivity of this procedure is very much dependent on the skill of the interpreter. Four of the 32 patients (12%) in the operated group had no significant injuries needing repair at surgery.

In contrast to diagnostic peritoneal lavage (DPL), CT scanning is more sensitive to retroperitoneal injuries, noninvasive, possibly capable of detecting injuries earlier in the posttraumatic period, able to pinpoint the location of the injury, and (with the use of contrast) useful in detecting lesions within the viscera. Computed tomography scanning for abdominal trauma may reduce the rate of nontherapeutic laparotomies. It is rapidly becoming the primary diagnostic study for stable patients with abdominal trauma. It may be that DPL, used selectively with CT scanning, may further improve its sensitivity. Further studies performed prospectively are needed to clarify the graver indications for these 2 procedures.—H.H. Osborn, M.D.

---

### Nonoperative Management of Adult Blunt Splenic Trauma: Criteria for Successful Outcome

Longo WE, Baker CC, McMillen MA, Modlin IM, Degutis LC, Zucker KA (Yale Univ)
*Ann Surg* 210:626–629, 1989                                        2–39

---

Nonoperative treatment of blunt splenic trauma in adults is controversial despite many reports advocating such management. To define criteria that may predict a successful outcome, data on all adult splenic injuries seen at a single institution over an 8-year period were retrospectively reviewed.

The injuries were documented by scintillation studies, CT, or at laparotomy. Of the 252 splenic injuries, 60 (24%) were treated initially without surgery. Management included bed rest, monitoring in the intensive care unit, frequent physical examinations, nasogastric tubes, serial hematocrits, and follow-up splenic imaging. Interval laparotomy was necessary in 5 of the 60 patients treated nonsurgically. Reasons for failure included blood loss greater than 4 units, enlarging splenic defects, or increasing peritoneal signs. Parameters predicting a successful outcome were localized trauma to the left flank or left side of the abdomen, hemodynamic stability, transfusion requirements of less than 4 units, rapid return of gastrointestinal tract function, age younger than 60 years, and early resolution of splenic defects on imaging studies. No morbidity or deaths resulted from delayed surgery. Blunt splenic trauma can be successfully managed without surgery in carefully selected adults.

▶ It is not surprising, in light of the great success with nonoperative management of splenic injuries in children, that some spleens can be saved in adults as well. On the other hand, the long-term adverse effect of splenectomy (in terms of postsplenectomy sepsis) is greatly reduced in adults; thus, the impetus to attempt conservative management is somewhat reduced. The authors of this series stress that careful patient selection (in their case, including only 24% of all patients with splenic injury) is a key element in the strategy and that nonoperative management should be attempted only in younger patients who are hemodynamically stable and who can be carefully, accurately, and repeatedly examined (i.e., patients with normal mental status who do not require general anesthesia because of some other injury). This also should be done only in a facility capable of close serial follow-up.—J.R. Hoffman, M.D.

---

**Evaluation of Computed Tomography and Diagnostic Peritoneal Lavage in Blunt Abdominal Trauma**
Meyer DM, Thal ER, Weigelt JA, Redman HC (Univ of Texas, Dallas)
*J Trauma* 29:1168–1172, 1989                                          2–40

---

The accuracy of CT compared with that of diagnostic peritoneal lavage (DPL) has been questioned in the assessment of blunt abdominal trauma. The accuracy of DPL and CT was evaluated in 301 hemodynamically stable patients aged 1 month–76 years (mean 26 years) who had sustained blunt abdominal injuries.

Patients were evaluated by CT using both oral and intravenous contrast medium, followed by DPL. Patients with an abnormal CT scan, an abnormal DPL, or both underwent celiotomy. Those with both a normal CT scan and a normal DPL were hospitalized for observation. The diagnostic results were compared with the intraoperative findings. Thirty patients were subsequently excluded from the final analysis.

Of the 271 evaluable patients, 194 had both a normal CT and a normal DPL and were considered true negatives. Fifty-one had both an abnormal CT and an abnormal DPL. All patients had injuries identified at operation. Seven patients had significant injuries at operation that had not been identified on CT scan. Nineteen had a normal CT and an abnormal DPL, and all had significant injury confirmed at operation. Five had an abnormal CT and a normal DPL; 3 of these patients had false negative DPL results. Two patients with normal CT scans and false positive DPL results experienced complications of DPL requiring operation.

Diagnostic peritoneal lavage had a sensitivity of 95.9% compared with 74.3% for CT; DPL had an accuracy of 98.2% compared with 92.6% for CT. Both had a specificity of 99%. The selection of 1 test over the other should be based on individual circumstances.

▶ As do all CT vs. DPL articles, and there have been many, this article illustrates that a key variable is the generation of the scanner and, more important, who reads the scan. Dr. Don Trunkey, in his review of this paper, emphasizes that it is unfair to compare CT and DPL in that they are entirely different tests.

Each has its own limitations that must be taken into consideration when results are evaluated. May the house officer who wants to send the patient home because the CT is normal be warned. The importance of the mechanism of injury, index of suspicion, need for observation, and serial examination in a well-monitored environment cannot be overemphasized.—J.T. Amsterdam, M.D.

---

**The Use of Serum Amylase and Lipase in Evaluating and Managing Blunt Abdominal Trauma**
Buechter KJ, Arnold M, Steele B, Martin L, Byers P, Gomez G, Zeppa R, Augenstein J (Univ of Miami)
*Am Surg* 56:204–208, 1990                                                        2–41

---

The diagnostic value of serum amylase determinations in the evaluation of blunt abdominal trauma (BAT) has long been controversial. Recent reports suggested that serum lipase may be a more specific and sensitive indicator of pancreatic disease than amylase, but the specificity of lipase determinations for pancreatic injury is unknown. It has further been suggested that elevation of both amylase and lipase levels probably indicates abdominal injury. Thus, the diagnostic value of amylase and lipase in the initial evaluation and subsequent management of BAT was investigated.

For 85 consecutive BAT patients aged 13–91 years who required hospital admission, serum amylase and lipase levels were measured during initial evaluation and resuscitation in the ED and on hospital days 1, 3, and 7. Thirty control patients with isolated head injuries, extremity fractures, or extremity soft tissue injuries without fracture also had initial serum amylase and lipase determinations while in the ED. A total of 522 enzyme determinations were done.

Eighteen patients had nonpancreatic intra-abdominal injuries, 63 had injuries that were not intra-abdominal, and 4 patients had no significant injuries. Only 1 patient had transection of the body of the pancreas in combination with an aortic injury. That patient died 12 hours after operation. Another 14 patients died of their injuries, yielding a total mortality of 17%. Autopies were performed on all 14 patients, but none had pancreatic injuries. Forty-five patients had at least 1 enzyme abnormality, but none of the patients without BAT had enzyme elevations at any time. Of the 70 surviving patients, 15 still had enzyme elevations at the time of hospital discharge. Therefore, serum amylase and lipase appear to be elevated randomly in patients with BAT, even if they do not have pancreatic injury. Neither amylase nor lipase values were correlated with type of injury or outcome. None of the controls had abnormal enzyme values.

Clinically significant blunt pancreatic injury is rare among patients with BAT. Serum amylase and lipase values are elevated randomly in patients with nonpancreatic BAT, both initially and during subsequent hospitalization. Therefore, neither initial nor serial lipase and amylase determinations are useful diagnostic tools in evaluating BAT.

▶ The serum amylase level contributes little to the acute care of the patient in the ED.

Many experts in health policy are now calling for health care rationing. They cite the high cost of medical care, which accounts for 12% of the gross national product. Other experts, however, state that we can afford adequate care if we will just stop delivering the 50% of health care that is not necessary. The authors of this paper conclude that the routine determination of serum lipase and amylase levels falls in the half of medical care that can be eliminated while maintaining high quality.—E.H. Taliaferro, M.D.

---

**Gastrointestinal Injuries in Childhood: Analysis of 53 Patients**
Grosfeld JL, Rescorla FJ, West KW, Vane DW (Indiana Univ, Indianapolis)
*J Pediatr Surg* 24:580–583, 1989                                                              2–42

---

Injuries of the stomach and small bowel in 53 children during 1972–1987 were reviewed. The mean age at injury was 8 years. Blunt trauma was responsible in 51 cases; 2 children had penetrating wounds. The jejunum and duodenum were the most common sites of injury, and jejunoileal perforation was the most frequent type of injury. Two patients had gastric injuries. Diagnoses were made by noting peritoneal irritation, using CT, and finding free air on radiography. Associated injuries were present in 40% of the children.

Nine of 16 duodenal hematomas were resolved without surgery, whereas 7 were evacuated in the course of other procedures. Twenty-three of 30 perforations were managed with simple closure; 7 jejunoileal perforations were resected. Five mesenteric avulsions required resection. A patient with eviscerated bowel had replacement of the bowel, and 1 with entrapped bowel underwent resection. Thirteen patients had complications, the most frequent being atelectasis, pseudocyst formation, and sepsis. One infant with a duodenal laceration died of head injuries.

Duodenal hematoma in children is managed conservatively, but prompt surgery is indicated for traumatic perforation and avulsion. Early diagnosis and modern pediatric anesthesia support will improve the survival of children with gastrointestinal injuries.

▶ The authors present a significant series of childhood gastrointestinal injuries. As one might expect, the majority occurred by a blunt-type etiology. In addition, a submucosal hematoma of the duodenum accounted for 30% of the injuries. This condition, occurring predominantly in the childhood population, can be nonoperatively managed in the majority of cases once the diagnosis is established. The diagnosis is best established by contrast ingestion with plain or CAT scanning of the abdomen. Of interest is the authors' statement that neither an abdominal CAT scan nor a diagnostic peritoneal lavage can be relied on for complete diagnosis in blunt traumatic situations. Repeated bedside evaluation provides the most consistent means to enhance diagnostic capabilities. (See also Abstracts 2–37 and 2–43.)—D.K. Wagner, M.D.

### Abdominal CT in Children With Neurologic Impairment Following Blunt Trauma: Abdominal CT in Comatose Children

Taylor GA, Eichelberger MR (Children's Hosp Natl Med Ctr, Washington, DC)
*Ann Surg* 210:229–233, 1989                                    2–43

To determine if children with severe neurologic impairment after blunt trauma are at increased risk for intra-abdominal injury compared with those who have little or no neurologic impairment, 310 injured boys and 172 injured girls aged 1 month–18 years with an average age of 7.7 years underwent CT scanning.

Mechanisms of injury included 376 motor vehicle accidents (78%), 60 falls, 24 assaults, 11 bicycle accidents, and 8 miscellaneous injuries. In 3 children, the mechanism of injury was not known. The children were divided into 2 groups based on Glasgow Coma Scale (GCS) scores: 90 children with GCS scores less than 8 had severe neurologic impairment, and 369 children had little or no neurologic impairment.

Lower GCS scores were associated with a progressively increasing risk of significant abdominal injury. Children with GCS scores less than 8 and signs suggestive of underlying abdominal injury were at higher risk for abdominal injury than those with a GCS score of 8 or greater. However, neurologic impairment alone was a low-yield indication for abdominal CT examination, because all 11 children with a GCS score of less than 8 as the only indication for abdominal CT examination had a normal abdominal CT scan. The prevalence and severity of associated chest injury was also higher in comatose children. The mortality rate among the comatose children was 24% compared with a 0.26% mortality rate among the children without coma. Abdominal surgery was necessary in 3 children (3.3%) with GCS scores less than 8 compared with 14 children (3.8%) with a GCS score of 8 or greater. The difference was statistically not significant.

Although children with severe neurologic impairment after injury are at higher risk for intra-abdominal injury than those without coma, neurologic impairment without concurrent abdominal signs is a low-yield indicator of underlying abdominal injury. Abdominal CT scanning should be reserved for children in whom there is a high clinical index of suspicion of significant abdominal trauma based on physical examination and the mechanism of injury.

▶ Hold thy horses! Yes, you did read that last paragraph correctly. The authors, based on their finding that all 11 patients with a GCS score of less than 8 and no signs of abdominal injury had normal CT scans, suggest foregoing CT in this group. How they can state this in face of their reference to another study by Beaver et al. (1), which showed a 22% incidence of abnormal findings in a similar, but larger group (n = 27), is beyond me. Perhaps the most significant information in this article is the relatively low rate of surgery required (3.3%) in the most severely neurologically affected group, those with GCS scores greater than 8.—R.M. McNamara, M.D.

*Reference*

1. Beaver BL, et al: *J Pediatr Surg* 22:1117, 1987.

## Abdominal Injuries Associated With the Use of Seatbelts

Appleby JP, Nagy AG (Univ of British Columbia, Vancouver)
*Am J Surg* 157:457–458, 1989                                    2–44

The Canadian government has legislated mandatory use of seat belts, and the government of British Columbia adopted this policy in 1977. The effects of seat belt restraints were investigated by review of the records of 562 patients injured in motor vehicle accidents who were admitted to the Vancouver General Hospital from January 1985 to January 1988. The use of seat belts was verified for 126 of these patients, 36 of whom were considered for laparotomy and were the subject of study.

The male/female ratio was equal, and the average patient age was 47. Of the 36 patients, 20 wore 3-point seat belts (lap and shoulder harness), 10 wore lap belts, and in 6 the type of belt was unidentified. Preoperative investigations included peritoneal lavage in 10 patients, abdominal CT in 2, and abdominal ultrasonography in 1. There was 1 death; there were 2 false negative results of peritoneal lavage. The other 23 patients underwent laparotomy.

Results demonstrated that gastrointestinal injuries occurred in 24 patients (67%). Of these 24, 14 had more than 1 injury, and 1 patient had 7 different intestinal injuries. Small bowel injuries were most frequent, requiring 11 small bowel resections. Duodenal injuries occurred in 2 patients. Other studies have reported gastric injuries, but none was noted in this series. Six colon resections were performed for perforated or ischemic colon injuries. Seven patients had nonperforated seromuscular-type injuries to the colon. This type of injury is rarely associated with the use of seat belts. Resection was not necessary, and most patients had repair by direct suture or omental patch. The associated injuries were head injuries, 8; orthopedic, 15; chest, 10; spinal, 9; and abdominal wall, 11. Intra-abdominal injuries included spleen, 12; liver, 6; diaphragm, 4; urinary bladder, 3; kidney, 2; and aorta, 2.

Physicians caring for trauma patients should be aware of some specific injuries that may be related to the use of seat belts. Abdominal wall bruising secondary to the use of seat belts should be regarded with suspicion because these patients have a high incidence of gastrointestinal injuries in addition to associated lumbar spine injuries.

▶ This study once again points out that seat belts do not confer immunity from injury, especially if one is traveling at high speed. The use of seat belts is associated with injury to hollow viscera primarily. The authors should be commended for drawing our attention to some unique injuries associated with the use of seat belts. They found a high incidence of lumbar spine fractures and many patients with major injury to the abdominal wall. Spine trauma was seen more commonly in patients wearing lap belts. These injuries should be looked for whenever a victim of a road traffic accident is evaluated. (See also Abstract 4–47.)—H.H. Osborn, M.D.

## Vascular Trauma

**Value of Plain Chest Film in Predicting Traumatic Aortic Rupture**
Savastano S, Feltrin GP, Miotto D, Chiesura-Corona M (Istituto di Radiologia dell' Università degli Studi, Padua, Italy)
*Ann Radiol* 32:196–200, 1989                                        2–45

Findings were reviewed on chest films of 26 patients with traumatic aortic rupture after blunt chest trauma and on films of 10 others whose findings on aortograms were normal.

The significant findings included mediastinal widening and abnormalities of the aortic knob (enlargement, obscuration, or an altered outline). The left pulmonary hilus was blurred in 8 patients with rupture but was not blurred in any of the control patients; however, it always was accompanied by other signs of hemomediastinum. Four or more findings of "left hemomediastinum" (mediastinal widening, aortic knob changes, tracheal and left main bronchus shift, hilar blurring, and left apical cap) were present only in patients with aortic rupture. Signs of left hemomediastinum were absent only in patients with normal findings on aortograms.

Angiography is not necessary in patients with blunt chest trauma whose chest radiographs show no signs of left hemomediastinum. If, however, mediastinal widening or aortic knob changes are present, aortography should be performed.

▶ This is not a complete study. The small numbers of patients and lack of controls invalidates the authors' conclusions, though accurate they may be.— G. Ordog, M.D.

**Aortic Rupture in Seat Belt Wearers**
Arajärvi E, Santavirta S, Tolonen J (Univ Central Hosp, Helsinki, Finland)
*J Thorac Cardiovasc Surg* 93:355–361, 1989                         2–46

Immediate death in traffic accidents is often the result of rupture of the aorta. To study the effect of seat belt wearing and mechanisms of injury, 68 persons wearing seat belts who died in traffic accidents with rupture of the thoracic aorta were compared with 72 unbelted persons with fatal aortic rupture from similar accidents.

The distal part of the descending aorta was the most common site of injury in seat belt wearers, especially in right front-seat passengers and those in frontal impact collisions. In unbelted persons, the ascending aorta was the usual site of rupture, especially among drivers. Lateral impact collisions caused ruptures in the isthmus region and in the ascending aorta in seat belt wearers.

In belted persons, the part of the car thought to cause injury was the seat belt in only 7% of cases; usually, some interior portion of the car was the cause. In unbelted persons, the most frequent cause of injury was the steering wheel.

The mechanism of injury in rupture of the isthmus region usually was rapid deceleration and, in lateral impact collisions, complex body movements. Fracture of the thoracic vertebra often led to rupture of the distal portion of the descending aorta. In unbelted persons, ascending aortic rupture was attributable to a blow to the thorax.

Aortic rupture plays a more important role in fatal chest trauma in seat belt wearers than was once thought. Seat belts fail to protect in lateral impact collisions. Steering wheels still cause injury in seat belt wearers.

▶ This study from Finland demonstrates a high incidence of aortic rupture in seat belt wearers in road traffic accidents. The authors do not say how information on the use of seat belts was obtained, but each accident was investigated by a special board.

Aortic ruptures in both those with and without seat belts were usually not at the isthmus. Thus, lesions in all segments of the aorta should be anticipated in those surviving high-speed car crashes. More than one mechanism may be involved in the genesis of aortic rupture in seat belt wearers. Chest compression on the steering wheel, in addition to sudden deceleration, may play a role. It may be that other protections besides seat belts, such as air bags, are necessary to more fully protect against these injuries.

The fact that so many seat belt users sustained aortic rupture should not deter or discourage us. Less than 20% of all those dying in fatal traffic accidents during the study period were belt wearers. Seat belts save lives.

Finland has had a mandatory seat belt law since 1975. We still don't have one. Only 25 states in the United States currently have laws requiring seat belts. (See also Abstract 2–44.)—H.H. Osborn, M.D.

---

## Traumatic Carotid Artery Dissection: Diagnosis and Treatment

Watridge CB, Muhlbauer MS, Lowery RD (Univ of Tennessee; Semmes-Murphey Clinic, Memphis)
*J Neurosurg* 71:854–857, 1989                                    2–47

---

Since an aggressive approach to diagnosing traumatic carotid dissection was adopted, 24 patients have had such a diagnosis in a 4-year period at 1 institution. Three fourths were aged 15–35 years. Motor-vehicle accidents were most often responsible. Patients generally were first seen with cerebral ischemic events including coma, lethargy, hemiparesis, aphasia, and Horner's syndrome. The average Glasgow Coma Scale score was 11. The initial CT scan was normal for two thirds of patients, but most of them eventually had hypodense areas consistent with cerebral infarcts. Six patients had bilateral carotid artery dissections.

Treatment was individualized, but a majority of patients were immediately heparinized. Seven patients received antiplatelet therapy only. None were operated on. Three patients had complications from heparin therapy, including 1 acute subdural hematoma. On follow-up after 3 weeks—3 years, 3 patients had normal neurologic findings, and 6 had only minimal sequelae and were independent. Nine patients had moderate residual deficits and were disabled. One patient was persistently vegetative, and 5 patients had died. Two deaths resulted from massive strokes caused by bilateral carotid dissection and total occlusion.

Carotid artery dissection is more frequent than previously realized. It should be considered in the treatment of deceleration injuries, especially focal neurologic deficits. Conservative management with anticoagulation is preferable to thromboendarterectomy for acute traumatic carotid artery dissection.

▶ The diagnosis of traumatic carotid artery dissection is often difficult, with a high degree of suspicion the most valuable diagnostic adjunct. Delay in diagnosis may be increased because of the availability and reliance on CAT scans in patients with neurologic alterations subsequent to a traumatic event. Before the availability of CAT scans, the more ready use of cerebral angiography provided a diagnostic evaluation of the extracranial vascular system. Consequently, in patients with a normal CAT scan and associated, persistent neurologic deficit, consideration for angiographic evaluation should be entertained. Of interest is the total absence of a bruit in all the reported cases of traumatic carotid artery dissection, effectively eliminating this physical finding as a diagnostic maneuver.—D.K. Wagner, M.D.

## Burns

**Full Skin Thickness Burns Caused by Contact With the Pavement in a Heat-Stroke Victim**
Vardy DA, Khoury M, Ben-Meir P, Ben-Yakar Y, Shoenfeld Y (Soroka Med Ctr, Ben-Gurion Univ of the Negev, Beer Sheva, Israel)
*Burns* 15:115–116, 1989                                                                    2–48

Burns from contact with the pavement are uncommon. An elderly patient was treated for burns as a complication of heat stroke when she fell on hot pavement.

Woman, 70, obese, with a previous history of heat stroke and mild coronary insufficiency, experienced another heat stroke on a hot summer day (43° C) while walking. She lay unconscious on the pavement for about 30 minutes. Deep thermal burns were seen on the posterior aspect of buttocks, thighs, and shins caused by contact with the hot pavement. The patient recovered rapidly after rehydration, vigorous cooling, and artificial respiration. Thermal burns were treated conservatively.

Heat stroke victims can sustain deep burns with prolonged contact with the hot pavement, particularly those who are immobile, obese, and poorly insulated. Paramedics should be aware of this complication and make sure that patients are not placed on hot pavements during resuscitation attempts. A previous history of heat stroke is another important risk factor for a second heat stroke, in addition to age, obesity, previous illness, incidental fever, drugs, dehydration, and physical effort.

▶ This paper points out the hazards of extremely high temperatures of asphalt during the summertime in warmer regions of the United States. Asphalt pavement is hotter than concrete pavement, approaching temperatures of 82° C.— E.J. Reisdorff, M.D.

---

**Car Radiator Burns: A Report on 72 Cases**
Al-Baker AA, Attalla MF, El-Ekiabi SA, Al Ghoul A (Hamad Med Corp, Doha, State of Qatar)
*Burns* 15:265–267, 1989                                                            2–49

---

The effects of scalds from sudden exposure to high-pressure steam and hot fluid droplets from car radiators were studied in 72 male patients, aged 11–58 years, over a 6-year period. The highest incidence was noted in the 20- to 35-year age group. Thirty-nine patients had burns of less than 5% of the body surface area (BSA); 30, 6%–10% of the BSA; and 3, more than 10% of the BSA. The exceptionally high summer temperatures in Qatar were significantly related to the incidence of this type of burn. The light summer clothing worn may have also been a contributing factor. There were 36 Asians, 28 Arabs, 2 Europeans, and 6 of other nationalities. The percentage of Asians was high because most hired drivers are Asian.

Most of the patients had injuries involving more than 1 anatomic area, with most of them in the right upper quadrant of the body. The right upper limbs were involved in 42 patients, the right side of the chest wall in 38, and the right side of the face in 25. Twelve patients had ear involvement, and 3 had conjunctival burns. Most burns were superficial and deep dermal; however, 5 patients required skin grafting.

Drivers lack a basic knowledge of safety precautions. Media stress on simple automobile safety is needed; however, in a multinational community, there are difficulties in publicizing an educational message.

▶ This retrospective survey describes the frequency and severity of scald burns caused by overheated car radiators in hospitalized patients in Qatar over a 6-year period. Predictably, the incidence of burns increased dramatically in the summer months.

Emergency physicians, especially those practicing in areas of the United States with a climate similar to Qatar, should take special note. Five of the cases reported (7%) required skin grafting.

Not enough information is included to determine the influence, if any, of various coolants and additives on the depth and extent of the burns.

Significantly, the advent of cars equipped with expansion (or overflow) tanks did nothing to change the incidence of this type of burn. A sustained public education covering automobile safety is necessary.—H.H. Osborn, M.D.

**Chemical Burns**

Herbert K, Lawrence JC (Birmingham Accident Hosp, Birmingham, England)

Burns 15:381–384, 1989                                                                    2–50

Chemical burns continue to be a significant cause of industrial burn injury. Chemical burns differ from thermal burns in that assessment of burn depth is often difficult, and the decision on whether to excise the wound is not always clear cut. The case reports of patients admitted to the Birmingham Accident Hospital with chemical burns during a 7-year study period were retrospectively studied.

Of 3,251 patients admitted to the burn unit during the study period, 100 (3.1%) had sustained chemical burns. However, 461 burns were sustained in industrial accidents, 16.5% of which were caused by chemicals, whereas chemicals accounted for only 0.9% of nonindustrial burns. Most chemical burn injuries involved less than 5% total body surface area, and none exceeded 20% total body surface area. Of the 100 patients with chemical burns, 89 were men and 11 were women. None of the patients was older than age 65. The face and neck were involved in 33 cases, followed by the trunk in 29 cases. Six patients sustained chemical burns to the eyes. Alkaline materials were involved in 37 accidents and acids in 28 accidents. In 15 cases, the nature of the corrosive material involved was not identified. Nineteen patients required split-skin grafts, and 12 patients underwent tangential excision plus split-thickness skin grafting. Eight patients underwent deroofing or excision of an abscess, and 4 patients underwent other surgical procedures. Burns caused by chemicals tended to be less severe than those seen in many thermal injuries.

Treatment of chemical burns can be divided into 3 stages: first aid at the accident site, complete medical assessment in the emergency department, and definitive treatment in a burn unit. Prompt and copious irrigation with water is the appropriate first aid therapy for almost all chemicals. Minimizing the time between contact with the chemical and irrigation is of the utmost importance. Oxygen therapy and intravenous fluid replacement should be instituted if the clinical situation warrants.

In view of the high incidence of chemical burn injuries for which no information on the involved chemical was available, all users of chemicals should be familiar with the name, nature, and dangers of the particular chemicals they are using at home or in the workplace.

▶ Interestingly, chemical burns were less severe than thermal burns. This is because many chemical and caustic skin injuries can be treated and prevented by adequate first aid measures. Immediate decontamination is the most important treatment. Ellenhorn (1) provides the best reference for this material. In summary: (1) corrosive substances should be irrigated copiously with water or saline within 10 minutes of exposure, and irrigation should continue for at least

15 minutes; (2) neutralizing substances should not be used on or in the body; (3) all contaminated clothing should be removed; (4) health personnel should wear impermeable gloves and gowns; (5) victims should be washed twice more with water and green soap to remove contaminants; (6) some chemicals require special treatment (lime, cement, lithium, sodium, phenols, phosphorus, hydrofluoric acid; see Ellenhorn and Barceloux [1]).—G. Ordog, M.D.

*Reference*

1. Ellenhorn MJ, Barceloux D: *Medical Toxicology: Diagnosis and Treatment of Human Poisoning.* New York, Elsevier North Holland, 1988.

## Fractures, Dislocations, and Musculoskeletal Trauma

### The Diagnosis and Treatment of the Dislocated Mandible
Luyk NH, Larsen PE (Univ of Otago, Dunedin, New Zealand; Ohio State Univ)
*Am J Emerg Med* 7:329–335, 1989                               2–51

The patient with mandibular dislocation is often seen first in the ED. In the most frequent type of dislocation, the mandibular condyle is displaced anteriorly to the articular eminence. Diagnosis is based on clinical signs such as pain, a preauricular depression, inability to close the mouth or move the mandible normally, and prognathism and is confirmed by panoramic radiography. Treatment consists of reduction.

*Technique.*—The patient is seated so that the mandible is below or at the level of the physician's forearm with elbow flexion at 90 degrees. The physician stands

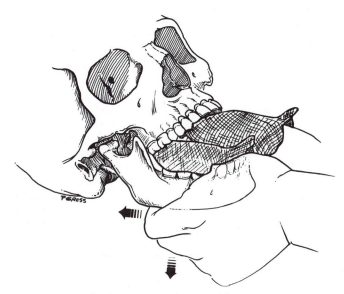

**Fig 2–5.**—Proper operator head positioning and vectors of forces *(arrows)* for reduction. (Courtesy of Luyk NH, Larsen PE: *Am J Emerg Med* 7:329–335, 1989.)

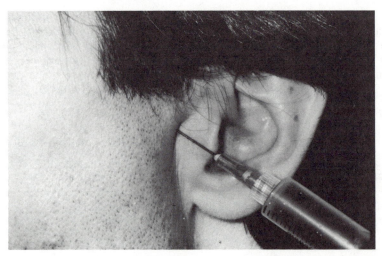

**Fig 2–6.**—Lateral facial photograph showing the preauricular depression associated with an anteriorly dislocated mandible and site of penetration and direction of advancement for the local anesthetic needle. (Courtesy of Luyk NH, Larsen PE: *Am J Emerg Med* 7:329–335, 1989.)

facing the patient with the thumbs, which are gloved, placed as far back on the molars as possible, with the fingers under the mandibular body and angle (Fig 2–5). Reduction is achieved by downward and backward thumb pressure. The patient's anxiety during reduction usually can be allayed by installation of 2 mL of local anesthetic solution into the joint capsule (Fig 2–6), but sedation with intravenously administered diazepam or even general anesthesia with muscle relaxation may be necessary.

Anterior mandibular dislocations are often seen in the ED. Usually, adequate management can be provided there by installation of local anesthesia and manual reduction. Other types of dislocation, such as posterior or lateral dislocations, are seen less often. There are treated by more complex methods.

▶ This is a review of the presentation and management of temporomandibular joint (TMJ) dislocations. The authors recommend using local anesthesia first and then sedation with intravenous diazepam. I personally prefer to use diazepam first since the patient often tenses and resists manipulation of the jaw before the relaxing effects of intravenous sedation. The pictures and diagrams used in this article are helpful guidelines in the reduction of anterior dislocation of the TMJ.—J.M. Mitchell, M.D.

---

**Atlanto-Axial Rotatory Fixation and Fracture of the Clavicle: An Association and a Classification**
Goddard NJ, Stabler J, Albert JS (Norfolk and Norwich Hosp; Queen Elizabeth Hosp, King's Lynn, England)
*J Bone Joint Surg (Br)* 72-B:72–75, 1990                                      2–52

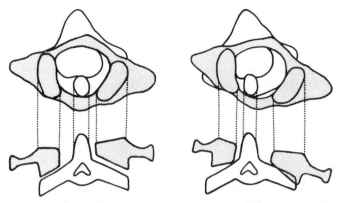

Fig 2−7.—Anteroposterior projection of C2 showing dislocation of C1. The left lateral mass of C1 is clearly seen, but the right lateral mass is tilted down and superimposed on C2, making it difficult to see. (Courtesy of Goddard NJ, Stabler J, Albert JS: *J Bone Joint Surg [Br]* 72-B:72−75, 1990.)

Atlantoaxial rotatory fixation (AARF) is an infrequent cause of childhood torticollis, usually associated with major injury or upper respiratory tract infection. Five children having AARF associated with clavicular fracture were reported.

Girl, 9 years, sustained a greenstick fracture of the left clavicle in a fall and, when seen 2 days later, had a torticollis with the head turned to the left and tilted to the right. Plain x-ray films were nonrevealing. A soft collar was applied, but repeated films 1 year later showed an atlantoaxial dislocation with the right lateral mass of the atlas rotated anteriorly on the axis (Fig 2−7). Skull traction was ineffective, and the dislocation proved irreducible at exploration. A Gallie fusion was done with the atlas fixed in the rotated position. Nine months later the girl held her head straight and had no facial asymmetry.

All 5 patients were girls aged 6−9 years who fell on their shoulders. It must not be assumed that torticollis is caused by sternomastoid spasm until CT has been used to rule out AARF. The diagnosis may be impossible to make from routine anteroposterior and lateral radiographs. Fluoroscopy may reveal AARF if a true anteroposterior view of C2 is obtained. Prompt treatment can be expected to permanently relieve the deformity.

▶ Virtually all plain radiographs in patients with torticollis reveal asymmetry of the lateral masses of C1 on C2. When the radiologist is confronted with these films and questioned about the presence of atlantoaxial rotary subluxation, they are unable to separate true pathology from rotational artifact. This paper supports that finding. However, it also suggests that further diagnostic studies (CT, fluoroscopy) in patients with persistent spasm can allow for a good outcome if performed within a reasonable period of time (2−3 weeks) following the injury. It should not be assumed that sternomastoid muscle spasm is solely a protective mechanism secondary to a clavicular fracture but that it may represent pathology of the cervical spine.— H. Unger, M.D.

---

**Scaphoid Tubercle Tenderness: A Better Indicator of Scaphoid Fractures?**
Freeland P (The Ulster Hosp, Dundonald, Northern Ireland)
*Arch Emerg Med* 6:46–50, 1989                                                  2–53

Tenderness in the anatomic snuff box (ASB) is generally accepted as an indicator of a possible scaphoid fracture. When the wrist is radially deviated, the longitudinal axis of the scaphoid lies in an anteroposterior plane, perpendicular to the other carpal bones, and the scaphoid tubercle (ST) can be easily and accurately palpated on the palmar aspect of the wrist. A prospective study was undertaken during a 10-month period to assess whether tenderness over the ST was superior to ASB tenderness for the identification of definite fractures.

Of the 246 patients with suspected scaphoid injury, 30 (12%) had definite fracture. As an indicator of definite scaphoid fracture, ST tenderness and ASB tenderness were similarly sensitive (87% vs. 90%), but ST tenderness was significantly more specific (57% vs. 40%). A small number of fractures were missed when ASB or ST tenderness alone was used as an indicator of fracture, but the presence of either ASB or ST tenderness had a sensitivity of 100% and a specificity of 40%.

The presence of either ASB or ST tenderness should be used to identify scaphoid fractures. Patients with neither ASB nor ST tenderness require symptomatic treatment only.

▶ Reading this paper stimulated me to review the important role of the scaphoid in wrist motion and stability. Scaphoid tubercle tenderness—a pearl worth remembering.— E. Ruiz, M.D.

---

**Fractures of the Scapula: A Retrospective Study of 40 Fractured Scapulae**
McGinnis M, Denton JR (Catholic Med Ctr of Brooklyn and Queens, New York)
*J Trauma* 29:1488–1493, 1989                                                  2–54

Scapular fractures are relatively rare because the scapula is protected by enveloping thick muscles. Consequently, fractures of the scapula occur only in association with other major injuries resulting from high-impact forces. Fractures of the scapula generally heal with little effect on the shoulder range of motion and with little permanent impairment. A large series of patients with scapular fractures was reviewed retrospectively and compared with those described in previous reports.

During a 4.5-year period, 39 patients aged 14–79 years were treated for 40 fractured scapulas. Many of the fractures involved more than 1 site, resulting in a total of 61 fracture sites. The mechanisms of injury included motor vehicle and motorcycle accidents in 69% of patients. Adequate follow-up data were obtained for 26 patients (67%). Follow-up ranged from 2 to 48 months. The average length of hospitalization was 16.5 days.

Patients generally did not require operation for the fractured scapula, but 40 operations were performed for associated injuries, some of which were life threatening. Scapular fractures usually were treated first with immobilization for 3–4 weeks or until the pain subsided and then with range-of-motion exercises. Rib fractures were the most common associated injury, occurring in approximately one half of patients. More than one fourth had a closed head injury. Clavicle fractures occurred in more than one fourth of the patients. Forty percent of the patients had either a pulmonary contusion, pneumothorax, or hemothorax. Spinal fractures occurred in 18% of patients. Only 3 patients had no associated injuries. The outcomes were considered good to excellent in 73% of patients and poor in 11%. Those with poor outcomes were multiply injured or elderly and unable to perform early range-of-motion exercises.

▶ The majority of patients with scapular fracture often require admission to the hospital for other reasons, and often the finding of a scapular fracture is incidental to the work-up of these patients. In this series of 3 patients discharged from the ED, 1 had a missed pneumothorax. With an average of 4.4 rib fractures occurring in 51% of the patients, careful scanning of the chest radiograph is mandatory in these patients. Fortunately, the scapular fracture itself does well with immobilization followed by range-of-motion exercises.—R.M. McNamara, M.D.

---

**An Isolated Capitate Fracture in a 9-Year-Old Boy**
Gibbon WW, Jackson A (Hope Hosp, Salford, England)
*Br J Radiol* 62:487–488, 1989                                                2–55

---

Capitate fractures are rare, but they are probably underdiagnosed in children. The diagnosis may require delayed radiographs, or if clinical suspicion is high, CT or radionuclide scanning may be helpful. Scaphoid tenderness should not lower suspicion of a possible capitate fracture. One such fracture was found in a boy aged 9 years.

Boy, 9 years, had fallen on his outstretched right hand while running and had tenderness and swelling over the dorsum of the wrist and mild tenderness in the anatomic snuffbox. Standard radiographs showed no fracture, and a plaster wrist cast was applied. Findings were again normal on repeat radiographs 10 days later; however, discomfort persisted. At 24 days capitate fracture was seen on radiographs as a band of sclerosis across the waist of the bone. Review of the previous films then showed a small break in the posterior cortex of the capitate on lateral projections.

In children the scaphoid is the carpal bone most frequently fractured. Capitate fractures are complicated relatively often, and the consequences are serious. Nonunion, avascular necrosis, instability in dorsiflexion, and capitolunate fusion all have been described.

▶ We are all aware of the necessity of ruling out scaphoid fracture in wrist and hand trauma, but there are other carpals at risk, as this case report reminds us. The symptoms of a fractured capitate may mimic those of a fractured scaphoid. Happily, this fracture is rare, and its initial management is similar to that of scaphoid fracture, as are, less happily, its complications.—J. Schoffstall, M.D.

---

**The Apical Oblique Radiograph in Examination of Acute Shoulder Trauma**
Sloth C, Lundgren Just S (Frederiksberg Hosp, Frederiksberg, Denmark)
*Eur J Radiol* 9:147–151, 1989                                         2–56

Anteroposterior (AP) and transthoracic (TT) views of the shoulder as obtained in radiologic assessment of acute shoulder trauma are often nondiagnostic. During a 6-month period, 125 patients with acute shoulder trauma underwent radiographic examination of the injured shoulder in standard AP and TT views, supplemented by an apical oblique (AO) projection.

For the AO view, the patient was placed facing the tube with the injured side rotated 45 degrees dorsally and the neck rotated contralaterally. The central beam was directed 45 degrees caudad and centered on the glenohumeral joint.

A total of 133 shoulder lesions were identified in 89 patients; the other 36 patients had normal findings. In 19 patients (15.2%), 24 lesions were found only on the AO view; another 15 lesions in 10 patients were demonstrated more clearly by the AO view than by the AP or TT views. The AO view provided additional diagnostic information in 29 patients (23.2%).

The inclusion of an AO projection increased the diagnostic sensitivity, particularly in patients with Hill-Sachs lesions, glenoid and coracoid fractures, posterior glenohumeral dislocations, acromioclavicular separations, and soft-tissue calcifications in the shoulder region. The AO projection is useful in the radiologic assessment of acute shoulder trauma; its routine use is recommended.

▶ This is a clearly written article, and the photographs of the radiographs have excellent definition with the pathology being the obvious event to the nonradiologist or nonorthopedist. This article demonstrates the superiority of the AO views over the TT view of the shoulder in detection of commonly radiographic missed posterior dislocations, acromioclavicular separations, and soft-tissue calcifications.—G.V. Anderson, M.D.

---

**The Ontario Cohort Study of Running-Related Injuries**
Walter SD, Hart LE, McIntosh JM, Sutton JR (McMaster Univ)
*Arch Intern Med* 149:2561–2564, 1989                                  2–57

Because few studies have examined the incidence and causes of running injuries, the frequency and types of injuries experienced by runners were investigated and risk factors were identified in 1,680 runners who participated in 2 community road race events. Both events included a longer and a shorter race.

All runners completed a baseline questionnaire, and as many as possible underwent a brief physical evaluation. The questionnaire covered training, running environment, use of stretching, warm-up, and cool-down exercises, other physical activities, occupational activity level, characteristics of shoes, height and weight, race participation, smoking status, and injuries during the previous year. Participants were followed up by telephone interviews at 4, 8, and 12 months after enrollment.

Of the runners, 48% had at least 1 injury; of these, 54% were new injuries, and the remainder were recurrences of previous injuries. Competitive runners had a substantially increased risk for new injuries compared with fitness runners. Excess risk was also associated with running more than 40 miles per week, running more miles per day on running days, length of the longest run during the week, number of days of running per week, and running year round. The relative risks for these variables were similar in men and women. Runners who never warmed up had less risk than those who did, and runners who sometimes stretched appeared to be at higher risk than those who usually or never did. An injury during the previous year was very predictive of a new injury. Tall men appeared to be at greater risk but not tall women. Factors such as pace, running surface, hill running, or intense training had little effect on the incidence of injury. Injury rates were similar for all age-sex groups and were unrelated to years of running experience.

Running is associated with a high incidence of injuries; however, many injuries might be prevented by a reduced training load. Running in moderation does not entail undue risk, but athletes who wish to train at high levels are at risk for more frequent injuries.

▶ There are a number of problems with this questionnaire survey of participants in 2 road races that should provoke caution in generalizing the findings. Most important, besides the large number of questionnaires unreturned or returned only long after the races, is the fact that many, many variables were sampled, without particular rationale; this should inevitably lead to "statistically significant findings" based on chance alone. Thus, tall men, but not tall women, or fat or thin men or women, supposedly had an increased risk of running injuries. Perhaps the authors would have found increased (or decreased) risk in green-eyed women, if they had only asked!—J.R. Hoffman, M.D.

---

**Injuries of the Knee Associated With Fractures of the Tibial Shaft: Detection by Examination Under Anesthesia: A Prospective Study**

Templeman DC, Marder RA (Hennepin County Med Ctr, Minneapolis; Univ of California, Davis Med Ctr, Sacramento)
*J Bone Joint Surg* 71A:1392–1395, 1989                                      2–58

To determine if ligamentous injuries of the knee are associated with fractures of the ipsilateral lower extremity, the knees of 50 patients with a fracture of the ipsilateral tibial shaft of varying severity were examined manually while the patients were under general anesthesia. An injury to at least 1 ligament of the knee resulting in increased laxity of 2+ or more was found in 11 patients (22%); 1 of the knees had dislocated. After stabilizing a fracture of the tibial shaft, clinicians must examine the knee thoroughly for associated ligamentous injuries.

▶ This article demonstrates that as with femoral shaft fractures, tibial fractures are not infrequently associated with important structural injuries in the knee. Although this may not significantly affect clinical decisions in emergency medicine, it is well worth our knowing.—J.R. Hoffman, M.D.

---

**Bilateral Spontaneous Rupture of the Quadriceps Tendons Misdiagnosed as a "Neurological Condition"**
Sagiv P, Gepstein R, Amdur B, Hallel T (Meir Gen Hosp, Kfar-Saba, Israel)
*J Am Geriatr Soc* 37:750–752, 1989                                        2–59

---

Bilateral spontaneous rupture of the quadriceps tendon is rare and occurs almost exclusively in older men. Only 17 such patients have been reported in the literature; often these patients are first misdiagnosed with a neurologic condition. A patient in whom the condition was initially misdiagnosed is presented.

Man, 78, was hospitalized with weakness in both legs after having fallen suddenly while walking in the street, and having been unable to stand up afterward. Neurologic examination revealed an absence of quadriceps reflexes and an inability to actively extend the knees. However, he had normal muscle strength in both legs, feet, and ankles. He had a history of chronic bronchitis, diaphragmatic hernia, and nephrolithiasis but was not taking steroids or any other medications at the time of this incident, and he had no history of knee pain or disability. Three days after admission, both knees appeared swollen, and an orthopedic surgeon was consulted. Examination revealed bilateral tenderness and hematomas in the suprapatellar region, and he was unable to actively extend the knees. Radiographic examination showed bilateral spontaneous tear of the quadriceps tendons, which was confirmed at operation. The avulsed tendons were reattached to the patella with nonabsorbable sutures using drill holes in the upper poles. Both knees showed full range of motion and good quadriceps muscular strength 4 months after surgery.

The following mechanism of trauma is suggested: The patient appears to trip and attempts to save himself from falling down. While the knees are bent and the feet are still fixed on the ground, a sudden, strong, and uncontrolled contraction of the quadriceps muscles occurs, causing the tendon to tear. Early surgical intervention allows direct suture of the tendon back to the patella, but a delayed diagnosis or operation will cause the quadriceps muscle to shorten, making direct suture of the tendon back to the patella impossible.

▶ Early diagnosis of this condition is important since the quadriceps muscle begins to contract immediately after tendon rupture. Early diagnosis in the ED results in early surgical intervention, and reattachment of the tendon to the patella can result in full functional recovery, even in a 78-year-old man.—G.V. Anderson, M.D.

---

**Acute Compartment Syndrome Following a Minor Athletic Injury**
Egan TD, Joyce SM (Univ of Utah)
*J Emerg Med* 7:353–357, 1989                                                    2–60

---

Acute compartment syndrome (ACS) is most commonly associated with fractures and other severe injuries. Acute comparment syndrome occurred in an athletic young man after a minor athletic injury.

Man, 23, had severe right calf pain after a twisting injury during a soccer game. Physical examination revealed no signs or symptoms of ACS, and the patient was discharged. He returned later with lateral and anterior compartment syndrome. Fasciotomy was performed, and follow-up showed partial loss of peroneal nerve and muscle function.

Although rare, ACS can occur after moderate exercise or minor athletic trauma, particularly in unconditioned individuals. A history of exertional muscle pain and presence of pain out of proportion to the apparent injury may be helpful in identifying these patients. The diagnosis can be confirmed by compartment pressure measurement. Prompt decompressive fasciotomy is indicated once the diagnosis is established.

▶ The emergency physician must think "compartment syndrome" in extremity trauma the way we "think ectopic" in women with lower abdominal pain. Unfortunately, the diagnosis may be more difficult to make. The cardinal symptom is pain out of proportion to that which might be weakness or numbness, or pain on passive flexion and extension. Since these symptoms may not be apparent on initial examination, careful discharge instruction must be given to the patient and close follow-up recommended. This holds true not only for blunt trauma and sprains but also for lacerations where unrecognized bleeding can cause similar symptoms after the patient leaves the ED. If, on presentation (or a return visit), a compartment syndrome is suspected, the pressures should be measured. The authors review a useful technique, but others are described (1).—J.T. Amsterdam, M.D.

*Reference*

1. Roberts J, Hedges J (eds): *Clinical Procedures in Emergency Medicine*, ed 2. Philadelphia, WB Saunders Co, 1990.

## Current Concepts in Pathophysiology and Diagnosis of Compartment Syndromes

Moore RE III, Friedman RJ (Med Univ of South Carolina, Charleston)
*J Emerg Med* 7:657–662, 1989                    2–61

Compartment syndrome results from an increase in local tissue pressure, which causes neurovascular compromise. The pressure may come from an increment in compartmental volume, tissue swelling or necrosis, or external sources. The increased pressure causes a decrement in arterial-venous pressure gradient, resulting in decreased blood flow. It may occur with fracture, burn, or other injury to the leg or forearm.

Early diagnosis is critical because neuromuscular tissue damage is not reversible after 8 hours without treatment, and neuromuscular function recovers best within 4 hours. Diagnosis is based on clinical grounds, but serial sensory testing is helpful in locating the compartment involved (table). When compartmental tissue pressure monitored by a portable system is 30 mm Hg or more and paresthesia extends distally, evaluation for emergency surgery is indicated. Treatment consists of fasciotomy with surgical decompression of all fascial compartments.

The emergency physician needs to be aware of the possibility of compartment syndrome when a leg or forearm has been injured and should monitor the extremity at risk. The diagnosis is best made before neurovascular dysfunction occurs and should be followed immediately by surgical decompression.

▶ This is a refreshing overview of compartment syndromes. Although most episodes of compartment syndrome are the result of injuries, they remind us that nontraumatic causes (spontaneous hemorrhage, weight lifting, reperfusion after ischemia) do exist. They emphasize the clinical diagnosis: Pain out of proportion to the suspected injury, a tense-appearing area over the compartment,

| Compartments of the Forearm | | |
| --- | --- | --- |
| Compartment | Nerve Supply | Nerve Distribution |
| Anterior compartment | Median nerve | Cutaneous to radial palm; motor to pronator teres, palmaris longus, flexor carpi radialis, and flexor digitorum superficialis |
| | Ulnar nerve | Cutaneous to hypothenar eminence and ulnar third of dorsal hand; Motor to flexor carpi ulnaris and medial portion of the flexor digitorum profundus |
| Lateral compartment | Radial nerve | Cutaneous to radial 2/3 of the dorsal hand; Motor to extensor carpi radialis longus |
| Posterior compartment | Deep branch of the radial nerve | Motor to supinator, abductor pollicis longus, and the extensor muscles of the forearm |

(Courtesy of Moore RE III, Friedman RJ: *J Emerg Med* 7:657–662, 1989.)

and sensory deficit are the basis for diagnosis. In a busy ED, x-ray findings alone may become the focus of the basis for clinical diagnosis.

Patients discharged with soft tissue injuries of the extremity need to be warned about the symptoms of compartment syndrome and, in particular, pain. Pain that is excruciating, out of proportion to the injury, or worsening with time should alert the physician and the patient to the potential complication of compartment syndrome. The scenario of a patient not seeking follow-up and taking large quantities of analgesics resulting in loss of limb function can be avoided by a good, careful examination on initial evaluation and very specific discharge instructions.—J.M. Mitchell, M.D.

---

**Plantar Puncture Wounds: Controversies and Treatment Recommendations**
Chisholm CD, Schlesser JF (Brooke Army Med Ctr, Fort Sam Houston; Womack Army Community Hosp, Fort Bragg, NC)
*Ann Emerg Med* 18:1352–1357, 1989                                      2–62

---

Patients often come to the ED with puncture wounds to the plantar surface of the foot, which are difficult to diagnose and treat because little has been published on the subject. Although superficial wounds have a low incidence of complications, difficulty in judging the depth of penetration and determining whether foreign bodies were retained renders such wounds high risk.

The pathophysiology and management of a puncture wound to the plantar surface of the foot depend on the material that punctured the foot, location of the wound, depth of penetration, time to initial examination, footwear, and the patient's underlying health status. Because superficial puncture wounds uniformly do well, depth of penetration probably is the most critical factor. Time to initial examination also is predictive of outcome because patients who are seen late usually have established or early subclinical infection with increasing pain, swelling, or drainage. *Pseudomonas aeruginosa* infection is the most devastating complication of puncture wounds; it can cause bone and joint destruction requiring extensive or repetitive débridement and may lead to amputation.

In patients treated early, the wound should be inspected and epidermal flaps should be trimmed where needed. Probing with a blunt-tipped instrument may help determine wound depth. Cleansing is appropriate, but irrigation into a closed space may be counterproductive. Tetanus vaccinations should be updated if needed. The patient should be made non-weight bearing and should be observed closely for 48 hours. Antibiotics should be given primarily for an established wound infection. If given for a dirty wound the initial dose should be administered intravenously.

Patients who come for treatment late should be treated similarly. However, because wound infection usually is established already, oral antibiotic therapy should be initiated. Ultrasonographic or CT examinations should be performed if a retained foreign body or a deep space infection is suspected. Bone scanning should be performed if osteomyelitis is suspected. If penetration of the joint space or plantar fascia is possible, particularly in wounds overlying the metatarsal heads, the patient should be referred to an orthopedic surgeon for appropriate follow-up evaluation.

▶ Puncture wounds of the foot have received significant notoriety because of the rare occurrence of *Pseudomonas* osteomyelitis. It is comforting to know that its estimated incidence is less than 1%. It seems clear from this review that the most effective management of plantar puncture wounds has yet to be defined. Some recommend more aggressive debridement and some, simple cleansing. I personally present the early patient (within 24 hours) with the option of "coring" or simple soaking, cleansing, and "see what happens" while describing the potential complications of the wound. Obviously, thus far, they all have chosen the latter. The late patients I treat depending on the presence or absence of cellulitis. Unfortunately, the major complication, *Pseudomonas* osteomyelitis, does not appear for several weeks, so the physician who initially saw the patient may never know there was a problem. Important in all cases is appropriate tetanus prophylaxis, non–weight bearing, and close follow-up in 48 hours. The role of prophylactic antibiotics and aggressive debridement needs further study.—J.M. Mitchell, M.D.

---

**Tendon Problems of the Foot and Ankle: The Spectrum From Peritendinitis to Rupture**
Plattner PF (San Leandro, Calif)
*Postgrad Med* 86:155–170, 1989                                    2–63

---

Eleven muscles originating in the leg have tendons that cross the ankle joint, and any of these may become inflamed or can rupture, sublux, or dislocate.

Achilles peritendinitis is an acute inflammatory process that is made worse by stair climbing or prolonged running. A chronic form also is seen. Complete rupture of this tendon is readily diagnosed if the condition is kept in mind and if the patient is seen early. Peritendinitis generally is managed nonoperatively with adjunctive anti-inflammatory medication. Some persons favor immediate repair of complete Achilles tendon rupture, whereas others recommend casting in a gravity equinus position for 8–12 weeks.

The tibialis posterior tendon also is subject to peritendinitis and rupture. Dysfunction of this tendon may be misdiagnosed as a chronic medial ankle sprain. Usually acute trauma is not described. Management most often involves rest and anti-inflammatory drugs or, if severe pain is present or the patient cannot walk, corrective surgery.

Persistent synovitis responds well to synovectomy. Complete rupture of the tendon can be treated with tendon reconstruction via a flexor digitorum longus transfer or with bony stabilization.

Inflammation and traumatic dislocation of the peroneal tendons are more frequent than recognized, but spontaneous rupture is rare. Peroneal peritendinitis usually is treated with rest, anti-inflammatory drugs, physical therapy, and possibly steroid injections. Acute dislocation can be managed nonoperatively, but most physicians believe that recurrent dislocation should be treated surgically. Either a soft-tissue procedure is done to reconstruct the peroneal retinaculum or a bony operation is done to deepen the retromalleolar groove.

▶ Injuries to the foot are most common in emergency medicine. The article is a nice review.—S. Repasky, D.O.

---

**Treatment of High-Pressure Water Gun Injection Injury of the Foot With Adjunctive Hyperbaric Oxygen: A Case Report**
Calhoun JH, Gogan WJ, Viegas SF, Mader JT (Univ of Texas, Galveston)
*Foot Ankle* 10:40–42, 1989                                                    2–64

---

Accidental high-pressure injection of paint, oil, grease, or water usually involves the hand but occasionally involves the foot. Hyperbaric oxygen therapy was used in 1 patient.

Man, 32, slipped when using a high-pressure water nozzle to clean a deck and accidentally injected his left forefoot. He had severe pain, a 3-cm wound at the base of the second toe, and crepitus from the ankle distally. Necrosis was minimal and little débridement was necessary, but pain persisted and crepitus extended into the calf. X-ray examination revealed subcutaneous gas extending from the foot to the popliteal fossa. Hyperbaric oxygen was administered at 2.5 atm, with immediate relief of pain and resolution of the soft tissue emphysema. The patient bore full weight 4 days after admission.

Hyperbaric oxygen therapy may have led to resorption of the injected oxygen and carbon dioxide, leaving nitrogen alone in the soft tissues, or ischemia may have been countered by hyperoxygenation and vasoconstriction. Patient discomfort is relieved by hyperbaric oxygenation, and hospital time is reduced.

▶ The increasing crepitation and pain that this patient demonstrated would be very concerning. Gas gangrene with or without a compartment syndrome would be a good possibility. Measuring compartment pressures and obtaining tissue for smear and culture would be indicated. Hyperbaric oxygenation should be considered an adjunct to surgical management as the title states.—E. Ruiz, M.D.

# 3 Organ System Emergencies

## Respiratory Emergencies

### Dystonia Presenting as Upper Airway Obstruction

Barach E, Dubin LM, Tomlanovich MC, Kottamasu S (Henry Ford Hosp, Detroit)
*J Emerg Med* 7:237–240, 1989                                          3–1

Dystonia is a common complication of neuroleptic medication, but it is not considered a life-threatening reaction. Dystonia with associated upper airway obstruction secondary to haloperidol abuse was encountered in a young woman.

Woman, 26, complained of difficulty breathing associated with head and neck dystonic reactions. Her symptoms abated spontaneously but recurred within 3 minutes, characterized by inspiratory stridor, peripheral cyanosis, and oculogyric crisis. Soft-tissue radiographs of the neck showed fullness or edema of the tongue, which was forced backward against the posterior pharynx, hypoaeration of the pharynx, and loss of cervical lordosis. The patient improved with intravenously administered diphenhydramine and intubation. Further questioning showed that she mistakenly took 4 10-mg haloperidol (Haldol) tablets as pain pills.

Asphyxiation caused by neuroleptic medications must be recognized, because failure to do so may result in unnecessary cricothyrotomy or even asphyxial death. In this case, asphyxiation is caused by dystonic activity of the pharyngeal muscles. Drug-induced dystonia is easily reversed with diphenhydramine.

▶ This report causes apprehension when haloperidol and phenothiazines are administered. It is noteworthy that the stridor disappeared within 60 seconds of intravenous administration of diphenhydramine.— E.J. Reisdorff, M.D.

### Stevens-Johnson Syndrome With Supraglottic Laryngeal Obstruction

Koch WM, McDonald GA (Univ Hosp, Boston Univ)
*Arch Otolaryngol Head Neck Surg* 115:1381–1383, 1989                  3–2

Stevens-Johnson syndrome (SJS), or erythema multiforme exudativum, is characterized by severe generalized cutaneous eruption with diffuse progressive oral lesions and ocular inflammations. Generally, there is a prodromal period with fever and symptoms of upper respiratory tract infection. A patient with SJS with acute obstruction of the upper airway is described.

*Case.*—Man, 36, had tachypnea and inspiratory stridor after a prodromal period of fever and symptoms of an upper respiratory tract infection. Physical examination showed white patchy exudates on the faucial arches and erythematous macular rash on the back, chest, and proximal extremities. Flexible fiberoptic examination of the larynx showed diffuse swelling of the supraglottic tissues with moderate erythema. An artificial airway was established because of the rapid progression of upper airway obstruction. The full clinical picture of SJS eventually developed.

This is the first reported case of SJS with early involvement of the supraglottic larynx. Physicians should be aware of this syndrome and should be prepared to manage the possible airway compromise.

▶ Given the pathophysiology of Stevens-Johnson syndrome, it is a bit surprising that severe upper respiratory tract symptoms are no more frequent than they actually are. The patient reported had airway symptoms of acute epiglottitis (supraglottis) with which every emergency physician should be familiar.—E.J. Lucid, M.D.

---

**Epiglottis: An Increasing Problem for Adults**
Sheikh KH, Mostow SR (Rose Med Ctr, Denver; Univ of Colorado)
*West J Med* 151:520–524, 1989                                      3–3

Recent reports suggest incidence of epiglottis, primarily a children's disease, is increasing among adults and is often misdiagnosed. Over a 2-year period, 9 adults with a mean age of 53 years were hospitalized with acute epiglottis confirmed by direct laryngoscopy, lateral neck radiograph, or both.

Acute epiglottis occurred from September to March in 89% of the patients. Intubation was necessary in 4 patients. The duration of symptoms was a mean 7.8 hours for intubated patients; the mean was 18.8 hours for patients not intubated. In 6 patients, the diagnoses were incorrect on first examination. All 8 patients who had laryngoscopy had typical findings; none had respiratory obstruction precipitated by the procedure. Blood cultures were positive in 5 patients, 4 for *Hemophilus influenzae* type b and 1 for *Streptococcus pneumoniae*. *Hemophilus influenzae* was resistant to ampicillin in 2 patients. All patients recovered after parenteral steroid treatment and appropriate antibiotics.

The diagnosis of epiglottis in adults is first clinical, then microbiologic. Awareness of epiglottis in adults is the most important step to correct diagnosis. Successful treatment requires early recognition.

▶ Epiglottitis, the disease that killed George Washington, was previously believed to be rare in adults; before 1969, only 37 cases had been reported in adults in the world's literature. It is unclear whether the increase in reports of this disease in the past 2 decades are the result of an increased awareness of it on the part of physicians or because of an increased prevalence or virulence of the organism that most commonly causes it, *H. influenzae.*

That two thirds of these cases were missed on initial presentation is not surprising; other series (1) report distressingly similar rates of misdiagnosis.

Emergency physicians must rule out this disease in patients who complain of a sore throat whose physical findings on oral examination are insufficient to explain their degree of pain. Laryngoscopy with a flexible laryngoscope or indirectly using a dental mirror is the diagnostic procedure of choice. Failing this, a lateral neck radiograph will often be helpful. Respiratory arrest precipitated by instrumenting the pharynx, an alleged complication in children, apparently does not happen in adults.

The reader should obtain a copy of this paper and read it in its entirety; it presents a good review of both the diagnosis and management of this difficult disease. (See also Abstract 4–57.)—J. Schoffstall, M.D.

*Reference*

1. Schabel SI, et al: *Radiology* 314:1133, 1986.

---

**Bilateral Vocal Cord Paralysis With Respiratory Failure: A Presenting Manifestation of Bronchogenic Carcinoma**
Baumann MH, Heffner JE (Univ of South Carolina, Charleston)
*Arch Intern Med* 149:1453–1454, 1989                                    3–4

---

Unilateral vocal cord paralysis and hoarseness caused by disruption of a recurrent laryngeal nerve by mediastinal tumor extension is a well-known manifestation of lung cancer. However, bilateral vocal cord paralysis is a much rarer and lesser known complication, which may turn into a life-threatening condition if not recognized and treated early. A patient with lung cancer had upper airway obstruction and hypercapnic respiratory failure resulting from bilateral vocal cord paralysis.

Man, 61, who had a 100-pack-year smoking history, was hospitalized with a 3-week history of progressive dyspnea. On admission, he had severe respiratory distress with inspiratory stridor and agitation, but he was able to speak short phrases in a normal voice. After intubation, the patient's stridor, dyspnea, and hypercapnia resolved completely. A chest radiograph showed dense infiltrates and volume loss in the left upper lobe. Computed tomography revealed a left lung mass extending into the right and left superior mediastinum involving the regions of both recurrent laryngeal nerves. Bronchoscopy and biopsy confirmed a diagnosis of squamous cell carcinoma. He underwent tracheotomy, which allowed spontaneous respiration without difficulty, but refused to undergo laryngeal operation to correct the underlying airway obstruction. Thoracic irradiation did not improve vocal cord dysfunction.

Both recurrent laryngeal nerves are vulnerable to disruption from invading mediastinal malignant neoplasms, but their concurrent disruption causing bilateral vocal cord paralysis is an uncommon but clinically important manifestation of bronchial cancer. The clinical presentation of bilateral involvement differs markedly from that of the more commonly encountered unilateral vocal cord paralysis in that patients with stridor retain a normal voice. The unusual paradox of a normal voice with stridor in patients with bilateral vocal cord paralysis may not be recognized immediately. However, a delay in urgent translaryngeal intubation may turn into a life-threatening situation.

▶ The circuitous course of the recurrent laryngeal nerves (especially on the left) makes them vulnerable to extension of mediastinal or pulmonary malignancies. Unilateral cord paralysis is more common, but hoarseness or a normal voice with stridor should cause the emergency physician to think of the possibility of malignancy involving the recurrent laryngeal nerve or "nerves." (See also Abstract 2–13.)—G.V. Andersen, M.D.

---

**Clinical Criteria for the Detection of Pneumonia in Adults: Guidelines for Ordering Chest Roentgenograms in the Emergency Department**
Gennis P, Gallagher J, Falvo C, Baker S, Than W (Bronx Municipal Hosp Ctr; New York Med College, Valhalla, NY; Albert Einstein College of Medicine, Bronx)
*J Emerg Med* 7:263–268, 1989                                          3–5

---

Emergency room physicians facing an adult with acute respiratory illness lack clinical guidelines on whether to order chest roentgenography for detection of pneumonia. To identify sensitive clinical criteria, 308 such adults who were nonasthmatic underwent prospective study. Definite or equivocal infiltrates were found in 38% and considered indicative of pneumonia.

Cough was equally prevalent in those with and without pneumonia. Of patients with pneumonia, 31% had no fever. Decreased breath sounds, rales, rhonchi, percussion dullness, wheezes, egobronchophony, and altered fremitus were present in less than 50% of patients with pneumonia. Abnormal auscultatory findings combined identified 78% of those with pneumonia. However, abnormal vital signs, that is, temperature more than 37.8° C, pulse more than 100 beats per min or respirations more than 20/minute, were present in 97% of patients with pneumonia. When chest x-ray films were reinterpreted blindly by a senior radiologist, the sensitivity of the vital sign abnormalities was retained.

Most cases of radiographically detectable pneumonia will be found if ED physicians restrict chest roentgenograms to patients who have 1 or more abnormal vital signs. This does not apply to persons with asthma, who often lack radiographic findings.

▶ The authors point out and document several relevant features regarding the diagnosis of pneumonia in the emergency setting: (1) in the absence of an abnormal vital sign, radiographic evidence of pneumonia is extremely rare; (2) the chest x-ray film beats the stethoscope in the adult patient, and the stethoscope excels over the chest x-ray film in infants and children; (3) no single symptom or sign was reliably predictive of radiographic evidence of pneumonia; and (4) using the chest radiograph as the gold standard for the diagnosis of pneumonia has limitations unless correlated with lower respiratory tract microscopic and culture results.— D.K. Wagner, M.D.

---

**The Value of Routine Admission Chest Radiographs in Adult Asthmatics**
Aronson S, Gennis P, Kelly D, Landis R, Gallagher J (Bronx Municipal Hosp, Albert Einstein College of Medicine, Bronx)
*Ann Emerg Med* 18:1206–1208, 1989                                              3–6

---

To assess the value of chest radiographs as a routine admission procedure in adult asthmatic patients, the charts of 102 adult patients hospitalized for acute bronchospasm were reviewed. Although the data were obtained prospectively, patients were classified as uncomplicated and complicated asthmatics retrospectively.

Of the 125 admissions in 102 patients, 81 were classified as uncomplicated and 44 as complicated. Chest radiographs affected management in 13 patients with complicated asthma, whereas none of the 81 radiographs in the uncomplicated group affected patient care; the difference was significant.

Routine admission chest radiographs in adult patients with uncomplicated asthma may not be necessary. A prospective study, which classifies patients as complicated or uncomplicated asthmatics, is warranted before concluding that routine radiographs can be safely abandoned in these patients.

▶ In our ever-increasing attempt to limit the cost of health care, the issue of the need for chest x-ray studies arises frequently. This paper attempts to look at the issue for adult asthmatics who require admission to the hospital. It points out that the need for these films in children with asthma has repeatedly been shown to be unnecessary. However, older adult asthmatics represent a very different group of patients, with other potential problems such as heart disease and chronic obstructive pulmonary disease. In 44 patients classified as complicated, the chest x-ray film altered therapy in 13 patients. This is clearly significant. I think the key point to be gained from this paper is that it may very well be true that uncomplicated asthmatics do not require a chest x-ray film, but we must be extremely careful in patients with complicating illnesses.— E.J. Lucid, M.D.

---

**Who Is Dying of Asthma and Why?**
Lanier B (Univ of Texas, Dallas)
*J Pediatr* 115:838–840, 1989                                              3–7

---

The number of deaths from asthma has been increasing, which may be because of insufficient assessment of the problem and delay in initiating treatment. Several steps to prevent such deaths can be taken.

Recognizing the child who is at high risk is important. The highest-risk asthma patient is a black, male, inner-city adolescent with fairly chronic asthma who is somewhat noncompliant, has little parental support, and has had an acute asthma attack in the preceding year.

To prevent fatalities, physicians should assess the extent of reversibility in the high-risk patient. Appropriate laboratory analyses include determination of serum theophylline levels, studies of pulmonary function before and after bronchodilator therapy, and assessment of peak flow rates. Reversibility trials of short periods of steroid therapy, as well as other therapeutic modalities, will show the pattern of asthma episodes and demonstrate optimal results to the patient, allowing for a long-term management plan, including regular follow-up visits and efforts to achieve patient compliance.

▶ It is most distressing to realize that despite all of the new drugs made available in the past 20 years for treatment of asthma, we are seeing an increasing death rate from the disease. This paper attempts to identify those children at high risk and notes that the highest-risk patient is a black, male, inner-city adolescent with chronic asthma. We should, however, be concerned about any child who is somewhat noncompliant, and in my experience, this is usually found to be an adolescent, just as is the case in juvenile diabetes. The patients identified as high risk frequently use the ED as their source of ongoing primary care, and it thus is imperative that we try to establish a rapport with these young people so that we can educate them about their disease and its proper management. This is not an easy task, especially in the environment that the physician and high-risk patient both find themselves—a busy, overstressed inner-city ED.

The article suggests having the patient involved in assessing the severity of this attack by performing peak flow studies routinely, thus giving objected evidence of the results of treatment to the patient. I agree with this approach. Clearly, an essential component of the management of such patients is a close working relationship between patient and physician. In our setting, it also requires a close working relationship among the patient, emergency physician, and pediatrician or internist. (See also Abstract 4–58.)—E.J. Lucid, M.D.

---

**Theophylline: Is It Obsolete for Asthma?**
Rooklin A (Crozer-Chester Med Ctr, Chester, Pa)
*J Pediatr* 115:841–845, 1989                                                    3–8

---

Theophylline is the drug most often used for treating moderate asthma in patients requiring daily medication, even though it may cause CNS and gastrointestinal tract side effects. In the hospital, selective $\beta_2$ agents have largely replaced theophylline, mostly because the latter produces caffeinelike symptoms, such as gastric distress, nervousness, and headache. However, use of aminophylline along with a selective $\beta_2$ agent may enhance bronchodilation.

Selection of the theophylline preparation requires understanding of the differences in preparation and of the more rapid absorption rates in children, especially those between 7 months and 9 years of age. In children who are vomiting, rectal suppositories are not recommended in view of their erratic absorption characteristics. Intravenous administration during brief hospitalization is probably safer in most patients. Finding the specific dosage needed usually requires measurement of serum theophylline levels.

Theophylline is not the best choice for children who have intermittent asthma symptoms, behavioral changes during theophylline therapy, a history of seizures, or in whom abdominal pain, gastroesophageal reflux, or headache develop. If theophylline levels are at or less than 15 μg/mL and symptoms arise only during strenuous exercise, the addition of a $\beta_2$ agent, cromolyn, or both before exercise is better than increasing serum levels of theophylline.

▶ This article is a well-written discussion of the appropriate use of theophylline in treating pediatric asthma, and the answer to the question of whether or not theophylline is obsolete is clearly no from this author's point of view. He gives a very clear discussion of the different types of theophylline preparations and guidelines for their use. He also discusses when not to use theophylline. Emphasis is placed on the importance of following blood levels of the drug while initiating therapy, during periods of rapid growth of the patient, and when the patient is taking drugs that alter the metabolism of theophylline, such as erythromycin and phenytoin. It is recommended for thorough reading by all emergency physicians.—E.J. Lucid, M.D.

---

**Alternative Approaches to Asthma**
Wynn SR (Fort Worth, Tex)
*J Pediatr* 115:846–849, 1989                                                    3–9

Because asthma is more than bronchospasm alone, agents used to control chronic asthma must also control inflammation. The mechanisms of action, clinical uses, and side effects of 3 types of anti-inflammatory agents used in children (corticosteroids, cromolyn sodium, and ipratroprium) were reviewed.

Corticosteroids prevent the formation of prostaglandins and leukotrienes, increase the number of β-adrenergic receptors on bronchial smooth muscle cells, and may decrease IgE levels and control production of mucus. Steroids appear to be beneficial when combined with bronchodilators for the treatment of acute, severe asthma. Inhaled steroids can reduce the use of oral doses of steroids. Multiple courses of prednisone have caused prolonged adrenal suppression. The effects of inhaled steroids are not clear, and caution is still needed when steroids are used.

Cromolyn sodium, now challenging theophylline as a first-line drug in the treatment of asthma, appears to play a central role in mitigating the immunopathogenesis of the disease. It prevents many forms of asthma, and is the only agent to consistently block the bronchoconstriction that is first triggered by allergen inhalation and then recurs within 4–8 hours. Cromolyn administered by a metered-dose inhaler is generally preferred by patients and is as safe and effective as the Spinhaler. It is most valuable when administered with a β-agonist. Children may not respond to cromolyn, however, if the trial period is inadequate, when the 4 times daily schedule is not maintained, or when it is given only on an as-needed basis for bronchodilation.

Ipratropium bromide, an anticholinergic drug chemically related to atropine, exerts its most important effect on the basic cholinergic hyperactivity of asthma. In 1 study, the combination of ipratropium with albuterol was more effective than either drug alone. Another promising drug, azelastine, may decrease underlying bronchial hyperreactivity.

▶ Of the 3 "anti-inflammatory" medications discussed in this article, corticosteroids and ipratropium are pertinent to emergency physicians. Further study is required on ipratropium, but it shows more promise when combined with a β-antagonist. Steroids have been shown to decrease admission rates for asthma when given early in emergency therapy (1).

I routinely administer steroids early in the ED therapy to all asthmatics without contraindications using doses of 1–2 mg/kg of intravenous methylprednisolone or oral prednisone.

A second valuable role of steroids is in preventing relapse after ED discharge. Fiel (2) demonstrated a decrease in relapse rates from 21% to 6% with a tapering dose of steroids. Why he used a taper and why many emergency physicians confuse themselves and their patients in trying to coordinate a 5-day taper is not clear to me. A 5-day course of 1 50-mg prednisone tablet daily is safe and does not require a taper.—R.M. McNamara, M.D.

*References*

1. Littenberg B, et al: *N Engl J Med* 314:150, 1986.
2. Fiel SB, et al: *Am J Med* 75:259, 1983.

---

**Nebulized Ipratropium in the Treatment of Acute Asthma**
Summers QA, Tarala RA (Royal Perth Hosp, Perth, Western Australia)
*Chest* 97:430–434, 1990                                      3–10

---

Ipratropium, a new anticholinergic antimuscarinic agent, has been shown to be an effective bronchodilator in acute asthma. Previous reports suggest that sequential administration of an adrenoreceptor agonist and an antimuscarinic agent is superior to either agent when given alone in patients with acute asthma. The efficacy of ipratropium and salbutamol was assessed in 117 patients with acute asthma who were randomly assigned to 1 of 3 treatment groups. Nebulized salbutamol, 5 mg, followed by ipratropium, .5 mg, was given to 40 patients; ipratropium, followed by salbutamol, was given to 41 patients; and both drugs adminis-tered together, followed by nebulized saline, were given to 36 patients. The patients received 2 nebulized treatments at an interval of 1 hour in this double-blind study.

Ipratropium was an effective bronchodilator when given as the initial treatment. However, ipratropium given after salbutamol was as effective as when given in combination with salbutamol. At 1 hour after treatment, there was no difference in peak expiratory flow rates between the combina-tion of drugs and either drug given separately. Ipratropium given after sal-butamol was not superior to saline solution after the combination of drugs.

The routine use of ipratropium in acute asthma remains to be estab-lished. Addition of ipratropium to salbutamol provides no additional benefit in the immediate treatment of acute asthma.

▶ As the authors point out, although anticholinergics have a theoretical basis for use in asthma, more studies are necessary to validate their routine inclusion in acute asthma therapy. Asthma remains an intensely personal problem. For some, anticholinergics may be personally quite rewarding.—D.K. Wagner, M.D.

---

**Frequency of Inhaled Metaproterenol in the Treatment of Acute Asthma Exacerbation**
Nelson MS, Hofstadter A, Parker J, Hargis C (Stanford Univ)
*Ann Emerg Med* 19:21–25, 1990                                                                3–11

Few studies address the optimum dose of an inhaled sympathomimetic drug in the treatment of acute asthma exacerbation. In a prospective, double-blind study during a 6-month period, the frequency of dosing of an inhaled β-agonist, metaproterenol, was studied in adult patients who went to the ED with an acute asthma exacerbation. Forty-one patients initially received 0.3 mL of nebulized metaproterenol, followed by 2 ad-ditional doses of either metaproterenol or saline every 20 minutes. Pul-monary function tests were performed at 30, 60, and 120 minutes after arrival.

Forced expiratory volume in 1 second did not differ significantly be-tween groups at 30 minutes, but there was an improved response in the metaproterenol group at 60 and 120 minutes after arrival. Total time spent in the ED and admission rates were approximately the same be-tween groups. The incidence of side effects was similar in both groups. Serum potassium levels were not affected by metaproterenol.

In patients with an acute asthma exacerbation, frequent dosing of neb-ulized metaproterenol produces a rapid and significant improvement without an increase in toxicity.

▶ The use of subcutaneous epinephrine for treatment of bronchospasm is dimin-ishing. The role of theophylline loading in the ED is also being challenged. There is greater reliance on β-adrenergic aerosolized agents. This study supports the use of an aerosol treatment as often as every 20–30 minutes. Aggressive, frequent use of nebulized adrenergic agents may be the cornerstone for treating exacerbations of asthma. From this study, it would appear that 3 β-adrenergic aerosol treatments during the first hour in the ED admission should be the first step in treating patients with acute bronchospasm.—E.J. Reisdorff, M.D.

---

**Glucagon as a Therapeutic Agent in the Treatment of Asthma**
Wilson JE, Nelson RN (Northeastern Ohio Univs, Akron; Ohio State Univ)
*J Emerg Med* 8:127–130, 1990                                              3–12

---

Because glucagon stimulates production of cyclic adenosine monophosphate (cAMP) and relaxes smooth muscle as a result, it might have a bronchodilator effect in asthmatic patients. Fourteen patients with mild to moderate acute bronchospastic airway disease had peak expiratory flow rates measured before and after the intravenous administration of 1 mg of glucagon.

The mean peak expiratory flow rate rose from 207 to 275 L/min after glucagon injection. Eight patients had an increase of more than 60 L/min 10 minutes after glucagon was administered. The mean increase in peak flow in responders was 113 L/min. No responding patient later had an exacerbation of bronchospasm. Responders had a much greater rise in blood glucose levels than did nonresponders. There were no adverse effects other than mild nausea.

Glucagon apparently has a favorable effect on asthmatic bronchospasm, and further studies are warranted. Studies of synergism between glucagon and other β-adrenergic agonists or methylxanthines would be of interest.

▶ The authors present a physiologic rationale for giving glucagon to the bronchospastic patient. Although the data show some improvement in their patient population, their subset is such as to include those less severely impaired by the disease process. As the authors conclude, further investigation is necessary to effectively evaluate glucagon and other agents used to control bronchospasm.—D.K. Wagner, M.D.

---

**Civilian Spontaneous Pneumothorax: Treatment Options and Long-Term Results**
O'Rourke JP, Yee ES (East Tennessee State Univ, Johnson City)
*Chest* 96:1302–1306, 1989                                                3–13

---

Records were reviewed for 130 patients seen in an 11-year period with 168 episodes of spontaneous pneumothorax and followed for a mean of 6.5 years. All were first seen with chest pain, dyspnea, or both. Nearly one third of the patients were aged more than 50 years, and at least three fourths of the patients smoked cigarettes. Associated lung disease was present in one third, including a large number with chronic obstructive pulmonary disease. Associated lung disease was most frequent in older patients.

Forty episodes were treated by observation alone, usually in a hospital; most of these patients had mild symptoms and less than 15% lung involvement. Nine patients admitted for observation later had chest tube thoracostomy. Thoracentesis was done in 6 instances, and chest tube thoracostomy was done 102 times. Twenty patients underwent thoracotomy, most often because of multiple ipsilateral episodes of pneumothorax. Mortality among all patients was 5%, and the complication rate among patients given chest tubes was 15%.

The most obvious differences between civilian and military patients with pneumothorax are greater age and associated lung disease in the civilian population. Spontaneous pneumothorax is not a totally benign disorder. Current techniques allow surgery to be considered even for older patients with associated lung disease. Patients who are not candidates for thoracotomy may be offered chemical pleurodesis. Observation alone is risky.

▶ The authors present data on unintentionally induced "spontaneous" pneumothorax. Conclusions were simple and straightforward: (1) closed thoracotomy is the treatment of choice; (2) open thoracotomy is indicated in cases with a persistent, pulmonic air leak; (3) needle aspiration should be considered for reexpansion only in stable patients without evidence of continued pleural leak; and (4) observation alone is rarely indicated. We would agree with all of those conclusions.—D.K. Wagner, M.D.

---

**Roentgenogram of the Month: A One-Sided Affair?**
Zwaveling JH, Gans SJM (Univ Hosp Utrecht, The Netherlands)
*Chest* 95:673–675, 1989                                                     3–14

---

Cardiogenic pulmonary edema usually appears as a bilateral butterfly or bat wing configuration on radiographs, with the periphery of the lung relatively clear. Unilateral distribution, which is uncommon, was observed in an elderly patient.

Woman, 78, was hospitalized with respiratory failure and coma. She was well until the day of hospitalization, when a nonproductive cough and progressive shortness of breath developed. She had no history of substernal or abdominal pain or preexisting respiratory disease. On the basis of a thorough examination, including a chest radiograph (Fig 3–1), a tentative diagnosis of pneumonia and sepsis was made. The patient was therefore treated with mechanical ventilation, erythromycin, gentamicin, and cefuroxime. Her failure to respond prompted a reconsideration of the initial diagnosis, and a new diagnosis of high-pressure pulmonary edema was made, followed by treatment with furosemide, nitroglycerin, and dobutamine. Within 48 hours, her chest radiograph cleared almost entirely,

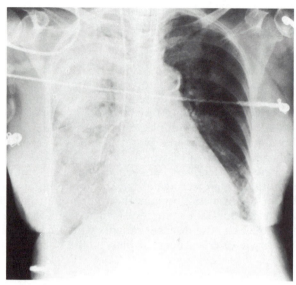

**Fig 3–1.**—Chest roentgenogram obtained on admission. (Courtesy of Zwaveling JH, Gans SJM: *Chest* 95:673–675, 1989.)

beginning at the subpleural space. A follow-up ECG was suggestive of anterior myocardial infarction. The final diagnosis was myocardial infarction with pulmonary edema and forward failure.

In this patient, who had unilateral abnormalities on the initial chest radiograph, the original diagnosis of pneumonia could not be maintained because of absence of fever, negative cultures, and complete resolution of the pulmonary infiltrates in 48 hours. The most likely cause of unilateral pulmonary edema was prolonged lateral decubitus position in the presence of cardiac failure before hospitalization.

▶ The authors' case points out the difficulties in reliance on the chest x-ray film to differentiate between a primary cardiac and primary pulmonic cause for a patient with respiratory failure. Both clinical and radiographic signs of failure require adequate parenchymal perfusion. Conditions such as local emphysema, unilateral pulmonary embolism, and congenital or acquired lobar deficits limit pulmonary perfusion and consequently cause signs of failure to be directed primarily to the opposite side. In addition, as in the authors' case, a persistent, dependent position may cause increased capillary pressure on the dependent side and, therefore, unilateral pulmonary signs and symptoms. Finally, a unilateral infectious process is certainly capable of tipping a cardiosensitive person into a symptomatic fluid overload picture. Moment-to-moment management with the early institution of wedge pressure monitoring is required in these confusing situations.—D.K. Wagner, M.D.

### Neurogenic Pulmonary Edema: New Concepts of an Old Disorder
Bekemeyer WB, Pinstein ML (Univ of Tennessee, Memphis)
*South Med J* 82:380–383, 1989                                    3–15

Neurogenic pulmonary edema (NPE) probably occurs much more often than is recognized or reported. It occurs in various settings, having in common an acute onset, such as head trauma, grand mal seizures, subarachnoid or intracerebral hemorrhage, and electroconvulsive therapy. An early or acute form of NPE and a delayed form are distinguished. Early NPE is heralded by dyspnea occurring minutes to hours after a neurologic event. The delayed form, occurring after a delay of 12 hours to several days, tends to be more insidious. The pathologic findings include alveolar edema and hemorrhage.

Lesions of the medulla or hypothalamus and intracranial hypertension can cause pulmonary edema in laboratory animals. Marked autonomic sympathetic discharge is a possible pathogenic factor. Delayed NPE may be the pathogenetic equivalent of adult respiratory distress syndrome.

If NPE is distinguished from other causes of diffuse pulmonary infiltration with profound hypoxemia, unnecessary antibiotic therapy and invasive procedures may be avoided. Supportive measures, including supplemental oxygen, are appropriate for both forms of NPE. Continuous positive airway pressure, mechanical ventilation, and positive end-expiratory pressure may be necessary. Diuresis can minimize hydrostatic edema formation. In addition, α-adrenergic blocking drugs may be useful.

▶ A diagnosis of exclusion is associated with common ER illnesses such as trauma or intracranial bleed. The onset may be rapid or insiduous but should be kept in mind as part of our differential diagnosis.—S. Repasky, D.O.

### Pulmonary Edema in the Renal Failure Patient
Gehm L, Propp DA (Lutheran Gen Hosp, Univ of Illinois Affiliated Hosps, Park Ridge)
*Am J Emerg Med* 7:336–339, 1989                                    3–16

Pulmonary edema is even more serious in association with renal failure. Congestive heart failure accounts for up to 30% of cardiovascular deaths in patients requiring hemodialysis.

Woman, 49, with renal failure for 12 years that required regular hemodialysis, complained of severe shortness of breath and reported having gained about 1.8 kg since the last dialysis. She had a history of hypertension, chronic bronchitis, and a failed renal transplant 10 years before. The patient was taking clonidine, diazepam, and supplemental calcium. Periorbital edema and coarse pulmonary rales were noted, as well as pitting pretibial edema. A chest radiograph revealed frank pulmonary edema. Trigeminy developed when dialysis was begun but responded to lidocaine. Pulmonary edema responded well to a single dialysis treatment, during which the patient lost about 2.7 kg. Subsequent ECGs showed an extensive subendocardial anterior myocardial infarction. The initial ECG had shown no ischemic changes.

Preload and afterload reduction should be pursued aggressively in cases of pulmonary edema associated with renal failure. Nitroprusside may be very useful in patients having markedly elevated left ventricular pressures. Vasodilation therapy may suffice, but if pulmonary edema is severe and renal failure is refractory, actual phlebotomy may be necessary. Peritoneal dialysis may be an option if hemodialysis is not immediately available.

▶ The patient in fulminant pulmonary edema is hypoxic and under extreme stress. Immediate nasotracheal or orotracheal intubation, followed by positive pressure ventilation with 100% oxygen, protects the patient from anoxic insult while allowing pharmacologic measures to work. Mask oxygen with continuous positive airway pressure is poorly tolerated under these conditions. The emergency physician has to make a quick judgment as to how hypoxic and stressed the patient is. If the patient is severely stressed, intubate. The indications for intubation were not discussed by the authors.—E. Ruiz, M.D.

## Cardiac Emergencies

DYSRHYTHMIAS

### Role of Transcutaneous Pacing in the Setting of a Failing Permanent Pacemaker

Kissoon N, Rosenberg HC, Kronick JB (Children's Hosp of Western Ontario, London)
*Pediatr Emerg Care* 5:178–180, 1989                                                    3–17

Transcutaneous pacing is a safe, rapid, and effective method for temporary cardiac pacing, particularly in children. Its use and potential hazard in a boy with a failing permanent pacemaker were reviewed.

Boy, 15 years, with acute symptomatic bradycardia caused by a failing permanent pacemaker, was paced transcutaneously in the ED. Despite application of maximal current output at a rate of 80, the patient remained symptomatic. Because his in situ pacemaker was generating regular electrical impulses without consistent capture and the ECG leads monitored electrical activity and not mechanical response, the use of the demand mode resulted in the transcutaneous device, sensing his pacemaker spikes as normal electrical impulses and, hence, failing to pace. With removal of the ECG leads, sensing was lost, and consistent ventricular pacing was achieved in an asynchronous mode. The patient improved.

The potential for asystole and ventricular dysrhythmia in this situation is significant; transcutaneous pacing is a potential lifesaving device in children.

▶ The external pacer electrodes picked up the output from the patient's non-capturing transvenous pacer and therefore would not generate any output. This problem should have been avoidable by setting the rate on the external pacer above the transvenous pacer rate. With an atrial-sensing ventricular pacemaker, the output rate on the pacemaker would have been variable, and perhaps the rate of 80 at which the external drive was set was too low. It is useful to know, however, that by removing the ECG leads, one can convert the external pacer to a nondemand mode.—W.P. Burdick, M.D.

---

**Efficacy and Safety of Intravenous Diltiazem for Treatment of Atrial Fibrillation and Atrial Flutter**
Salerno DM, Dias VC, Kleiger RE, Tschida VH, Sung RJ, Sami M, Giorgi LV, Diltiazem–Atrial Fibrillation/Flutter Study Group (Univ of Minnesota; Marion Labs, Kansas City, Mo; Jewish Hosp, St Louis; United Hosp, St Paul; San Francisco Gen Hosp; et al)
*Am J Cardiol* 63:1046–1051, 1989                                            3–18

---

The calcium antagonist diltiazem, given orally, reportedly is effective against atrial arrhythmias. In a multicenter double-blind, placebo-controlled study, the effects of intravenously administered diltiazem and an identical placebo on atrial fibrillation and atrial flutter were compared in 113 patients. All patients had a ventricular rate of at least 120 beats per minute and a systolic blood pressure of 90 mm Hg or more without severe heart failure. The initial dose of diltiazem was 0.25 mg/kg in 2 minutes, and a dose of 0.35 mg/kg was given 15 minutes later if necessary.

The total rate of response to diltiazem was 93%, whereas only 12% of patients responded to placebo administration. When patients in the placebo group received open-label diltiazem, 94% of patients were effectively treated. Patients with atrial fibrillation and atrial flutter had comparable response rates. The mean fall in systolic blood pressure after diltiazem was 8%. No patient had symptomatic hypotension, and none had chest pain.

Intravenously administered diltiazem was significantly more effective than a placebo in patients with atrial fibrillation or atrial flutter. Diltiazem may prove useful for controlling the heart rate in this setting, because class I antiarrhythmic drugs act slowly unless infused, and the risk of side effects probably is greater than that from diltiazem.

▶ This study, sponsored by Marion Laboratories, the sole producer of diltiazem, showed that this slow-channel calcium blocker is better than placebo for slowing ventricular response in atrial fibrillation—no great surprise. Hypotension occurred as frequently as with verapamil. Both drugs, however, are in for a strong challenge from adenosine in the treatment of supraventricular tachycardia (SVT). Adenosine, which acts by a vagotonic mechanism, has a half-life of about 6 seconds and does not cause hypotension. It is also safe in patients who have bypass tracts since it does not enhance conduction through this pathway. The short half-life may result in a higher rate of SVT recurrence. I suspect upcoming trials of adenosine vs. slow-channel calcium blockers (and esmolol, the short-acting β-blocker) will change the way we treat supraventricular tachycardias. (See also Abstract 3–19.)—W.P. Burdick, M.D.

## Esmolol Versus Verapamil in the Acute Treatment of Atrial Fibrillation or Atrial Flutter

Platia EV, Michelson EL, Porterfield JK, Das G (Washington Hosp Ctr, Washington, DC; Lankenau Med Research Ctr, Philadelphia; Johns Hopkins Hosp; Univ of North Dakota, Fargo)

*Am J Cardiol* 63:925–929, 1989
    3–19

Esmolol, an ultrashort-acting β-blocking agent, has been effective in treating patients with atrial fibrillation or atrial flutter with a rapid ventricular response. Its effect in acute management of such patients was compared with that of verapamil. Forty-five patients were stratified as having new-onset (<48 hours) or old-onset (>48 hours) atrial fibrillation or flutter with rapid ventricular rate and were randomly assigned to receive either esmolol or verapamil intravenously.

Patients receiving esmolol experienced a decline in heart rate from 139 to 100 beats per minute, and those given verapamil had a decline from 142 to 97 beats per minute. The decline in both groups was significant. Among patients with arrhythmia of recent onset, conversion to sinus rhythm occurred in 50% of those receiving esmolol and 12% of those receiving verapamil. Concurrent digoxin treatment did not significantly influence results. Mild hypotension affected both groups of patients.

Esmolol compares favorably with verapamil in acute treatment of patients with atrial fibrillation or flutter and a rapid ventricular response. It is significantly more likely to effect conversion to sinus rhythm in arrhythmia of new onset. Administration of digoxin does not cause adverse interactions.

▶ Esmolol is preferable to verapamil for emergency physicians for practical reasons. Hypotension may complicate the use of either drug. Verapamil may be contraindicated in atrial fibrillation associated with Wolff-Parkinson-White syndrome. Esmolol offers the attractive feature of ready reversibility, and it can be used with relative safety in tachyarrhythmias.

Care should be taken when esmolol is stopped that a rebound tachycardia not develop. Addition of a secondary drug such as digoxin or a long-acting β-blocker should be considered.

The article demonstrates a significant advantage of esmolol over verapamil in acute onset atrial fibrillation or flutter. The authors do not differentiate between flutter or fibrillation for purposes of the study. Such a breakdown would be of interest, because flutter is generally considered a more easily converted rhythm.

We must remember that cardioversion remains the treatment of choice in patients in shock or with evidence of cardiac or cerebral ischemia.—J.E. Clinton, M.D.

**Estimating the Duration of Ventricular Fibrillation**
Brown CG, Dzwonczyk R, Werman HA, Hamlin RL (Ohio State Univ)
*Ann Emerg Med* 18:1181–1185, 1989                                                3–20

The chance of successful resuscitation declines as the interval from the onset of ventricular fibrillation (VF) and the application of defibrillation lengthens. Data from animal studies suggest that success is more likely after prolonged arrest when drug therapy is given before defibrillation; accurate estimates of downtime therefore could be most helpful. Whether changes in the frequency or amplitude of the VF ECG signal during cardiac arrest can be used to estimate downtime was investigated.

Total power and the frequency distribution of power were determined during VF in swine. The median frequency of the power spectrum served to track power distribution. Median frequency was less variable between animals than was total power. A mathematical model of median frequency estimated downtime to within 1.3 minutes of actual downtime after 1–10 minutes of VF in additional animals.

The median frequency of the VF ECG signal may be used to estimate downtime when the efficacy of various interventions is studied. Downtime estimates can be available in about 8 seconds, with updates every 4 seconds.

▶ The authors have tested the fascinating hypothesis that downtime may be predicted from an ECG tracing. If this were true in human beings, testing of time-dependent resuscitation protocols would be possible.

The authors have shown that median frequency of ventricular fibrillation signal can be used to estimate downtime within the first 10 minutes in swine with electrically induced VF..

A needed next step with this model is demonstration of a difference in outcome with differing therapy determined by median frequency of the VF signal and time. If such a difference is demonstrable in swine, a human trial should be carried out.—J.E. Clinton, M.D.

---

**The Emerging Role of Echocardiography in the Emergency Department**
Hauser AM (William Beaumont Hosp, Royal Oak, Mich)
*Ann Emerg Med* 18:1298–1303, 1989                                                3–21

Echocardiography has become an important diagnostic tool in the evaluation of the heart. However, echocardiography remains primarily a tool of the cardiologist, because the anatomic and physiologic complexity of the dynamically beating heart and its wide range of normal and abnormal appearances requires expert analysis of the echocardiogram.

In the EDs of large institutions, cardiologists are available to administer and interpret this examination. In the EDs of smaller institutions, echocardiography commonly is underused because cardiologists are not always available and emergency physicians lack the skill to record and interpret echocardiograms. It would therefore be useful for emergency physicians to obtain a minimum familiarity with the technique sufficient to recognize potentially life-threatening disorders. This would permit triage of patients with chest pain, hypotension, or dyspnea in the ED.

Echocardiography most often is used in the ED to evaluate left ventricular contraction. Definitive assessment of left ventricular function is important in acute myocardial infarction because prognosis is most closely tied to the extent of left ventricular functional impairment. Evaluation of the echocardiogram is superior to assessment of the clinical Killip classification and provides the most accurate prediction of death or major complication after acute myocardial infarction. An echocardiogram that shows normal left ventricular wall motion during chest pain is a strong predictor of a nonischemic cause and, consequently, of low risk.

With the overwhelming evidence that thrombolytic agents reduce patient mortality and morbidity resulting from acute myocardial infarction, emergency decision making has become vitally important in determining outcome. Because the efficacy of thrombolysis in acute myocardial infarction is closely linked to the time between onset of ischemia and treatment, emergency physicians face increased pressure to make early and accurate diagnoses. The electrocardiogram may not provide an accurate indication of the degree of ongoing ischemia. Incorporation of cardiac ultrasound training in emergency medicine residency programs therefore appears warranted. The support of an experienced echocardiographer for expert review is essential to maintaining quality control and ongoing education for emergency physicians who want to perform echocardiographic examinations.

▶ Echocardiography in the ED has limited applicability, and routine inclusion in emergency medicine residency training is not practical at this point. Detection of wall motion abnormalities does not necessarily indicate an acute process, and even if this was clinically suspected to be acute, it is unlikely that thrombolytes would be administered to a patient without ST segment elevation. In the resuscitation of clinical electromechanical dissociation, the presence of wall motion may indicate a better prognosis and is another useful feature of echocardiography in the ED.—R.M. McNamara, M.D.

---

**Effect of Intravenous Magnesium Sulfate on Supraventricular Tachycardia**
Wesley RC Jr, Haines DE, Lerman BB, DiMarco JP, Crampton RS (Univ of Virginia, Charlottesville)
*Am J Cardiol* 63:1129–1131, 1989                                              3–22

---

The effect of magnesium sulfate ($MgSO_4$) in the treatment of supraventricular tachycardia (SVT) has not been systematically studied. The efficacy and clinical tolerance of $MgSO_4$ in the treatment of SVT were assessed in 10 patients with spontaneous (n = 5) or induced (n = 5) episodes of SVT. All patients had regular narrow complex tachycardia consistent with atrioventricular nodal or atrioventricular reciprocation reentry by electrophysiologic data or ECG data. Magnesium sulfate (2 g) was administered as a rapid intravenous bolus.

Intravenous $MgSO_4$ terminated SVT in 7 of 10 patients at 31 seconds postinjection. Termination was mediated by block in the atrioventricular node in 6 patients and by block in an accessory pathway conduction in 1 patient. In the other 3 patients, $MgSO_4$ restored the efficacy of carotid sinus massage during SVT despite treatment with terbutaline in 1. Another patient showed transient slowing of tachycardia with $MgSO_4$, and $MgSO_4$ failed to produce an electrophysiologic effect in 1 patient. Side effects included transient sensations of warmth and flushing, nausea, and vomiting. Except for 1 case of mild hypotension, no other significant changes in blood pressure were seen.

Rapid intravenous injection of $MgSO_4$ terminates or slows SVT when the atrioventricular node is a part of the reentrant circuit. The effect of $MgSO_4$ may be mediated by alterations in slow calcium channel kinetics or even enhanced parasympathetic tone.

► Magnesium is one of the most useful cardiovascular medications as both an antiarrhythmic and an antihypertensive. The authors demonstrate the use of intravenous $MgSO_4$ for treating SVT. It has also been shown to be effective in the treatment of quinidine toxicity, torsade de pointes, and digoxin toxicity (especially in the acute overdose). Magnesium sulfate should be used with caution in the hypotensive patient or the patient with renal failure. Recently, magnesium has also been advocated in the treatment of pulmonary bronchospasm.—E.J. Reisdorff, M.D.

ISCHEMIA/INFARCTION

**Chest Pain Evaluation Unit: A Cost-Effective Approach for Ruling Out Acute Myocardial Infarction**
De Leon AC Jr, Farmer CA, King G, Manternach J, Ritter D (St John Med Ctr, Tulsa)
*South Med J* 82:1083–1089, 1989                                      3–23

It is difficult to identify those patients who come to an ED with acute chest pain who are at low risk for myocardial infarction (MI). A substantial number of such patients are admitted to coronary care units where myocardial necrosis is subsequently ruled out by serial creatine kinase (CK) isozyme measurement. The accuracy of measuring CK-B subunit activity in serum after immunoinhibition of M subunit activity in the diagnosis of MI has been previously described (Figs 3–2 and 3–3). The safety and effectiveness of monitoring patients suspected of having MI for up to 20 hours in a chest pain evaluation unit (CPEU) where they are subjected to a diagnostic cardiac profile of CK measurement were assessed.

The diagnostic cardiac profile involved taking 3 serial blood samples from the patient suspected of having MI. The initial blood sample was tested for total CK, total lactate dehydrogenase (LD), and CK-B concen-

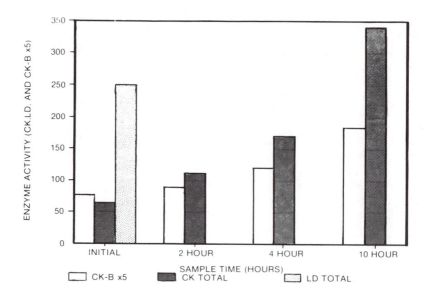

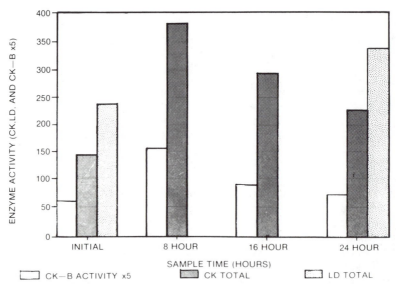

**Fig 3–2.—Top,** serial enzyme studies at 2-hour intervals show initial normal CK-B × 5 *(clear bars)*, total CK *(dark bars)*, and total LD *(stippled bar)*. Concurrent rise of CK-B and total CK at 2 and 4 hours is confirmed by further rise at tenth hour in case of non-Q-wave MI. CK-B has been magnified 5 times actual value for better illustration of changes. **Bottom,** serial enzyme studies at 8-hour intervals show CK-B × 5 *(clear bars)* peaking at 8 hours, then declining; CK total *(dark bars)* after similar rise and fall; and total LD *(stippled bars)* at initial and 24-hour samples showing expected slower rise of LD in acute MI. In this case example, single CK electrophoresis would be done on 8-hour sample, and 1 LD electrophoresis on the 24-hour sample. (Courtesy of De Leon AC Jr, Farmer CA, King G, et al: *South Med J* 82:1083–1089, 1989.)

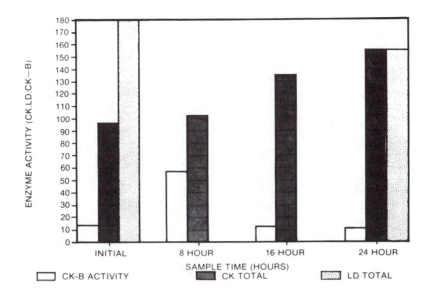

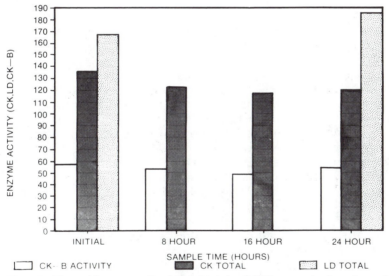

**Fig 3–3.—Top,** serial enzyme studies show isolated rise of CK-B as a result of superimposed CK-BB release on 8-hour sample *(clear bars)*. Rising total CK *(dark bars)* results from CK-MM release. Notice discordance of CK-B and CK changes and differing temporal pattern compared with those in patient who has had myocardial infarction. **Bottom,** serial enzyme studies show persistently elevated CK-B *(clear bars)* of essentially unchanged magnitude over 24-hour period. This is not consistent with CK-MB kinetics, and represents macro-CK. (Courtesy of De Leon AC Jr, Farmer CA, King G, et al: *South Med J* 82:1083–1089, 1989.)

trations. The second blood sample was tested for total CK and CK-B. The third blood sample was tested for total CK, total LD, and CK-B. Standard serial CK and LD measurements were also performed for comparison.

Of 798 patients admitted to the ED with symptoms of acute MI but no diagnostic electrocardiographic changes, 495 were placed in the CPEU and followed up with the cardiac profile enzyme screen for up to 20 hours. On the basis of the screening results, 327 of the 495 patients could be sent home without hospital admission after MI had been conclusively ruled out. Of the 168 patients who were hospitalized, only 30 had subsequent enzyme evidence of myocardial necrosis. The use of serial enzyme testing in the CPEU resulted in an 80% reduction in the cost of ruling out acute MI for the 327 patients not admitted.

The use of a CPEU is more cost effective than any other hospital admission alternative. Furthermore, while awaiting results of the cardiac enzyme profile, patients and their families can be readily engaged in discussions on the importance of reducing the risk of MI by appropriate behavior and life-style modification.

▶ The authors present an interesting and well-documented study in which chest pain patients were evaluated in an observation setting adjacent to the emergency center. Subsequent admission to the hospital or discharge occurred during an 11.1-hour average period of time. Essential to the study was the utilization of a cardiac profile enzyme screen consisting of CK-B, CK, and LD enzyme evaluation. The rise and fall of CK-B levels was correlated to the more traditional CK-MB determinations in a statistically satisfactory fashion. By the use of the less complicated and less expensive CK-B screening test, evaluation every 2 hours was possible with a vector determination of enzyme change occurring over a 12-hour period of time. As observation medicine becomes more a part of many emergency center's activities, such protocols have enormous potential. The increased risk of sending out a patient with a potentially treatable, evolving MI are markedly diminished as a broader screen of patients is allowed to have the 12-hour evaluation occur. Of note is the fact that only 6% of patients admitted to the CPEU were shown to eventually show enzyme evidence of myocardial necrosis, indicative of the generous criteria used for admission to the CPEU. (See also Abstract 4–31.)—D.K. Wagner, M.D.

---

## Clinical Correlates of Acute Right Ventricular Infarction in Acute Inferior Myocardial Infarction

Sinha N, Ahuja RC, Saran RK, Jain GC (Sanjay Gandhi Post-Graduate Inst of Med Sciences, Lucknow, India; KG's Med College, Lucknow)
*Int J Cardiol* 24:55–61, 1989                                    3–24

---

Acute myocardial infarction (MI) is generally viewed as an infarction of part of the left ventricle. Isolated right ventricular (RV) infarction is extremely rare and has been of interest mainly to pathologists looking at autopsy specimens. Yet the clinical recognition of RV infarction is important because it occurs in 25%–53% of patients with inferior MI. When present, RV infarction may dominate the clinical picture and hemodynamic consequences. The ECG changes in patients with RV infarction were correlated with the clinical features and course during hospitalization.

The study population consisted of 42 men and 8 women aged 35–70 years with ECG evidence of inferior MI. None of the patients had a history of a previous MI. A 16-lead ECG had been recorded at the time of hospital admission and was repeated at 24, 48, and 72 hours after the onset of symptoms and daily thereafter until discharge. Right ventricular infarction was diagnosed by the presence of ST-segment elevation of at least 1 mm in 1 or more right precordial leads. Clinical and ECG features of patients with RV infarction were compared with those having only inferior MI.

Twenty of the 50 patients with inferior MI had ECG evidence of RV infarction, of whom 5 had ST-segment elevation in a single right precordial lead and 15 had ST-segment elevation in 2 or more right precordial leads. These ECG changes resolved within 72 hours in 90% of the patients. A comparison of the clinical features showed that giddiness and hiccups were significantly more common in patients with RV infarction. There was no difference between patients with and without RV infarction in the occurrence of other symptoms (e.g., chest pain, referred pain, nausea, vomiting, restlessness, choking, suffocation, syncope, palpitation, or breathlessness). Signs of RV dysfunction—raised jugular venous pressure, Kussmaul's sign, hypotension excluding cardiogenic shock, and right-sided third heart sound in the absence of clinical left ventricular failure were seen either exclusively or more commonly in patients with RV infarction; 11 of 20 patients had 2 or more of these signs.

In most patients with hemodynamically significant RV infarction, the diagnosis can be made on the basis of a combination of clinical signs and ST elevation of at least 1 mm in 2 or more right precordial leads.

▶ The authors present convincing evidence that the bedside diagnosis of right ventricular infarction can be accurately carried out without the need for extensive hemodynamic monitoring and evaluation. Specifically, raised jugulovenous pressure, hypotension without cardiogenic shock, and right-sided third sounds without left ventricular failure were noted in two thirds of such patients. Because a more complicated course can be anticipated in patients with right ventricular failure, it is useful to identify these characteristics early on. The ability to provide clinically significant information with limited bedside data is a unique skill of the emergency physician that demands embellishment whenever possible. The authors provide 1 such way.—D.K. Wagner, M.D.

---

## Unexpected Sudden Death During Acute Myocardial Infarction: Role of Primary Electromechanical Dissociation

Bellotto F, Valente S, Buja GF, Martini B, Scattolin G, Resta M, Maddalena F, Dalla Volta S (Padua Univ, Italy)
*Int J Cardiol* 24:77–81, 1989                                                3–25

The introduction of intravenous thrombolytic therapy and new forms of instrumentation has significantly reduced the mortality rate of acute myocardial infarction (AMI). Electromechanical dissociation (EMD) in AMI remains a relatively frequent cause of sudden death, but this entity has not been well reported in the literature. The clinical and pathologic features of EMD as a cause of death during AMI were reviewed retrospectively.

During an 8-year study period, 993 consecutive patients were admitted to the coronary care unit (CCU) with unequivocal AMI, 128 of whom died in the CCU during continuous ECG monitoring, for a mortality rate of 12.8%. Of these 128 patients, 85 (66.4%) died of cardiogenic shock, 4 (3.1%) of uncontrollable ventricular fibrillation, 7 (5.5%) of asystole, and 32 (25%) of EMD. Electromechanical dissociation was defined as the sudden disappearance of an effective arterial pressure in the presence of adequate ECG complexes. Autopsy was performed on 84 patients, 23 of whom died with EMD; 12 (52.2%) patients died of secondary EMD as confirmed by a finding at autopsy of cardiac rupture and hemopericardium. Primary EMD was diagnosed in the remaining 11 patients, because anatomic findings directly responsible for death were not identified; the 8 men and 3 women who died of primary EMD had a mean age of 67.4 years. A recurrence of chest pain was experienced immediately before the sudden disappearance of vital signs in 8 of 12 patients with EMD and 6 of 11 patients with primary EMD. Evaluation of the terminal ECG event showed ventricular fibrillation in 54.5% of the patients who died of primary EMD. Asystole was recorded in all 12 patients who died of cardiac rupture. Inferior myocardial infarcts were found in only 5 of the 11 patients who died of primary EMD; the other 6 patients had subendocardial or anterolateral infarcts with a more extensive area of necrosis than had been suggested by the clinical picture.

Although the pathophysiology of primary EMD is not completely understood, these findings suggest that recurrence of global or local ischemia may play a more important role than cardiovascular inhibitory reflexes.

▶ The purpose of this article is to draw attention to the incidence of EMD as a cause of death from acute MI and to point out the difference between the primary EMD and secondary EMD caused by cardiac rupture, and so forth. Primary EMD is a poorly understood phenomenon and has virtually no adequate treatment. It represents "cardiogenic shock" at its most extreme. Unfortunately, it is not a rare cause of death from AMI, and much remains to be learned about it.— E.J. Lucid, M.D.

---

**Clinical Characteristics and Outcome of Acute Myocardial Infarction in Patients With Initially Normal or Nonspecific Electrocardiograms: A Report From the Multicenter Chest Pain Study**

Rouan GW, Lee TH, Cook EF, Brand DA, Weisberg MC, Goldman L (Brigham

and Women's Hosp, Boston; Univ of Cincinnati Hosp; Yale–New Haven Hosp;
Danbury Hosp, Conn; Milford Hosp, Milford, Conn; et al)
*Am J Cardiol* 64:1087–1092, 1989                                        3–26

The initial ECGs in patients coming to an ED with symptoms and signs
of acute myocardial infarction (AMI) may be normal or nonspecific in
6%–20% of patients and diagnostic of AMI in 18%–65% of patients.
Serial ECGs eventually will reveal abnormalities in 83%–93% of patients, but these data are not available to the ED clinician who needs to
select the proper treatment for these patients. The prevalence and characteristics of 7,115 patients with AMI who came to the ED with initially
normal or nonspecific ECGs were determined.

The patients, aged 30 years or older, came to the ED with unexplained
chest pain and had initial ECGs performed there. A total of 1,024 (14%)
had a diagnosis of AMI. Initial ECGs were normal or nondiagnostic in
107 (17%) of the 1,024 and highly suggestive of AMI in 811 patients
(79%).

The patients with AMI with normal or nonspecific ECGs were as likely
to be older than 60 years, to be men, to have chest pressure, and to have
a typical pattern of pain radiation, as were patients with AMI with highly
suggestive ECGs. However, those with normal ECGs were less likely to
have a previous history of AMI or angina or associated diaphoresis. Patients with AMI with initially normal or nonspecific ECGs had significantly lower mean peak creatine kinase levels than those with initial
ECGs highly suggestive of AMI. Only 6% of patients with AMI admitted
with a normal or nonspecific ECG died compared with 12% of those admitted with highly suggestive initial ECGs. Another 13 patients with
AMI with initially normal or nonspecific ECGs were released mistakenly
after initial evaluation, 3 of whom died after being released. In comparison, only 8 patients with highly suggestive initial ECGs were released
mistakenly after initial evaluation, 2 of whom died. The overall prevalence of AMI among all patients with initially normal or nonspecific
ECGs was 3%. Thus, patients with AMI with initially normal or nonspecific ECGs may have a less severe short-term clinical outcome.

▶ In the evaluation of the patient with chest pain, a normal or nonspecific initial
ECG is not a ticket out the door. Up to 3% of these people will have an AMI
with a mortality rate that is 6%. Clinical judgment is paramount in identifying
these patients but unfortunately is not perfect, as in this study, where 12% of
those with AMI or initially nondiagnostic ECGs were appropriately discharged.
Although of no proved efficacy, I routinely observe a patient in whom the nature of the chest pain does not allow for a comfortable disposition decision for
4 hours, after which time an ECG is repeated. The use of enzymes is controversial but seems most likely to benefit patients who come to the ED several
hours after the onset of chest pain. If you are lucky enough to have a rapid laboratory turnaround, enzyme studies may be useful during prolonged observation in the ED.
A missed AMI in the ED frequently resulted from improper ECG interpreta-

tion. In this study, 1% of patients with highly suggestive ECGs were discharged. If you are going to practice in the ED your ECG skills must be impeccable.— R.M. McNamara, M.D.

---

**Meta-Analytic Evidence Against Prophylactic Use of Lidocaine in Acute Myocardial Infarction**
Hine LK, Laird N, Hewitt P, Chalmers TC (Harvard School of Public Health; Boston VA Med Ctr; Mt Sinai School of Medicine)
*Arch Intern Med* 149:2694–2698, 1989                                    3–27

---

About one half of the deaths from coronary heart disease in the United States result from ventricular arrhythmias complicating acute myocardial infarction (AMI). To prevent such arrhythmias, many coronary care units administer prophylactic lidocaine. Yet the value of lidocaine in preventing mortality has not been confirmed in randomized control trials (RCTs). A meta-analysis was conducted of death rates in 14 RCTs in which prophylactic lidocaine was administered to patients with proved or suspected AMI.

Six prehospital-phase and 8 hospital-phase RCTs were selected and reviewed in a blinded fashion. The prehospital-phase trials involved a single-bolus administration; the hospital-phase trials consisted of bolus plus continuous infusion. The 14 trials included more than 9,000 patients. Mortality data were evaluated according to therapy type, reporting interval, and patient category.

No meaningful mortality effect was noted with prehospital administration of lidocaine. Results for only those patients with subsequently confirmed AMI were similar to those in the intention-to-treat group. During the treatment period, patients who received lidocaine in the hospital-phase RCTs had a statistically significant increase in mortality.

Lidocaine reduces episodes of primary ventricular fibrillation. However, this effect does not bring about improved survival. Prophylactic lidocaine may be harmful to some patients later shown not to have had AMI.

▶ The use of lidocaine prophylactically in all patients suspected of having an AMI began rather by default in the early 1970s. With the development of coronary care units in the 1960s, lidocaine was used in those patients with AMI who developed "warning arrhythmias," ventricular, premature heartbeats that were believed to herald the potential onset of ventricular fibrillation (VF). When the warning arrhythmia theory was not substantiated clinically, prophylactic lidocaine became advocated in all cases of suspected MI. This analysis of the RCTs of routine prophylactic lidocaine solidifies the present understanding of its role in the management of AMI: It may reduce VF, but this is not translated into improved mortality in the current setting of cardiac monitoring and readily accessible defibrillation, and there may indeed be significant adverse effects to its use. The role of nonprophylactic lidocaine in patients with ventricular arrhythmias and AMI has not been fully studied. It is interesting that the in-hospital trials analyzed occurred from 1970 to 1974. Where I trained in the late 1970s, prophylactic lidocaine was adamantly advocated in all coronary care unit patients with suspected AMI. Done earlier, this present analysis would have discouraged this practice. The analysis of the prehospital studies done utilizing single-dose therapy of prophylactic lidocaine mirrors that of the in-hospital trials. Energies directed at the prehospital care of AMI are probably better directed at the development of emergency medical technicians' (EMTs') defibrillator capability than at the ability for basic EMTs to administer prophylactic lidocaine.—J.M. Mitchell, M.D.

---

## Risk of Adverse Outcome in Patients Admitted to the Coronary Care Unit With Suspected Unstable Angina Pectoris

Wilcox I, Freedman SB, McCredie RJ, Carter GS, Kelly DT, Harris PJ (Royal Prince Alfred Hosp, Sydney, Australia)
*Am J Cardiol* 64:845–848, 1989                                        3–28

Unstable angina pectoris has become the most frequent indication for admission to many coronary care units, and most of these admissions are for suspected rather than definite unstable angina. To compare the prognoses of patients with suspected and definite unstable angina, 196 patients consecutively admitted to a coronary care unit were followed up prospectively to determine their outcome in the hospital and in the first 4 months after discharge. On the basis of the patient's history, description of chest pain, and ECG recorded during pain, the patients were classified clinically within 24 hours of admission as having either definite unstable angina (with symptoms characteristic of unstable angina, n = 113) or suspected unstable angina (with symptoms not characteristic of unstable angina, n = 83).

In the hospital, 3 patients had nonfatal myocardial infarctions and 2 died. During a mean follow-up of 4.2 months, 6 additional patients had a nonfatal myocardial infarction, 4 died, and 22 were readmitted with definite unstable angina. Patients with unsuspected unstable angina had a significantly lower incidence of nonfatal myocardial infarction or death during both the primary hospital admission and at follow-up than those with definite unstable angina. In addition, significantly fewer patients with suspected unstable angina were readmitted with a recurrence of definite unstable angina.

Patients admitted with suspected unstable angina have a benign prognosis and are at low risk of adverse outcome. These patients can be identified by a careful clinical evaluation performed within 24 hours of admission.

▶ The authors are careful to stress that the differentiation of the patients into the suspected unstable angina and definite unstable angina categories was made after only 24 hours in the coronary care unit. This study has no bearing on whether or not to admit patients in either group.—E. Ruiz, M.D.

### Acute Myocardial Infarction: Subtleties of Diagnosis in the Emergency Department

Bresler MJ, Gibler WB (Stanford Univ, Vanderbilt Univ)
*Ann Emerg Med* 19(suppl):4–15, 1990                                      3–29

It often is quite difficult to make a definitive diagnosis of acute myocardial infarction (AMI) in the ED. The ECG is diagnostic initially in only about one half of all patients. Apart from ischemic disorders such as unstable angina, pulmonary embolism, pericarditis, and aortic dissection may masquerade as AMI. Costochondritis also should be considered. The presence of radiating pressure-like pain that is not reproducible suggests AMI, especially if accompanied by autonomic symptoms.

The absence of diagnostic change on the initial ECG does not exclude AMI. A false positive diagnosis of acute injury may result from ST segment elevation in an area of past Q wave infarction; ST-segment depression may be the only ECG abnormality in AMI, especially subendocardial infarction. The diagnosis may be obscured by an intraventricular conduction disorder that either predates infarction or results from it. The finding of Q waves should not rule out thrombolytic therapy in the presence of continuing ischemia.

The usual serum protein markers, total creatine phosphokinase (CPK) and lactate dehydrogenase, are of limited use in the emergency setting because they may not become abnormal for some hours after the onset of AMI. Myoglobin and CPK-MM isoforms are under study for use in the early diagnosis of myocardial cell death. In addition, more rapid and sensitive methods to detect serum CPK-MB are now available.

▶ Making the diagnosis of AMI in the ED continues to be difficult. Aside from being clinically astute, the emergency physician must document thoroughly and provide for reliable follow-up. A rapid, reliable laboratory test is probably "pie in the sky."—E. Ruiz, M.D.

### How Many Myocardial Infarctions Should We Rule Out?

Wears RL, Li S, Hernandez JD, Luten RC, Vukich DJ (Univ of Florida, Jacksonville)
*Ann Emerg Med* 18:953–963, 1989                                      3–30

To be sure that virtually all of those with acute myocardial infarction (AMI) are hospitalized, many patients without infarction are admitted. Because more than two thirds of admissions to coronary care units are false positives, computer simulation methods were used to determine the results of 4 different admitting strategies on costs and outcome. Strategies included admissions to a coronary care unit, an intermediate care unit, and routine ward care, as well as outpatient follow-up.

At nearly any probability level of AMI, substituting less intensive for more intensive strategies saved money but increased mortality and lowered life expectancy. When the most effective strategies for progressively lower-risk patients were invoked up to a cutoff value for the added cost per additional life saved ($1–$2 million), the acceptable proportion of false positive admissions appeared to be as high as 70%–80%.

Clinicians today may operate closer to the optimal decision point than previously claimed. No current means of assigning patients to risk categories has the requisite discriminatory power. At present, false positive rates lower than 70%–80% might indicate an excessively restrictive admitting policy.

▶ As this paper points out, it is dangerous to strictly apply data generated by mathematical modeling to patient care. The plethora of variables considered in this abstraction, as well as those not (i.e., induced costs), make it clear that cost effectiveness in the management of potential ischemic chest pain may not be easily determined. Any future arguments that favor fewer patient admissions to the hospital for potential ischemic chest pain must be based on pure objective data. It is not possible to do that at the present, and consequently, the false positive admission rate for AMI (as high as 70%–80%) may be totally appropriate.—H. Unger, M.D.

---

### The Utility of the Presence or Absence of Chest Pain in Patients With Suspected Acute Myocardial Infarction

Fesmire FM, Wears RL (Univ Hosp of Jacksonville)
*Am J Emerg Med* 7:372–377, 1989                                    3–31

Many researchers have investigated the spectrum of symptomatic to silent myocardial ischemia in patients with coronary artery disease. The incidence of silent myocardial ischemia in patients with significant coronary artery disease ranges from 30% to 90%. Many patients with coronary artery disease have intermittent symptomatic and asymptomatic ischemic episodes. Long-term follow-up studies in patients with pure silent myocardial ischemia suggest that these patients have a worse long-term prognosis than those with symptomatic myocardial ischemia.

The hypothesis that chest pain that persists on the patient's arrival in the ED or recurs during the initial ED evaluation is a useful predictor of acute myocardial infarction (AMI) and complications of coronary ischemia was tested in 424 patients admitted from the ED for suspected AMI, 92 (22%) of whom had a diagnosis of AMI. Of the 424 patients, 290 had chest pain before arrival in the ED that persisted or recurred during the initial ED evaluation, 76 had pain before arrival that ceased spontaneously before arrival and did not recur during the ED evaluation, and 58 patients never experienced chest pain.

Patients with suspected AMI whose chest pain persisted or recurred during the initial ED evaluation had a 2.3 times greater risk of interventions, a 1.7 times greater risk of complications, a 3.8 times greater risk of life-threatening complications, and a 2.4 times greater risk of AMI compared with patients whose chest pain spontaneously resolved before arrival in the ED. Patients with suspected AMI who never experienced chest pain had a risk of death 3 times higher than patients whose chest pain persisted or recurred in the ED, and a risk of death 7.9 times higher than patients whose chest pain resolved before arrival in the ED. Patients who never had chest pain also had a risk of interventions 2.1 times greater and a risk of life-threatening complications 5.2 times greater than those whose chest pain resolved before arrival in the ED. Thus, patients with chest pain that resolved spontaneously before arrival in the ED had a better in-hospital prognosis than those whose chest pain persisted or recurred in the ED or those who never had chest pain.

▶ The authors present a large amount of data in an attempt to subset persistent or recurrent chest pain in the emergency center. The authors' data may seem to confirm the obvious, namely, that patients who have stabilized their MI before arrival in the emergency center, have a better prognosis than those who have not. However, their data does tend to dispel the concern that silent myocardial ischemia commonly occurs subsequent to hospitalization. If the problem of silent myocardial ischemia persists, this is, by definition, excluded from patients who have chest pain.— D.K. Wagner, M.D.

---

**Usefulness of Two-Dimensional Echocardiography for Immediate Detection of Myocardial Ischemia in the Emergency Room**
Peels CH, Visser CA, Funke Kupper AJ, Visser FC, Roos JP (Free Univ Hosp, Amsterdam; Interuniversity Cardiology Inst, Utrecht, The Netherlands)
*Am J Cardiol* 65:687–691, 1990                                                  3–32

---

Many patients with acute chest pain who do not have acute infarction are admitted to coronary care, whereas some are inappropriately discharged from emergency rooms. Two-dimensional echocardiography, which readily demonstrates regional asynergy, might help predict the presence or absence of coronary artery disease in patients with nondiagnostic ECGs. Forty-three such patients with acute chest pain were examined. None had a previous infarct or known coronary artery disease.

Coronary angiography, done within 3 weeks of echocardiography, showed coronary artery disease in 25 patients. Coronary disease was present in 85% of 26 patients with regional asynergy and in 3 of the 17 with normal ECGs. The positive predictive accuracy of the study was 85%, and its negative predictive accuracy was 82%. Regional asynergy had a negative predictive accuracy of 94% for infarction, but its positive predictive accuracy was only 46%.

Two-dimensional echocardiography can identify coronary artery disease in patients with acute chest pain and nondiagnostic ECGs. In addition, it can accurately rule out acute myocardial infarction (AMI) in such patients.

▶ The authors conclude that 2-dimensional echocardiography evaluation during acute chest pain can accurately rule in patients with coronary artery disease and rule out those with AMI. Would that this were the missing diagnostic piece in that often difficult diagnostic dilemma. Their data would suggest that 2-dimensional echocardiography remains a useful adjunct in determining the presence or absence of abnormal myocardial motion, but its use as a definitive decision maker is not acceptable to most emergency physicians.—D.K. Wagner, M.D.

---

**Initial ECG in Q Wave and Non-Q Wave Myocardial Infarction**
Fesmire FM, Percy RF, Wears RL, MacMath TL (Univ Hosp of Jacksonville; Univ of Florida, Jacksonville)
*Ann Emerg Med* 18:741–746, 1989                                                    3–33

Little progress has been made in diagnosing acute myocardial infarction (AMI) in the emergency department setting. Initial ECGs in 440 patients admitted with suspected AMI were reviewed, with emphasis on differences between Q-wave and non-Q-wave infarcts. One hundred patients had a diagnosis of AMI. Forty percent of all patients required at least 1 intervention, and 26% had complications. Overall mortality was 7%.

Acute injury was the most sensitive and specific ECG interpretation, and it had a positive predictive value for AMI of 84%. The value for ischemia was only 39%. Serial ECG studies indicated Q-wave infarction in 43 patients and non-Q-wave infarction in 50. Nearly twice as many patients with a Q-wave infarction had acute injury as the initial ECG interpretation. Only 17% of those with Q-wave infarction had an initial interpretation of ischemia or left ventricular hypertrophy with strain, compared with 36% of patients having non-Q-wave infarction. Complications and life-threatening complications were more frequent in patients with Q-wave infarction.

The initial ECG is not sufficiently sensitive or specific for diagnosing AMI. Early thrombolytic therapy will reach only a minority of patients who could benefit from it on the basis of current criteria. Prospective studies are needed to evaluate early treatment in selected patients having acute ST-segment depression or ischemic T-wave inversion.

▶ Definitive diagnosis of the AMI in the ED remains a frustrating task. The best that the emergency physician can do is to follow a standard of appropriate care. Two factors that complicate the ability to diagnose an AMI includes the Bayer et al. study, which shows only 38% of patients greater than 85 years old complain of chest discomfort with an MI (1). In addition, McNamara et al. (2) demonstrated the inconsistency of patients' histories when given simple questions, which caused a 57% difference in the overall impression by physicians concerning patients with known coronary artery disease.—E.J. Reisdorff, M.D.

*References*

1. Bayer AJ, et al: *J Am Geriatr Soc* 34:263, 1986.
2. McNamara AM, et al: *Proceedings*, UAEM, May 26, 1989, Cincinnati.

THROMBOLYTIC THERAPY

**Potential Use of Thrombolytic Therapy Before Hospitalization**
Kennedy JW, Weaver WD (Univ of Washington)
*Am J Cardiol* 64:8A–11A, 1989                                    3–34

Results of recent clinical studies suggest that very early reperfusion therapy offers the greatest opportunity for both maximal myocardial salvage and reduction in mortality from acute myocardial infarction (AMI). Three trials of thrombolytic therapy in AMI up to 12 hours after symptom onset were conducted to measure the mean time from onset of chest pain to hospital arrival and mean time to therapy.

Intracoronary streptokinase (SK), intravenous streptokinase, and tissue plasminogen activator (t-PA) were used for thrombolysis. These trials showed a progressive shortening of the time between symptom onset and hospital arrival. The mean time from symptom onset to hospital arrival was 133 minutes for intracoronary SK, 107 minutes for intravenous SK, and 93 minutes for t-PA. The mean time from symptom onset to therapy was 274 minutes for intracoronary SK, 209 minutes for intravenous SK, and 139 minutes for t-PA.

The Seattle Myocardial Infarction, Triage and Intervention (MITI) trial is evaluating the safety and efficacy of thrombolytic therapy initiated by paramedics in the prehospital setting. Phase I studies show that more than half of the patients with AMI who use the emergency medical service can receive thrombolytic therapy within the first hour of symptoms, substantially sooner than in the hospital. Phase II will compare the use of intravenous t-PA in the field with hospital management in a nonrandomized trial over the next 2 years. It is anticipated that earlier therapy in the field will increase the rate of reperfusion, will reduce infarct size, will reduce the incidence of low cardiac output and shock, and may reduce shock. The widespread use of prehospital thrombolytic therapy must await the outcome of this and other ongoing studies.

▶ Of the first 1,871 patients in phase I of this study, the most common reason for exclusion was advanced age (>74 years) in 35% and pain beginning more than 6 hours in 16%. Therefore, a major problem in the initiation of thrombolytic therapy by current guidelines is still failure of the patient to seek medical attention. However, one half of the patients studied called within 30 minutes of the onset of the pain, so field intervention would still be a possibility. Phase II of the study both identifies who should be a candidate for thrombolytic therapy and randomizes which patients are started on therapy in the ED. Results are pending. Intuitively, one would think that early administration in the field might vary in importance depending on average transport time. Administration in the field might have more significance when the closest hospital is 30 minutes away vs. 5 minutes. In either case, early identification of potential candidates helps the ED prepare for arrival.—J.T. Amsterdam, M.D.

**Informed Consent in Emergency Research: Prehospital Thrombolytic Therapy for Acute Myocardial Infarction**

Grim PS, Singer PA, Gramelspacher GP, Feldman T, Childers RW, Siegler M (Univ of Chicago Hosps, Yale Univ)

*JAMA* 262:252–255, 1989                                    3–35

The availability of thrombolytic therapy for myocardial infarction raises the question of whether conscious patients in the midst of a medical emergency can provide adequate informed consent for a clinical research protocol. Federal regulations for clinical research fail to provide clear guidelines on emergency research in conscious patients. Some consequently avoid such research, but others omit the consent process, obtain deferred consent, or obtain customary consent.

An alternative approach is suggested using as an example a pilot trial of prehospital thrombolytic therapy for myocardial infarction. A 2-step consent process can allow emergency research to take place while protecting the right of the emergency research subjects. The paramedic reads aloud a brief statement requesting consent to administer a loading dose of tissue plasminogen activator (t-PA). After the patient signs a form and receives medication, the investigator gives the patient a standard consent form in the ED and answers any questions the patient may have.

This procedure allows prehospital treatment to be offered to patients who may benefit, and the patient's autonomy is respected. The quality of consent is commensurate with the assumed risk. In a general sense fundamental agreement is needed on what principles should guide emergency research in our society.

▶ The first sentence of this abstract is confused. It is not "the availability of thrombolytic therapy" that "raises the question of whether conscious patients in the midst of a medical emergency can provide adequate informed consent." This issue has always been present and always will be present in virtually all emergency medicine research.

Thrombolytic therapy actually has little to do with the issue. The problem here is not only whether informed consent is possible in a medical emergency but also that no physician is present when the consent is given. The t-PA is being given by paramedics who may not be informed enough about the benefits and dangers of t-PA to adequately instruct the patient, an issue that this article largely skirts. This initial sentence should be rewritten.

The authors raise a very important issue in emergency medicine research, whether true, informed consent is possible in the patient who is having an acute medical emergency—and this includes most potential emergency medicine research subjects—whose judgment may be clouded by fear, hope, or pain and who lack the time to consider the issues fully and consult his or her family. Their research protocol faces an additional difficulty, that of obtaining consent without a physician present. The authors present a good summary of the current state of thought of the federal agencies, medical ethicists, and emergency medicine researchers.

Their solution, however, strikes me as seriously flawed. They settle for a poor-quality initial consent, because "quality of consent is commensurate with assumed risk." If I were the patient, I wouldn't think much of being poorly informed just because the proposed experimental treatment was thought to be low risk. Other solutions such as phone consent through a physician, better education of the paramedics, or a physician on scene to obtain consent should have been explored.

These are living issues that have yet to be resolved satisfactorily. Many, many more papers will see print over the next few years before we thrash our way through them. Stay tuned.—J. Schoffstall, M.D.

---

**Pharmacodynamics of Thrombolysis With Recombinant Tissue-Type Plasminogen Activator: Correlation with Characteristics of and Clinical Outcomes in Patients With Acute Myocardial Infarction**
Stump DC, Califf RM, Topol EJ, Sigmon K, Thornton D, Masek R, Anderson L, Collen D, Thrombolysis and Angioplasty in Myocardial Infarction (TAMI) Study Group (Univ of Vermont; Duke Univ; Univ of Michigan; Riverside Methodist Hosp, Columbus, Ohio; Christ Hosp, Cincinnati)
*Circulation* 80:1222–1230, 1989                                    3–36

---

The major limitation in the use of thrombolytic therapy (including recombinant tissue plasminogen activator [t-PA] therapy) in acute myocardial infarction (AMI) is hemorrhagic side effects. The alterations in the coagulation system induced by recombinant t-PA in 386 patients with AMI were investigated for effects on patient outcome.

Plasma recombinant t-PA levels peaked at 2.1 ± 3.1 μg/mL. Fibrinogen levels, as measured by coagulation rate, decreased from 3.0 ± 0.9 to 1.4 ± 0.75 g/L; as measured by sulfite precipitation, fibrinogen levels decreased from 3.2 ± 1.0 to 1.8 ± 0.92 g/L. Trough levels of fibrinogen were associated with peak serum levels, 230 ± 470 μg/mL, of fibrinogen degradation products. Trough fibrinogen levels were not correlated with patency at 90 minutes or risk of reocclusion within 10 days. The risk of coronary artery reocclusion was inversely correlated with baseline functional fibrinogen level, magnitude of decline to trough level, and peak levels of fibrinogen degradation products. Quantitative blood loss correlated with all systemic fibrinogenolysis markers. Patients at risk for systemic fibrinogenolysis were older women with low body weight. Plasma levels of t-PA were greater in nonoperated patients with major bleeding.

Changes in coagulation parameters are highly variable in patients with MI treated with recombinant t-PA. However, these data may be useful in determining which patients are good candidates for alternative administration schemes.

▶ This article is very interesting, but it doesn't provide a lot of useful information for emergency physicians. One thing that is quite evident from this paper is that there is a great deal of variability in fibrinogen levels and systemic fibrinolysis. The authors do suggest that these data might be useful for deciding if additional therapy, such as heparin, is necessary after t-PA, but this is rarely a decision made by the emergency physician.—W.H. Spivey, M.D.

---

**Reperfusion, Patency and Reocclusion With Anistreplase (APSAC) in Acute Myocardial Infarction**
Anderson JL (Univ of Utah)
*Am J Cardiol* 64:12A–17A, 1989                                               3–37

---

Because the reestablishment of coronary blood flow is central to the benefit of thrombolytic therapy, measurements of reperfusion, patency, and reocclusion rates are essential in the evaluation of new thrombolytic therapies. Adequate trials have been performed to evaluate these rates for anisoylated plasminogen streptokinase activator complex (APSAC, anistreplase), a new second-generation thrombolytic agent. The results of recent clinical trials comparing ASPAC with control or placebo therapies to assess absolute efficacy and with streptokinase (SK) to assess relative efficacy were reviewed.

These trials suggest that APSAC, given within 4 hours, has similar reperfusion efficacy as intracoronary streptokinase. In 5 studies involving 177 patients with symptoms of acute myocardial infarction (AMI) for less than 6 hours, angiographic reperfusion (30 units over 2–5 minutes) was achieved in 55% of patients after APSAC. The perfusion rates of APSAC showed a dependence on time to treatment, with earlier treatment resulting in higher reperfusion success. In addition, reperfusion efficacy of APSAC appeared to be superior to intravenous SK. In 3 studies of patency rates, 74 (69%) of 177 treated with APSAC showed open infarct-related artery 1–4 hours after therapy. Using early peaking (≤15 hours) of the creatine kinase curve as indicator, a patency rate of 63% was observed among 387 patients treated with APSAC.

Reocclusion and reinfarction rates after APSAC are low. In 6 studies, angiography repeated within 1–3 days after initial treatment showed reocclusion in 6 (6.9%) of 87 patients with initially patent arteries after APSAC. Reinfarction, evaluated clinically among 1,058 patients given APSAC, occurred within 3 days of therapy in 3.7% and at any time during the convalescent period in 8.5%. Based on this overall assessment of APSAC and its ease of administration, APSAC may be the preferred agent for AMI thrombolysis.

▶ This article nicely defines the concept of reperfusion and patency, which is important in the evaluation of any thrombolytic agent. Reperfusion requires initial confirmation of coronary occlusion (by performing angiography) and subsequent demonstration of reperfusion after therapy (again by angiography). Patency refers to angiographic confirmation of coronary perfusion after (but not before) therapy. Patency rates are usually higher than perfusion rates. Because of the need for angiography to assess reperfusion, most studies have looked at indirect measures of patency. On one hand, APSAC has proven to be an effective thrombolytic and has the advantage of easy administration. Conversely, it has the disadvantage of full commitment once treatment has been initiated. As with most fields of medicine, the use of APSAC is a question of cost/risk-benefit ratio.—J.T. Amsterdam, M.D.

---

**Nonthrombolytic Intervention in Acute Myocardial Infarction**
Kirshenbaum JM (Brigham and Women's Hosp, Boston; Harvard Med School, Boston)
*Am J Cardiol* 64:25B–28B, 1989                                          3–38

Only 20%–30% of patients with acute myocardial infarction (AMI) are appropriate candidates for thrombolytic therapy. Alternative interventions for the other patients in whom thrombolytic therapy is inappropriate after AMI were reviewed.

Several pharmacologic agents have been studied for their ability to decrease mortality and preserve left ventricular function through reduction of infarct size, including β-blockers, calcium antagonists, and nitrates; the most successful of these agents are the β-blockers. When administered within the first 24 hours of the patient's admission to the coronary care unit, β-blockers can reduce overall morbidity and mortality within the first 7 days by about 15%. Maintenance therapy with an oral β-blocker can reduce mortality within the next 3 years by about 25%.

Patients with relative contraindications to β-blockers may be given esmolol, a unique cardioselective $\beta_1$-adrenergic receptor blocker. When injected intravenously, its half-life is only 9 minutes. In a study assessing the efficacy of esmolol in patients with AMI who had relative contraindications to the conventional β-blockers, esmolol (50–150 μg/kg per minute) produced the same effect on heart rate in patients with left ventricular dysfunction as in patients with atrial tachyarrhythmias. A dose-dependent reduction in blood pressure was also noted. There were no changes in pulmonary capillary wedge pressure during esmolol infusion. Although esmolol infusion causes a modest decline in left ventricular ejection fraction, a rapid return of left ventricular ejection fraction to baseline values within 60 minutes of termination of the infusion was demonstrated. Esmolol may also be used in screening patients for subsequent therapy with β-blockers. Patients who tolerate the esmolol infusion can be given a long-acting β-blocker. In patients who exhibit intolerance to esmolol, the infusion can be stopped and baseline hemodynamic parameters are restored within 15–20 minutes.

▶ With so much emphasis on thrombolytics, the emergency physician must not forget other modalities in the treatment of MI. Although it is unclear whether β-blockers need to be initiated routinely in the ED, clearly patients with a hyperdynamic state undergoing an MI might benefit. Esmolol, an intravenous β-blocker with a short half-life given as an infusion, is an ideal agent for the emergency physician. One need not be committed to therapy for many hours if the patient reacts adversely or if the consultant would prefer that a β-blocker not be used. As well, in a busy ED, where some patients with MIs stay for many hours, one does not have to remember to keep rebolusing the IV β-blocker.—J.T. Amsterdam, M.D.

---

**A New Thrombolytic Regimen for Acute Myocardial Infarction Using Combination Half-Dose. Tissue-Type Plasminogen Activator With Full Dose Streptokinase: A Pilot Study**
Grines CL, Nissen SE, Booth DC, Branco MC, Gurley JC, Bennett KA, DeMaria AN, Kentucky Acute Myocardial Infarction Trial (Univ of Kentucky)
*J Am Coll Cardiol* 14:573–580, 1989                                                          3–39

Recombinant tissue plasminogen activator (t-PA) is more effective than streptokinase in achieving infarct vessel patency. However, early reocclusion is frequent, probably because of the brief half-life of recombinant t-PA. Forty patients with acute myocardial infarction were given a 1-hour infusion of 50 mg of rt-PA combined with 1.5 million units of streptokinase within 6 hours (mean 3.6 hours) of the onset of symptoms.

At 90 minutes, 30 patients had a patent infarct vessel. Angioplasty succeeded in 9 of the remaining patients. There was 1 hospital death. Fifteen percent of patients required transfusion. There were 3 documented reocclusions of the infarct vessel. Both regional wall motion and ejection fraction improved in the first week. The cost of treatment was about one half that of full-dose recombinant t-PA and one third the cost of urokinase.

▶ This is a very interesting attempt to look at a combination of thrombolytic agents that will not only enhance efficacy but also reduce cost. Although not always a major consideration for the physician, cost is a major issue for the hospital facing fixed reimbursement. At the same time, despite the pitches from aggressive salespeople, it is recognized that the various thrombolytics have their advantages and disadvantages. This study is an attempt to look at maximizing benefit and reducing cost. Major clinical trials in the United States will focus on a single agent vs. a single agent for the thrombolytics in addition to adjunct therapy, so it might be some time before a large clinical trial investigates this concept.—J.T. Amsterdam, M.D.

---

**Low Dose Urokinase Preactivated Natural Prourokinase for Thrombolysis in Acute Myocardial Infarction**
Dietrich CLG, Fischer K, Barthels M, Polensky U, Reil G-H, Daniel WG, Welzel D, Lichtlen PR (Hannover Med School; Vinzenz Hosp, Hannover; Sandoz AG, Nuremberg, Germany)
*Am J Cardiol* 63:1025–1031, 1989                                                          3–40

Prourokinase is a new physiologic plasminogen activator, which, unlike other plasminogen activators, has a long lag phase before it reaches its final thrombolytic activity. By inducing minimal free-fibrinolytic activity with low-dose urokinase, this lag phase can be overcome and the rate of thrombolysis with prourokinase can be strongly accelerated. In an open-label, nonrandomized dose-finding study, the thrombolytic potency of a combination of 250,000 IU of urokinase and 2 doses of prourokinase, 4.5 or 6.5 megaunits, was evaluated in 31 patients with acute myocardial infarction. Fifteen patients received 4.5 megaunits (group I) and 16 received 6.5 megaunits (group II) of prourokinase.

Coronary angiograms performed within 1 hour after thrombolysis showed a patent infarct-related coronary artery in 33% (5 of 15) of group I patients compared with 75% (12 of 16) of group II patients; the difference was significant. Angiograms performed on the second day after thrombolysis revealed reocclusion in 23% (4 of 17). Reocclusion rate was significantly higher in group I (3 of 5, 60%) than group II (1 of 12, 8%) patients. Hemostatic monitoring in both groups showed slight to moderate consumption of fibrinogen, plasminogen and $\alpha_2$-antiplasmin, and an increase in D-dimers, the split products of cross-linked fibrin. Bleeding complications were more frequent in group II patients, but bleeding was generally mild and related to puncture sites, except for 1 patient with mild oozing from the gums. There were no major hemorrhages. Other complications, such as cardiogenic shock and acute renal failure, occurred in 2 patients, both directly related to treatment failure.

Low-dose urokinase preactivation enhances the thrombolytic potency of prourokinase without affecting its high fibrin specificity. Previous studies have shown that low-dose urokinase preactivation reduces by 50% the prourokinase doses required for effective thrombolysis. Thus, the combination of 250,000 IU of urokinase and 6.5 megaunits of prourokinase is an ideal regimen for thrombolysis in patients with acute myocardial infarction. The low number of patients in this study precludes definite judgment of the hemorrhagic risk.

▶ This article examines the concept of combination therapy using other thrombolytic agents that are available for clinical investigation. The information in this article is less practical than that reviewed in Abstract 3–39. In addition, there is no analysis of cost (and urokinase is not inexpensive).—J.T. Amsterdam, M.D.

---

### An Analysis of Time Delays Preceding Thrombolysis for Acute Myocardial Infarction

Sharkey SW, Brunette DD, Ruiz E, Hession WT, Wysham DG, Goldenberg IF, Hodges M (Univ of Minnesota; Hennepin County Med Ctr, Minneapolis)
*JAMA* 262:3171–3174, 1989                3–41

---

Early administration of thrombolytic agents in acute myocardial infarction (AMI) is essential to successful treatment. Previous studies indicate that coronary artery thrombi are most susceptible to lysis if the thrombolytic drug is infused within 3 hours of the onset of symptoms. As part of the Thrombolysis in Myocardial Infarction (TIMI) II trial, a study was conducted to identify the time delays encountered during implementation of intravenous tissue plasminogen activator (t-PA) therapy.

During a 2-year period, 236 patients with AMI were treated with t-PA

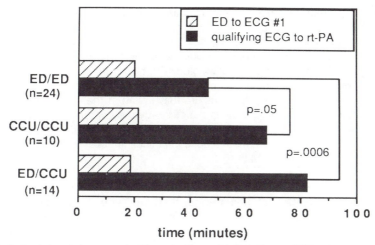

Fig 3–4.—In-hospital stays at the Hennepin County Medical Center. *CCU*, coronary care unit. (Courtesy of Sharkey SW, Brunette DD, Ruiz E, et al: *JAMA* 262:3171–3174, 1989.)

at 2 teaching hospitals and 2 private hospitals that participated in the TIMI II trial. The average time from symptom onset to treatment with t-PA was 153 minutes; the average interval from symptom onset to arrival at the ED was 65 minutes; and from ED arrival to initiation of t-PA was 81 minutes. After ED arrival, patients waited for an average of 19.9 minutes for an initial ECG and another 70 minutes after an AMI diagnosis was confirmed by ECG before t-PA therapy was initiated.

A detailed analysis of time delays was performed for 50 patients with AMI who were taken to 1 of the teaching hospitals. The interval between initial ECG and initiation of t-PA therapy was 46.8 minutes if t-PA was first administered in the ED and 82.1 minutes if the patient was first transferred to the coronary care unit (Fig 3–4). Most of the delay was thus encountered once the patient was already in the hospital. Factors contributing to the delay included securing additional peripheral intravenous access, determining arterial blood gas concentrations, obtaining blood samples for admission laboratory data, obtaining a chest radiograph, administering morphine and lidocaine, waiting for approval of administration of the thrombolytic agent, and waiting for the drug to arrive from the pharmacy. To overcome in-hospital time delays in administering thrombolytic drugs to AMI patients, the decision to use these drugs should be made by the primary care physician in the ED.

▶ For patients with MI to be treated efficiently once they arrive in the ED, several steps are essential. First, there must be a high-sensitivity (even at the cost of low specificity) triage screen for patients complaining of chest pain. Patients triaged into the ED then need an ECG as part of their initial nursing evaluation. A physician must be shown the ECG, and if acute changes are seen, he or she must evaluate the patient immediately. No more than 10 minutes should have elapsed by this point, and after 5 to 10 minutes of physician assessment, the decision to initiate thrombolytic therapy can be made. Tissue plasminogen activator or streptokinase and heparin must then be immediately available. Thrombolytic therapy must be stocked in the ED, and though consultation with a cardiologist is desirable, lytic therapy should be initiated while the call is going out to the cardiologist. Waiting for a cardiologist to return the call is not acceptable practice, except in ambiguous or complicated cases. It is, therefore, mandatory that emergency medicine physicians are fully aware of the indications and contraindications for therapy as well as the currently recommended treatment protocol. These need to be periodically reviewed and updated in a collaborative effort with the cardiology staff, because practices in this field are constantly evolving.—W.P. Burdick, M.D.

---

### Single-Bolus Injection of Recombinant Tissue-Type Plasminogen Activator in Acute Myocardial Infarction

Tebbe U, Tanswell P, Seifried E, Feuerer W, Scholz K-H, Herrmann KS (Georg-August Univ of Goettingen; Univ of Ulm, Germany)
*Am J Cardiol* 64:448–453, 1989                                                            3–42

---

Fibrinolysis of coronary artery occlusion related to myocardial infarct has been achieved with an infusion of recombinant tissue plasminogen activator (t-PA) lasting several hours. Infusion of a single bolus of recombinant t-PA, if safe and effective, would simplify the therapeutic regimen. Single boluses of 50 mg of recombinant t-PA were administered over 2 minutes to 20 patients with myocardial infarction (MI) to examine the efficacy and safety of this regimen.

One hour after administration, coronary angiography revealed patent infarct-related arteries in 75% of the patients. Reperfusion was achieved in the remaining patients with coronary angioplasty and intracoronary fibrinolysis. In 2 patients, bypass grafting of the coronary artery was required. After 1 day, angiograms showed reocclusion in 4 of 18 patients. One death from intracranial hemorrhage occurred. The mean peak concentration of recombinant t-PA was 9.8 μg/mL, and the total plasma clearance was 476 mL/min.

The administration of 50-mg boluses of recombinant t-PA to MI patients results in patency rates and kinetics similar to those of conventional recombinant t-PA infusion regimens. Final assessment of the safety and efficacy of this regimen requires the results of a large-scale clinical trial.

▶ This article discusses the use of a 50-mg single-bolus injection of t-PA as opposed to giving the total of 100 mg over 90 minutes. It was hoped that the single-bolus injection would result in the same long-term patency of the coronary artery as the longer period of infusion. However, it appears that a larger dose of drug may be necessary to accomplish this, thus potentially increasing the risk of bleeding. This was a very small study utilizing only 20 patients, and much larger studies need to be done. At this particular time, the use of all thrombolytics by emergency physicians should be done in accordance with guidelines agreed on by all physicians in a given institution who are caring for these patients. Each institution has different capabilities with regard to the availability of catheterization facilities, and I believe the final answer that can be uniformly applied to all patients has still not been found. The management of MI patients has become a team approach, and as emergency physicians, we must be a part of this team.—E.J. Lucid, M.D.

---

**Bleeding During Thrombolytic Therapy for Acute Myocardial Infarction: Mechanisms and Management**
Sane DC, Califf RM, Topol EJ, Stump DC, Mark DB, Greenberg CS (Duke Univ; Univ of Michigan; Univ of Vermont)
*Ann Intern Med* 111:1010–1022, 1989                                    3–43

---

Increasing evidence from large clinical trials indicates that the use of thrombolytic therapy early in the onset of acute myocardial infarction (AMI) decreases mortality. However, concern about hemorrhagic complications with thrombolytic therapy remains. Although bleeding is usually mild and easily treatable, it can occasionally be devastating.

More than 70% of bleeding episodes occur at vascular puncture sites. Hypofibrinogenemia and elevation of fibrinogen degradation products have been correlated weakly with the risk of hemorrhage. Although depletion of factors V and VIII may occur, the role of such depletion in bleeding has not been established. Whereas several in vitro trials have detected plasmin-induced platelet dysfunction with thrombolytic agents, clinical data are not yet available. The role of platelet inhibition should not be overlooked, because many patients with bleeding episodes are treated successfully with antiplatelet agents.

Most patients with bleeding complications associated with thrombolytic therapy can be managed without transfusion therapy through interruption of thrombolytic and anticoagulant therapy, volume replacement, and application of manual pressure to an incompetent vessel. Protamine sulfate may be given to neutralize the effects of heparin administered within 4 hours of the onset of bleeding. Blood products for treating the occasional patient with uncontrolled massive bleeding should be used with caution. A typical strategy for the management of major bleeding that causes hemodynamic compromise but is not immediately life threatening starts with the use of cryoprecipitate. A target fibrinogen level of 1 g/L after cryoprecipitate infusion is desirable. If the patient is still bleeding, 2 units of fresh frozen plasma may be administered. If hemorrhage still is not stopped, 10 units of platelets are administered. Antifibrinolytic agents such as ε-aminocaproic acid and tranexamic acid should be reserved until last bleeding because serious thrombotic complications have been reported with these agents.

Historically, patients with bleeding have been managed by hematologists. The current use of thrombolytic agents in the treatment of AMI has created an unusual clinical setting in which general internists and cardiologists must make life-saving decisions about bleeding complications.

▶ This excellent review article is a must for anyone involved in the aftercare of patients who have received thrombolytic therapy. Several important points are pertinent to the emergency physician. First, appropriate screening of patients is mandatory. Once patients are selected, the following guidelines are helpful: Avoid unnecessary invasive procedures, use external pacemakers when possible, avoid arterial lines and cervical central venous lines whenever possible, limit phlebotomy, avoid nasal intubators, and compress vascular access sites for longer periods than usual.—R.M. McNamara, M.D.

---

**Intracranial Hemorrhage After Use of Tissue Plasminogen Activator for Coronary Thrombolysis**
Kase CS, O'Neal AM, Fisher M, Girgis GN, Ordia JI (Boston Univ; Univ of Massachusetts, Worcester; Waltham-Weston Hosp, Waltham, Mass)
*Ann Intern Med* 112:17–21, 1990                                              3–44

---

Six patients, none of them hypertensive when admitted, had intracranial hemorrhage after receiving tissue plasminogen activator (t-PA) for thrombolysis. Three patients were from a center in which 60 patients received t-PA in a 1-year period.

Woman, 67, previously treated for hypertension, had a diagnosis of inferior myocardial infarct. After normal coagulation values were documented, the patient was given 6 mg of t-PA 4 hours after the onset of chest pain, with a total dosage of 100 mg in 6 hours. An intravenous bolus injection of 5,000 units of heparin was given, followed by an infusion of 1000 units/hour. The heparin dose was reduced when a partial thromboplastin time (PTT) of 81 seconds was found. Dysarthric speech and right hemiparesis were noted 8 hours after the start of t-PA treatment. The highest blood pressure had been 164/100 mm Hg. Computed tomography showed several areas of intracerebral hemorrhage. Blood was evacuated at craniotomy; no vascular malformation was seen. The patient was left with moderate spastic hemiparesis.

Up to one third of patients given t-PA have hemorrhagic complications, mostly bleeding at vascular accession sites. All of the patients discussed bled after receiving a full dose of 100 mg of t-PA. All had an excessively prolonged PTT. Hemorrhages predominated in the subcortical white matter of the hemispheres but also occurred in deep ganglionic areas, as in anticoagulant-related intracerebral hemorrhage. No patient had received aspirin before or after t-PA.

It is possible that the combined use of t-PA and heparin raises the risk of intracerebral bleeding.

▶ This report casts doubt on the low rate of intracranial hemorrhage cited in many thrombolytic studies. The recent GISSI trial reports a rate of hemorrhagic cerebral events at 0.4%. This trial reports a 5% incidence; the experience at our institution is consistent with this higher rate of intracerebral hemorrhage. It is interesting that in all patients, intracranial hemorrhage occurred 3–17 hours after an infusion of heparin was started, and all patients had an excessively prolonged activated PTT. This confuses the issue as to whether the bleeding was a result of the t-PA, heparin, or a combination of both. The majority of patients who had intracranial hemorrhage had an activated PTT greater than 150 seconds. Careful titration of the heparin infusion is essential. It would appear that with t-PA, heparin increases reperfusion and decreases reocclusion rates.

In addition, there is no effective way at the bedside to objectively monitor the hematologic influence of t-PA. One center has developed a clot lysis time monitor that gives rapid results. Preliminary data show that those patients who are going to reperfuse have clot lysis times of 516 seconds, and those patients who do not reperfuse with fixed-dose t-PA have a clot lysis time of more than 800 seconds. This device could be used to monitor risk of bleeding as well as modify t-PA dosing to achieve maximal reperfusion rates.—E.J. Reisdorff, M.D.

---

**Thrombolytic Therapy in the Emergency Department: A New Treatment Modality for Acute Myocardial Infarction**
Muller HA, Aghababian R, Smith M (Pennsylvania State Univ; Univ of Massachusetts; George Washington Univ)
*Ann Emerg Med* (Suppl) 18:4–15, 1989                                              3–45

---

Thrombolytic therapy lowers mortality in patients with acute myocardial infarction (AMI) and is reasonably safe if proper precautions are observed. Intravenous streptokinase or tissue plasminogen activator (t-PA) can be started quickly in the ED after expeditious evaluation. Time wasted is muscle lost. Five large-scale trials indicate a clear reduction in mortality with intravenous t-PA or streptokinase.

A growing consensus indicates that the decision to use thrombolytic therapy should be made by the emergency physician at the bedside, but a cardiologist should become involved as soon as possible, especially if refractory pain or serious arrhythmia is noted. Indications for thrombolytic therapy include chest pain or equivalent symptoms within 6 hours of presentation, ST-segment elevation of 1 mm or more, and lack of a pain response and ST-segment elevation to nitroglycerin.

The risk of intracranial bleeding is increased in patients with a history of recent intracranial or intraspinal surgery or trauma, an intracranial tumor or aneurysm, a history of stroke, or severe uncontrolled hypertension. Treatment also is contraindicated by a bleeding diathesis and by surgery or biopsy in the preceding 8 weeks. Invasive procedures should be minimized. Use of a controlled infusion device is recommended strongly.

▶ Limited echocardiography performed by emergency physicians will become a standard adjunctive tool in helping make the decision to use thrombolytic therapy. Nonclotted pericardial effusions are easy to see with ultrasound. Clotted blood in the pericardial sac is harder to appreciate. A dissecting aneurysm usually cannot be detected unless it has ruptured into the pericardial sac. The rapid evaluation of AMI patients is now essential. Emergency physicians must become experts in this process, and learning to use and interpret ultrasound instruments will become a requirement in the near future.—E. Ruiz, M.D.

## Gastrointestinal and Urogenital Emergencies

### The Role of Contrast Radiography in Presumed Bowel Obstruction

Riveron FA, Obeid FN, Horst HM, Sorensen VJ, Bivins BA (Henry Ford Hosp, Detroit)
*Surgery* 106:496–501, 1989                                                    3–46

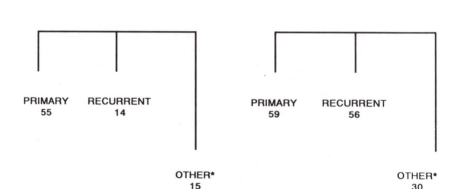

300 PATIENTS WITH THE ADMITTING
DIAGNOSIS OF BOWEL OBSTRUCTION

FINAL DIAGNOSIS
NO SBO IN 71

FINAL DIAGNOSIS
SBO IN 229

NO CONTRAST
84 (36.7%)

CONTRAST
145 (63.3%)

PRIMARY
55

RECURRENT
14

PRIMARY
59

RECURRENT
56

OTHER*
15

OTHER*
30

\* OTHER- Crohn's disease, carcinomatosis, previous
   abdominal/pelvic irradiation and hernias

Fig 3–5.—Three different subgroups of patients with final diagnosis of small-bowel obstruction. (Courtesy of Riveron FA, Obeid FN, Horst HM, et al: *Surgery* 106:496–501, 1989.)

Contrast radiography is increasingly used in diagnosis of acute small-bowel obstruction, but its value remains controversial. In an assessment of the role of contrast radiography in diagnosis, 300 patients with an admitting diagnosis of small-bowel obstruction were reviewed. The observations from clinical examination and plain abdominal films were helpful enough to be a basis for a final diagnosis of small-bowel obstruction in 84. Contrast studies, either upper gastrointestinal series, barium enema, or both, were employed in 145 patients (Fig 3–5).

Of the 145, there were 2 instances of false positive results and 3 instances of false negative results. Contrast radiography revealed no evidence of obstruction in 77 patients, low-grade or moderate obstruction in 21, Crohn's disease in 8, carcinoma or radiation changes in 16, and incarcerated ventral hernia in 1. In 22 patients, contrast studies confirmed high-grade or complete obstruction that warranted early operation. No morbidity was attributable directly to the contrast studies. The mortality rate was 7.6% in those who had such studies and 6% in the others.

Contrast radiography is a safe and effective means of increasing diagnostic accuracy when the diagnosis of small-bowel obstruction is equivocal. In such cases the studies should be performed early to differentiate between patients who need early operative intervention and those who can have conservative management.

▶ Contrast radiography may serve as an adjunct in the diagnostic evaluation of small-bowel obstruction in those patients with inconclusive findings. Likely, it will be administered 10–12 hours into the course of a bowel obstruction that has not improved with suction or has not clearly defined itself as being complete in nature. As observational emergency medicine becomes more in vogue and patients are observed 12–24 hours in the ED, this adjunctive study, in consultation with the surgeon, may become a tool for the emergency physician.— H. Unger, M.D.

**Sonographic Diagnosis of Perforation in Patients With Acute Appendicitis**
Borushok KF, Jeffrey RB Jr, Laing FC, Townsend RR (Univ of California, San Francisco; Stanford Univ)
*AJR* 154:275–278, 1990                                      3–47

The sonographic diagnosis of appendicitis may be difficult in patients with perforation. In a retrospective study, graded compression sonograms in 100 patients with surgically confirmed acute appendicitis were reviewed to evaluate sonographic findings associated with appendiceal perforation.

Perforation had occurred in 22 patients. Three sonographic findings were significantly associated with appendiceal perforation: loculated pericecal fluid, prominent pericecal fat, and circumferential loss of the echogenic submucosal layer of the appendix. The specificity for perforation was 100% for loculated pericecal fluid, 81% for prominent pericecal fat, and 68% for circumferential loss of the echogenic submucosal layer of the appendix. No single finding had a sensitivity greater than 59%. The combination of 1 or more of these findings increased sensitivity to 86%, but the specificity was only 60%.

Recognizing sonographic features of appendiceal perforation is important. In a patient without a sonographically visible appendix, the presence of prominent pericecal fat, and/or loculated pericecal fluid, is an important indirect clue to the diagnosis of perforating appendicitis.

▶ In patients where perforation is already suspected, ultrasound can help determine the size and location of the abscess or phlegmon and thus help plan the therapy. This will not affect the ED evaluation of most early appendicitis patients. (See also Abstract 4–100.)—T. Stair, M.D.

---

**Acute Abdominal Pain: The Value of Liver Function Tests in Suspected Cholelithiasis**
Dunlop MG, King PM, Gunn AA (Bangour Gen Hosp, Broxburn, Scotland)
*J R Coll Surg Edinb* 34:124–127, 1989                    3–48

---

The value of biochemical liver function tests in the diagnosis of acute cholecystitis is unclear. To evaluate the role of such tests when acute cholecystitis is suspected, 311 patients with a tentative diagnosis of acute cholecystitis during a 4-year period were studied prospectively.

Acute cholecystitis was confirmed in 73.6%. Liver function tests were performed in 270 patients, with a final diagnosis of cholecystitis in 76.3%. Some abnormality of liver function was evident in 57.8% of the 64 with other diagnoses and 69.9% of those with confirmed cholecystitis (table). The predictive value of a normal test result was 30.3%, and that of an abnormal test result was 79.6%. The frequency of liver function abnormalities was significantly greater in patients with stones in the common bile duct than in those with a normal duct, but abnormal results of

| Abnormality of Liver Function Tests Related to Diagnostic Category in 270 Patients | | |
|---|---|---|
| | Final diagnosis | |
| Test abnormal | Cholecystitis (*n* = 206) | Other (*n* = 64) |
| Bilirubin | 110 | 24 |
| Alanine aminotransferase | 95 | 21 |
| Alkaline phosphatase | 107 | 23 |
| All three tests | 69 | 13 |
| Any test | 144 | 37 |

(Courtesy of Dunlop MG, King PM, Gunn AA: *J R Coll Surg Edinb* 34:124–127, 1989.)

liver function tests had only a 45.7% predictive value, and abnormal test results had an 87% predictive value for ductal calculi.

Liver function tests have little diagnostic value in patients with suspected acute cholecystitis but help in determining direction of further investigation. When acute cholecystitis is diagnosed provisionally, initial supine abdominal and erect chest radiography, urinalysis, and serum amylase determination should be performed and followed by ultrasonography. If cholecystitis is confirmed, liver function tests will help in guiding management.

▶ Liver function tests are not proved to be helpful in the diagnosis of acute cholecystitis in 311 patients in this study. The authors recommend that in cases of suspected acute cholecystitis, initial plain films, serum amylase determination, and urinalysis be performed, followed by ultrasonography and liver function tests, at the earliest opportunity. If ultrasonography is unavailable, the patient could be studied by oral or intravenous cholangiography. Ultrasonography is readily available in our facility between 8:00 AM and 11:00 PM and for severe cases can be obtained at any time. At some facilities, screening ultrasonography by emergency physicians is becoming a diagnostic tool in the ED. In the patient with right upper quadrant pain and tenderness, I use liver function tests to diagnose hepatocellular disease, but I do not delay obtaining ultrasonography based on these results. My personal experience is that except in the rare case of radiopaque gallstones or in the patient with significant peritoneal signs, the plain films of the abdomen are not helpful in the diagnosis of cholecystitis. This study confirms what many of us have already experienced clinically, that is, symptoms of cholelithiasis and cholecystitis occur commonly without abnormalities in liver function test results and speaks for the ready availability of ultrasound in the emergency center.—J.M. Mitchell, M.D.

---

**Prognosis of Abdominal Aortic Aneurysms: A Population-Based Study**
Nevitt MP, Ballard DJ, Hallett JW Jr (Mayo Clinic and Found; Northeastern Ohio Univ, Rootstown)
*N Engl J Med* 321:1009–1014, 1989                                    3–49

---

The mean rate of expansion for small abdominal aortic aneurysms, based on case-series studies from referral centers, indicates a mean rate of expansion of 0.4–0.5 cm/year and a risk of rupture of 6%/year. These data have influenced the recent recommendations for a more aggressive screening and elective repair of aneurysms. Because these studies are subject to considerable bias, a population-based study was made among residents of Rochester, Minnesota in whom an abdominal aortic aneurysm was initially diagnosed from 1951 to 1984 to determine the rate of change in the size and risk of rupture of abdominal aortic aneurysms.

Of the 370 residents with an abdominal aortic aneurysm, 181 had aneurysms documented by ultrasound examination. Of the 103 patients who had more than 1 ultrasound study of the initially unruptured aneurysm, 17% showed no change or reported a decrease in the diameter of the aneurysm, 59% had an increase of less than 0.4 cm/year, and 24% had an increase of 0.4 cm or more/year. The overall median rate of increase in the diameter of the aneurysm was 0.21 cm/year.

Among 176 patients who initially had an unruptured aneurysm, 11 had a rupture. The cumulative incidence of rupture was 6% after 5 years and 8% after 10 years. However, the risk of rupture after 5 years was 0% for the 130 patients with an aneurysm less than 5 cm in diameter compared with 25% for the 46 patients with an aneurysm 5 cm or more in diameter. All ruptured aneurysms measured 5 cm or more in diameter at the time of the rupture.

These population-based data challenge the validity of previous estimates of the rate of expansion and risk of rupture of aneurysms. The risk of rupture is considerably lower than previously reported in aneurysms less than 5 cm in diameter, whereas aneurysms that are 5 cm or more in diameter are associated with a clinically important risk of rupture and should be considered for elective repair.

▶ The importance of this study to the emergency physician is that ED patients with abdominal aneurysms of 5.0 cm or more should be referred for elective repair.—G.V. Anderson, M.D.

---

### The Presentation and Management of the Acute Abdomen in the Patient With Sickle-Cell Anemia
Baumgartner F, Klein S (Harbor-UCLA Med Ctr, Torrance, Calif)
*Am Surg* 55:660–664, 1989                                              3–50

The differentiation between acute surgical abdominal pain and painful vaso-occlusive episodes from a sickle crisis may prove difficult. Factors that may differentiate these 2 disorders were retrospectively studied in 53 patients with sickle cell anemia who had abdominal pain. Their genotypes were SS (62%), SC (15%), SA (11.5%), and S-other (11.5%). Seventy percent were women. Mean age of the patients was 23 years.

Abdominal pain was caused by a sickle crisis in 57% of patients, surgical abdomen in 23%, and a nonsurgical genitourinary disorder in 20%. Of the 12 patients with surgical abdomen, 9 (75%) had cholecystitis and 4 (33%) had acute appendicitis (1 patient had both). Vaso-occlusive crises were characterized as diffuse (50%), associated with remote pain such as limbs and chest (77%), and relieved with hydration and oxygen (97%) within 48 hours. Abdominal pain of sickle cell crisis often was precipitated by an upper respiratory tract infection and simulated previous crises in 70% of patients. In contrast, surgical abdomens tended to deviate from the pattern of sickle cell crises and did not resolve with hydration and oxygen. Temperatures in patients with sickle cell crises generally were lower than those in patients with surgical abdomen. The leukocyte count was ineffective in differentiating vaso-occlusive pain from surgical abdominal pain but was significantly higher for renal pathology. Liver function tests were ineffective in distinguishing between vaso-occlusive pain and surgical pain.

The history and physical examination are the primary factors that distinguish between vaso-occlusive crises and a surgical abdomen. Specifically, a localized pain, deviation from patterns of previous crises, lack of a precipitating event and remote pain, and lack of pain relief with hydration and oxygen suggest an acute surgical abdomen. Laboratory tests are less effective in differentiating between the 2 entities.

▶ This is a very important review, especially for those who see a large number of patients with sickle cell disease. Deviation from the typical crisis pattern is a red flag that needs to be investigated. Failure to improve with conventional therapy is another red flag. Unfortunately, the difficulty in diagnosing the acute abdomen is increased by the fact that often the sickle cell patient is not a good historian, some are "frequent fliers" to the ED, seeking narcotics, and their story is suspect; frequently these patients are given sedating drugs that might alter the physical examination. All patients should be given the benefit of the doubt; one should obtain a good history and perform a complete physical examination before administering potent analgesics. If analgesics are required, a titrated low intravenous dose to gain patient control is preferable to a large intramuscular dose with unknown effect. Deviation from the patient's normal pattern should be given serious consideration, and these patients should be admitted for observation and serially examined for localized tenderness. Early surgical consultation is warranted. (See also Abstract 4–76.)—J.T. Amsterdam, M.D.

---

**Torsion of the Spermatic Cord in Adults**
Witherington R, Jarrell TS (Med College of Georgia, Augusta)
*J Urol* 143:62–63, 1990                                         3–51

---

Intravaginal torsion of the spermatic cord is a true surgical emergency; delay for more than 8–12 hours often leads to loss of the testicle. The condition is considered infrequent in adults and may be misdiagnosed as epididymitis. At 1 center, 33 cases of intravaginal torsion were confirmed operatively in 1970–1986.

Thirteen patients (39%) were more than 20 years of age. Five patients were older than 30 years. Seven men reported episodes of testicular pain that had ended spontaneously. All had pain and swelling when first seen; pain had begun suddenly in most patients. In 9 patients, pain had been present longer than 12 hours. A few patients had low-grade fever, nausea and vomiting, or voiding symptoms. Erythema or edema of the hemiscrotum was noted in 8 patients, and frank scrotal suppuration was noted in 1. Results of 4 of 5 nuclide tests revealed a hypovascular testicle.

Four men whose condition was diagnosed early underwent bilateral orchiopexy; their testicles have remained normal. Eight of the 9 having delayed exploration had nonviable testicles and underwent unilateral orchiectomy and contralateral orchiopexy. One patient had bilateral orchiopexy with long-term salvage of the testis. The overall salvage rate was 38%.

At least one third of the cases of spermatic cord torsion appear to occur in adults, and the condition should be suspected in men with acute testicular pain and swelling. Timely diagnosis is critical. Small silk sutures are preferable to absorbable sutures for orchiopexy for these patients.

▶ The differentiation of epididymitis from testicular torsion is usually not difficult, based on history and physical findings. However, when the diagnosis is questionable, a urologic consultation should be freely obtained. Often, the only way to make a firm diagnosis is to operate and see.—E. Ruiz, M.D.

## Neurologic Emergencies

### Pneumocephalus Associated With Nasal Continuous Positive Airway Pressure in a Patient With Sleep Apnea Syndrome

Jarjour NN, Wilson P (Univ of Wisconsin)
*Chest* 96:1425–1426, 1989                                      3–52

Nasal continuous positive airway pressure (CPAP) is used to maintain continuous positive pressure along the upper airway, preventing occlusion by the tongue and soft palate. In 1 patient a CSF leak, seizures, and pneumocephalus developed after the application of nasal CPAP for obstructive sleep apnea syndrome.

Woman, 55, had a history of obesity, daytime hypersomnolence, and snoring and underwent polysomnography, which documented obstructive sleep apnea syndrome. She also had moderate chronic obstructive lung disease, chiefly of the bronchitic type, and sinusitis. Nasal CPAP at 12.5 cm $H_2O$ dramatically improved the patient's sleep, but significant oxygen desaturation persisted, necessitating oxygen at a flow rate of 1 L/minute. Clear nasal discharge was noted when the CPAP mask was applied, and the patient had a grand mal seizure. Sinus x-ray films showed pneumocephalus. Rhinorrhea ceased after bed rest and lumbar catheter drainage of CSF were instituted. The patient stopped using nasal CPAP, and the pneumocephalus was resolved.

Perhaps 5% of patients with sleep apnea syndrome do not tolerate CPAP therapy for various reasons. Complications include ear pain and conjunctivitis, which may be caused by barotrauma to the inner ear or the conjunctiva. Leakage of CSF should be considered when patients with persistent nasal discharge are treated, especially if new neurologic abnormalities develop.

▶ The authors report on pneumocephalus as a complication of CPAP therapy. This has previously been reported as a complication of face mask resuscitation. Although a complication such as this can be considered acceptable in the face of a life-saving resuscitative event, it is wise to remember its possibility so that appropriate, preventive measures may be instituted in patients with postresuscitative neurologic symptomatology. The current usage of CAT scans in such patients will provide early diagnosis of the condition.—D.K. Wagner, M.D.

## Glucocorticoid Treatment Does Not Improve Neurological Recovery Following Cardiac Arrest

Jastremski M, Sutton-Tyrrell K, Vaagenes P, Abramson N, Heiselman D, Safar P, Brain Resuscitation Clinical Trial I Study Group (Univ of Pittsburgh)
*JAMA* 262:3427–3430, 1989                                              3–53

Glucocorticoids commonly are used after global brain ischemia, but their efficacy for this indication has not been confirmed. The multicenter Brain Resuscitation Clinical Trial I evaluated the effect of high-dose thiopental sodium therapy on neurologic outcome after global brain ischemia. The database of this trial was used to review retrospectively the effects of glucocorticoids on mortality and neurologic outcome after global brain ischemia in 262 initially comatose cardiac arrest survivors who made no purposeful response to pain 10–50 minutes after restoration of spontaneous circulation.

The brain-oriented intensive care treatment protocol left the use of glucocorticoids to the discretion of the hospital investigators. A total of 192 patients received steroids within the first 8 hours of restoration of spontaneous circulation. One patient was subsequently excluded from analysis. Of the 191 steroid-treated patients, 67 received a low dose of steroids, 58 received a medium dose, and 66 received a high dose.

Of these 191 patients, 171 were still alive at 24 hours. Of these, 140 (82%) had received multiple doses of steroids during the first day after resuscitation. No statistically significant differences were noted in mortality or neurologic outcomes among patients who never received steroids, those who received only a single early dose, and those who received multiple doses within the first 24 hours after global brain ischemia. Because the use of glucocorticoids has the potential for causing serious toxicity and because none of the steroid regimens statistically improved survival or neurologic recovery when compared with no steroid use, the routine clinical practice of giving glucocorticoids after global brain ischemia is not justified.

▶ As a retrospective study, this work cannot be viewed as conclusive regarding the role of steroids following anoxic brain injury, but it certainly suggests their routine use is questionable. The main flaw in this study is that the authors were unable to separate out patients who received steroids very early (within 1 hour) after restoration of circulation. Evaluation of any intervention to ameliorate anoxic brain injury is best studied as close as possible to restoration of circulation.—R.M. McNamara, M.D.

## Acute Transient Memory Loss

Vinson DC (Univ of Missouri, Columbia)
*Am Fam Physician* 39:249–254, May 1989                    3–54

Anterograde amnesia is the inability to form new memories. Alcoholic blackout, benzodiazepine-induced amnesia, and transient global amnesia are 3 disorders that result in acute transient memory loss. These conditions may prove difficult to diagnose because the memory loss is not usually accompanied by other neurologic impairment symptoms.

Detailed psychometric testing may be necessary to differentiate among some memory disorders, such as early Alzheimer's disease, Korsakoff's syndrome, and depression. In acute anterograde amnesia, the memory impairment can usually be detected easily with the patient being given 3 simple, unrelated words, such as "window, apple, chair." A few minutes later the patient with anterograde amnesia will be unable to recall the words.

In management of anterograde amnesia in the intoxicated patient, instructions on the patient's care should be given to family members or those caring for the patient. Counseling should be postponed until the patient is sober. In benzodiazepine-induced amnesia, the patient should be monitored for subtle impairment in learning new material, and the response to benzodiazepine therapy should be checked. In transient global amnesia, witnesses should be questioned on the occurrence of the episode. If possible, a neurologic examination should be performed during the amnestic spell. An electroencephalogram and a CT scan are often helpful. If the results are normal, the patient should be reassured.

Blackouts are not necessarily a sign of alcoholism and are not always a symptom of advanced disease. The frequency of blackouts may be helpful in clarifying a diagnosis of alcoholism. Family physicians should be aware of the possibility of anterograde amnesia in intoxicated patients.

Oral medication with benzodiazepines, especially in the elderly and in patients with significant illness, may cause less profound degrees of anterograde amnesia. In these patients, the benzodiazepine-induced memory impairment may be confused with dementia or delirium. If memory is impaired out of proportion to other cognitive deficits, benzodiazepine therapy should be discontinued.

The cause of transient global amnesia remains unknown, although three major etiologic theories have been advanced: (1) it is a form of transient ischemic cerebrovascular disease, (2) seizure disorder is a possible cause, and (3) an association between transient global amnesia and migraine has appeared in many case reports. However, migraine is not a common cause of this memory disorder. Permanent memory loss from transient global amnesia alone seems to be unlikely. In the absence of other signs of ischemia, transient global amnesia most likely needs no therapy, although this point requires more rigorous study.

▶ This article is not very helpful to emergency practitioners. Although transient anterograde amnesia is a problem to be taken seriously, the entities discussed are rather uncommon and should remain diagnoses of exclusion. Far more common, and potentially more serious, are the various conditions that can cause transient memory loss with or without a change in mental status; hypoglycemia, seizure disorder, drug overdose, head injury, psychogenic fugue state, transient ischemic attack (TIA), and malingering.

Transient global amnesia (memory loss with an intact intellect) is an entity that is generally accepted by the medical community, but it remains a theoretical instruct, and its cause or causes are obscure. Even in the absence of neurologic findings or a change in mental status, a structural lesion affecting the lymph system, TIA, or psychomotor seizure must be ruled out. Since an EEG cannot easily be obtained in the ED, an admission and thorough work-up may be warranted contrary to the advice of the author.— H.H. Osborn, M.D.

---

**A Directed Approach to the Dizzy Patient**
Herr RD, Zun L, Mathews JJ (Univ of Utah; Northwestern Univ)
*Ann Emerg Med* 18:664–672, 1989                    3–55

---

Diagnosis of the dizzy patient is complicated by the many possible causes, and a wide range of diagnostic approaches and tests have been proposed. A prospective survey was conducted of 125 consecutive patients seen in a 16-month period with a chief complaint of feeling dizzy, lightheaded, or faint. The study included 73 women and 51 men with a mean age of 47 years. Of the patients, 72% were available for follow-up at 4 weeks.

Peripheral vestibular disorder accounted for 43% of diagnoses; 5 of these patients were hospitalized. The best predictors were a positive Nylen-Barany test result, vertigo, and vomiting. Causes of dizziness were considered serious in 38 patients. Medication-related causes, arrhythmia, and seizures were most frequent; 20 of these patients required hospitalization for medical reasons. Serious causes were more frequent in older patients, those without vertigo, and those with neurologic abnormality.

Routine glucose testing seems warranted in these patients. Cardiac rhythm should be monitored in patients aged older than 45 years. Carotid stimulation testing, the Romberg test, mental status examination, blood count, and serum electrolyte and blood urea nitrogen estimates may be used in a directed way based on a brief history. Potassium should be estimated in patients who are admitted and those taking antihypertensive medication.

▶ The authors' hypothesis was that certain historical and laboratory data obtained in the ED will predict whether a "dizzy" patient will turn out to have a "serious" problem. One key to the validity of a study like this is that it is prospective, with few exclusions, and a demonstrated equivalence of the excluded patients. Unfortunately, in this study, more than half (54%) of the patients with dizziness are neither included nor described. This is a crippling flow that leaves a cloud of uncertainty over the results.

Another key to a valid study of this kind is good follow-up and a compulsive definition of diagnoses. The patients should have been followed up by independent physicians and subjected to a battery of tests such as audiometry, electronystagmography, and Holter monitoring so that unambiguous, unbiased etiologies could be determined with a solid endpoint like this. The investigator could have then looked at the mitral data and tested their hypotheses. In the study by Drachman and Hart (1) there were few exclusions, and the diagnoses were painstakingly defined and thoroughly pursued for each patient. That is why the Drachman and Hart study is a classic.—W.P. Burdick, M.D.

*Reference*

1. Drachman DA, Hart CW: *Neurology* 22:323, 1972.

## The Administration of Rectal Diazepam for Acute Management of Seizures
Seigler RS (The Childrens Hosp of the Greenville Hosp System, Greenville, SC)
*J Emerg Med* 8:155–159, 1990                                               3–56

Intravenous diazepam is commonly used as a first-line therapy in the emergency management of seizures, but intravenous access in patients having seizures, particularly children, is often difficult. In studies seeking an alternate route of diazepam administration, the efficacies of intramuscular diazepam and diazepam suppositories have been inconsistent. Literature was reviewed to determine the efficacy of intravenous diazepam solution administered rectally in the emergency treatment of seizures.

Eighteen studies involved a total of 755 patients who received 840 doses of intravenous diazepam solution. Four studies were done exclusively with adults, and 14 studies involved children only. The diazepam dosages in these studies ranged from .12 mg/kg of body weight per dose to 30 mg per dose. The appropriate dose is probably .5–1 mg/kg of body weight. Intravenous diazepam solution was administered rectally with disposable plastic syringes attached to plastic or rubber catheters or with a bulb-syringe type tube with a blunt tip. In 1 study, a 1-cc disposable insulin syringe was used without a needle or catheter attached.

All 3 studies that examined the effect of rectally administered intravenous diazepam solution on electroencephalographic (EEG) activity found it to be rapidly effective. In 1 of the pediatric studies, 7 of 9 patients ceased fast activity on the EEG in less than 5 minutes. The observed EEG changes after rectal administration of intravenous diazepam solution were essentially the same as those observed after intravenous administration. Although intravenously administered diazepam is associated with CNS side effects and cardiovascular depression, the incidence of side effects was very low when intravenous solution was administered rectally.

Serum diazepam concentrations after rectal administration of intravenous diazepam solution were measured in 13 studies. The precise serum diazepam concentration needed to stop seizure activity is not known, and therapeutic serum concentrations in these studies varied widely, ranging from 754 to 98.5 ng/mL at 4 minutes.

This literature review indicates that rectal administration of intravenous diazepam solution in the emergency treatment of seizures is safe, effective, and simple to use. Administration of intravenous diazepam solution via the rectal route is the best alternative for patients having seizures in whom intravenous access cannot be obtained.

▶ This article addresses 1 of the most frustrating situations in emergency medicine: the seizing child, the sweating physician, and the worried cast of parents and staff. A new way to deliver diazepam (Valium), a way that is rapid, safe, simple, and effective, is a hard-to-beat combination. Perhaps the new way should be the first way. Then, intravenous administration can be reserved for a second-line approach.— E.H. Taliaferro, M.D.

---

**Compliance With a Standard for the Emergency Department Management of Epileptics Who Present After an Uncomplicated Convulsion**
Baraff LJ, Schriger DL, Starkman S (Univ of California, Los Angeles)
*Ann Emerg Med* 19:367–372, 1990                                3–57

---

Charts were reviewed retrospectively to determine whether emergency treatment of uncomplicated convulsions in patients with epilepsy met a defined clinical standard and whether the degree of compliance with this standard was related to a treating physician's specialty or postgraduate year of training.

The clinical standard included 7 essential and 7 desirable items obtained from a patient's history and physical examination. The only laboratory tests considered necessary were the measurement of anticonvulsant drug levels if patients were taking such medications, and the measurement of serum glucose levels if not part of a routine chemistry profile. A CT head scan was deemed appropriate only for patients whose neurologic status either deteriorated or failed to return to baseline within 60 minutes or for patients who had scalp lacerations that required suturing. Each medical record was assigned a performance score, with 28 considered a perfect score.

The record sample documented 100 consecutive visits to the ED by 82 epileptic patients, aged 18–88 years, who had treatment for uncomplicated convulsions. Time in the ED ranged from 8 to 539 minutes (median 174.5 minutes). Medical record scores ranged from 7 to 82 (median 43). Charges for ancillary services ranged from $0 to $1,774 (median $181.50). Only 27.4% of these charges were for diagnostic tests deemed appropriate. Charges for unnecessary ancillary services ranged from $0 to $1,722 (median $131). The relationship between time spent in the ED and charges for ancillary services was significant, confirming that waiting for the results of tests leads to longer ED times. Performance of resident physicians differed significantly by specialty, with residents in emergency medicine ordering fewer unnecessary diagnostic tests than residents in internal medicine. However, median charges for ancillary services did not differ significantly by postgraduate year of resident training.

Compliance with a clinical standard for the treatment of epileptic patients who arrive at an ED after uncomplicated convulsions did not meet expectations. Resident physicians still order far too many unnecessary diagnostic tests for a common complaint for which specific treatment guidelines are well defined. That resident physicians specializing in emergency medicine performed better than those specializing in internal medicine perhaps reflects the emphasis placed on cost containment in the ED curriculum.

▶ Performance standard and clinical indicators are the theme of the nineties: the current—the latest major effort to curb the runaway medical costs while providing quality care.

This article provides a tool to study charting compliance to defined clinical standards. The methodology delineated in the article can be readily adapted for ongoing quality assurance professional activities in every ED.

The article addresses the secret to change—feedback. Without feedback, practice continues unaltered and proves what the piano teacher knows: Practice does not make perfect; practice makes permanent.—E.H. Taliaferro, M.D.

---

### Utility of Laboratory Studies in the Emergency Department Patient With a New-Onset Seizure

Turnbull TL, Vanden Hoek TL, Howes DS, Eisner RF (Univ of Illinois, Chicago; Univ of Chicago; Univ of California, Los Angeles)
*Ann Emerg Med* 19:373–377, 1990                                                   3–58

Extensive routine laboratory testing often is advocated to evaluate adult patients seen in the ED with a first seizure. Because few data support the need for such testing, a prospective study evaluated the utility of a laboratory testing protocol for such patients.

One hundred thirty-six patients with a mean age of 45 years were evaluated in an ED for a first seizure. Laboratory evaluation included complete blood cell count, serum electrolyte values, blood urea nitrogen value, and serum creatinine, glucose, calcium, and magnesium levels. The most common seizure etiologies obtained from histories and physical examination were idiopathic, alcohol withdrawal, and cerebral infarct, accounting for 71.3% of all cases. Only 11 patients had significant laboratory abnormalities considered the sole or contributory cause of their seizures. Four patients had hypoglycemia, 4 had hyperglycemia, 2 had hypocalcemia, and 1 had hypomagnesemia. For only 2 patients with hypoglycemia were abnormal laboratory findings not suspected on the basis of history and physical examination.

Thus, the incidence of new-onset seizures caused by correctable metabolic abnormalities is low. With the exception of a routine serum glucose determination, the extensive ED laboratory testing done to evaluate a new-onset seizure is unnecessary. Further ordering of tests for a patient with new-onset seizure should be guided by the patient's medical history and physical examination.

▶ The value of this paper is that it reports a prospective study to eliminate unnecessary laboratory tests for the patient with new-onset seizure. The conclusion of the authors is that extensive, routine laboratory examination, with the exception of serum glucose level, can be eliminated in these patients.

This study is ideal for prospective inclusion into departmental quality assurance activities. The authors' conclusions should be validated in your patient setting before blanket adoption.—E.H. Taliaferro, M.D.

---

**Use of High Dose Naloxone in Acute Stroke: Possible Side-Effects**
Barsan WG, Olinger CP, Adams HP Jr, Brott TG, Eberle R, Biller J, Biros M, Marler J (Univ of Cincinnati; Univ of Iowa; Natl Inst of Neurological Disorders and Stroke, Bethesda, Md)
*Crit Care Med* 17:762–767, 1989                                3–59

---

Data on high doses of naloxone in human beings are limited. To evaluate the potential efficacy and toxicity of high-dose naloxone in acute stroke, 36 patients aged 35–85 years with acute ischemic cerebral infarction were treated with a naloxone loading dose of 160 mg/m$^2$ (4 mg/kg), followed by a 24-hour continuous nalaxone infusion at a rate of 80 mg/m$^2$ (2 mg/kg/hour).

There were no significant changes in group mean arterial pressure, respiratory rate, or heart rate in response to the loading dose or infusion, although clinically significant changes occurred in 4 patients. Adverse reactions possibly related to naloxone were observed in 23 patients, the most common of which were nausea (20), bradycardia, hypotension, or both (3), myoclonus (1), and hypertension (1). Naloxone was discontinued in 7 patients for possible adverse reactions. All side effects were alleviated by medication or discontinuance of naloxone. There were no deaths attributable to naloxone.

High-dose naloxone appears to be well tolerated in most elderly patients with acute cerebral infarction. The most serious side effect is hypotension and bradycardia.

▶ The rationale for the therapeutic benefit of using naloxone in the ED setting for the management of acute ischemic cerebral infarction ("acute stroke") is not apparent in this article. So why use a preparation that has "possible side effects"?—G.V. Anderson, M.D.

---

**An Analysis of Time of Presentation After Stroke**
Alberts MJ, Bertels C, Dawson DV (Duke Univ)
*JAMA* 263:65–68, 1990                                3–60

---

Several agents for the early treatment of stroke are now under clinical investigation. However, for these drugs to be effective, most need to be administered shortly after the onset of stroke. Large numbers of patients with acute stroke will be needed for ongoing and future trials, but few studies have investigated the time delay between stroke onset and initiation of medical care. The delay between stroke onset and initiation of treatment was investigated using data obtained from 584 patients entered into a stroke registry during a 14-month period.

Time of presentation data were not available for 24 patients; of the 560 remaining patients, 103 had an in-hospital stroke. A total of 457 patients with out-of-hospital stroke formed the basis for this analysis. For all stroke types, only 192 (42%) patients were seen within 24 hours of stroke onset, 116 (25%) were seen within 48 hours, and 149 (33%) were seen after 48 hours. By 48 hours after stroke onset, only 67% of patients had been seen for treatment. Analysis by type of stroke revealed that 176 (64%) of 276 patients with infarcts, 44 (54%) of 88 patients with stroke in evolution, and 25 (54%) of 46 patients with subarachnoid hemorrhage were not seen for treatment within 24 hours of stroke onset. However, 34 (63%) of 54 patients with intracerebral hemorrhage were seen within 24 hours.

Delays in seeking medical treatment after stroke may be attributable to the patient's general lack of awareness about the symptoms of stroke and lack of recognition of early signs of stroke by medical personnel. Because the development of new treatments for stroke may be hampered by this delay of patients with stroke, better education of both patients and physicians is needed to improve recognition of stroke symptoms and reduce the delay in obtaining treatment.

▶ This article is an interesting statement regarding medical care in the United States. Our system has advanced to the point where we can now treat and cure many diseases once thought hopeless, yet we cannot educate people sufficiently to allow them to benefit from such advances.— R.M. McNamara, M.D.

---

### Comparison of Cerebral Angiography and Transcranial Doppler Sonography in Acute Stroke

Zanette EM, Fieschi C, Bozzao L, Roberti C, Toni D, Argentino C, Lenzi GL (Univ "La Sapienza," Rome)
*Stroke* 20:899–903, 1989                     3–61

---

A noninvasive way of detecting intracranial arterial occlusion at an early stage and following its response to treatment would be most helpful. Thus, transcranial Doppler (TCD) ultrasonography was compared with digital intra-arterial angiography in 48 patients with acute focal deficits caused by hemispheric cerebral ischemia. The patients, all with carotid involvement, were seen within 4 hours of the onset of symptoms.

Doppler studies failed in 9 cases because of an undetectable temporal window. When angiography showed occlusion of the carotid siphon or the middle cerebral artery at its origin, TCD ultrasonography failed to demonstrate the middle cerebral artery. When occlusion was in the terminal tract of the main middle cerebral artery or a terminal branch, the TCD study showed reduced flow velocity and an asymmetric appearance. Increased flow velocity in the anterior or posterior cerebral artery, usually in the symptomatic hemisphere, often accompanied pathology of the middle cerebral artery.

Doppler studies were technically not feasible in nearly one fifth of cases in this series. Nevertheless, TCD ultrasonography is a useful bedside method of monitoring the patency of intracranial arteries in the acute phase of stroke. Middle cerebral artery pathology may be assessed more reliably if collateral paths are present.

▶ The authors present yet another indication for noninvasive bedside evaluation of acute vascular compromise. Whether their level of sophisticated evaluation can be carried out in other settings is unclear, nor is the degree to which the study is operator dependent identified. Noninvasive ultrasonic evaluation in the emergency center for selected conditions is rapidly expanding. Where this study fits on that list is unclear, but it warrants continued evaluation and observation.—D.K. Wagner, M.D.

---

### Intracerebral Hemorrhage in Young Adults

Bell MC, Olshaker JS, Osborn RE (Naval Hosp, San Diego)
*Ann Emerg Med* 18:1230–1232, 1989                                    3–62

---

Nontraumatic intracerebral hemorrhage is rare in younger adults and children. The cause and predisposing factors may be elusive, and the signs and symptoms can be atypical or subtle. Rapid assessment and referral to a neurosurgeon are crucial. Two patients with intracerebral hemorrhage were seen at an ED.

Man, 32, arrived at the ED complaining of numbness in the right side of his body and face that had persisted for 24 hours. He did not have any current or antecedent headache; weakness; visual, hearing, or speech difficulty; or recent trauma or illness. His medical history was unremarkable. He was taking no medications, did not use illicit drugs, and had no allergies. He smoked tobacco and sometimes drank alcohol. On physical examination, he was alert, fully oriented, cooperative, and in no apparent distress. A neurologic examination demonstrated hypesthesia to light touch and pinprick on his right side. He had mild facial asymmetry, but his cranial nerve function was intact. Results of laboratory tests, serum tests, an ECG, and a chest radiograph were normal. Computed tomography of the head showed a 2.5-cm acute hematoma in the region of the left lentiform nucleus, and a mild amount of circumferential edema; the patient was hospitalized. A repeated CT scan appeared unchanged 11 days later. Magnetic resonance imaging showed an acute hematoma. A vascular malformation was identified medial to the hematoma within the internal capsule. Cerebral angiography revealed a venous angioma involving the basal ganglia region and draining into the adjacent internal cerebral vein. The patient was discharged with a mild right hemihypesthesia and hemiparesis 19 days after admission.

In treating young adults, physicians must maintain a high index of suspicion and consider intercerebral hemorrhage before signs and symptoms are attributed to a less malignant process.

► Although emergency physicians should not interpret these case reports to mean that the next young adult patients they see with subjective sensory findings have intracerebral hemorrhage, this does stress that even subtle focal neurologic findings require serious investigation.—J.R. Hoffman, M.D.

---

**Recognition of Subarachnoid Hemorrhage**
Fontanarosa PB (Northeastern Ohio Univ, Akron; Akron City Hosp, Ohio)
*Ann Emerg Med* 18:1199–1205, 1989                          3–63

---

Early recognition and prompt intervention are crucial in reducing the mortality and morbidity from subarachnoid hemorrhage (SAH) and its acute complications. To characterize the clinical presentation and diagnostic features of patients who come to the ED with nontraumatic, spontaneous SAH, data on 109 patients with proved SAH who came to an ED within a 5-year period were reviewed.

The most common historical features were headache, nausea or vomiting, and loss of consciousness. Nonexertional activities preceded SAH more often than exertional activities. Sixty-four percent of the patients had neurologic findings, which consisted mainly of altered levels of consciousness. Thirty-five percent had nuchal rigidity. Ninety-six emergency cranial CT scans were done, of which 91 were diagnostic, yielding a sensitivity of 95%. Lumbar puncture of 2 patients with normal CT findings revealed bloody spinal fluid. Emergency physicians' overall diagnostic accuracy was 85%. The correct diagnosis was delayed primarily among patients with headaches and normal neurologic results.

Emergency physicians must recognize the clinical features of nontraumatic, spontaneous SAH. An accurate, prompt diagnosis, appropriate supportive therapy, and timely neurosurgical consultations are vital in such cases. A significant number of patients may first be seen with atypical complaints or symptoms of the aneurysmal warning leak syndrome. Liberal use of cranial CT and, when indicated, selective lumbar puncture will improve detection of SAH.

► One of the greatest fears of an emergency physician is that he or she will fail to diagnose SAH. We treat hundreds of patients every year for headaches, and thankfully only a few have SAH. However, it requires a high index of suspicion to make this diagnosis in many of the patients who have it. This article emphasizes that as high as 60% of the patients have a "warning leak" before a catastrophic bleed. Our goal is to make this diagnosis early, and we must be sensitive to the potential for this problem in every patient with the complaint of headache. Clinical judgment is extremely important. Not every patient with a headache needs a CAT scan. We must take a careful history on these patients.

It is important to emphasize that 5% of these patients will have a normal CAT scan and will require a lumbar puncture to make the diagnosis. This is particularly true of patients with normal neurologic examination, thus making a very high index of suspicion on the physician's part all the more necessary.

This article is well worth reviewing by all emergency physicians.—E.J. Lucid, M.D.

## Endocrine, Metabolic, Hypertensive, and Hematologic Emergencies

**Lithium Toxicity and Myxedema Coma in an Elderly Woman**
Santiago R, Rashkin MC (Univ of Cincinnati)
*J Emerg Med* 8:63–66, 1990                                           3–64

Thyroid diseases occur more often in elderly than in younger adults. Hypothyroidism as a side effect of lithium therapy is a well-recognized complication. However, myxedema coma after lithium intoxication has not previously been documented.

Woman, 71, was taken to the ED for evaluation because she had become incoherent. The patient had been chronically treated with lithium and trifluoperazine for an unspecified psychiatric condition and had recently begun taking a combination diuretic of hydrochlorothiazide and triamterene to treat her hypertension. She had also been taking naproxen for arthritis. Laboratory evaluation revealed chronic lithium toxicity and mild dehydration. She was placed on a monitored bed and treated with forced alkaline diuresis for 2 days. Plasma lithium values dropped gradually from 2.48 mEq/L at admission to 1 mEq/L on day 4. Her condition appeared to be stable during the first 3 days of admission. However, on day 4 she was suddenly noted to have no spontaneous respirations, and she became bradycardic with an undetectable pulse. She was resuscitated and transferred to the intensive care unit where she was diagnosed with third-degree heart block. A transvenous pacemaker was inserted. The patient was comatose with a Glasgow Coma Scale score of 8. Thyroid function tests drawn on admission showed a thyroxine value of 1 $\mu$g/dL and a triiodothyronine resin uptake of 84%. She was given 500 $\mu$g of intravenous levothyroxine and 50 $\mu$g daily for an additional 2 doses, after which she was maintained on oral thyroid therapy. At the time of discharge, the patient was alert, oriented, and ambulatory and had returned to her baseline mental status.

Because the typical signs and symptoms of hypothyroidism in the elderly may be either absent or misinterpreted as age-related changes, dementia, or depression, the diagnosis of lithium toxicity may not be recognized in elderly patients. A careful differential diagnosis in an elderly patient with vague symptoms suggesting dementia or depression who is taking lithium for recurrent affective disorder cannot be overemphasized.

► This case report was justified by the assumption that hypothyroidism might have been caused by lithium therapy. We in the ED can easily miss hypothyroidism during other illnesses, especially the elderly (e.g., hypothermia, stroke, overdose as in this case). Thyroid hormone levels are not often available immediately, and I have occasionally empirically administered .2 mg of thyroxine to hypothermia patients.—T. Stair, M.D.

---

### Acute Porphyria in the Emergency Department
Karcz A, Farkas PS (Lahey Clin Med Ctr, Burlington, Mass; Mercy Hosp, Springfield, Mass)
*J Emerg Med* 7:279–285, 1989                                                    3–65

---

Although abdominal pain is a frequent complaint in patients admitted to the ED, porphyria is seldom considered in the assessment of these patients. In acute hepatic porphyria, clinical manifestations are a result of generalized neurologic impairment. Abdominal pain, ileus, tachycardia, postural hypotension, and diaphoresis are the result of autonomic dysfunction. Peripheral sensory and motor neuropathies may be present, and CNS involvement can result in seizures, behavioral abnormalities, and changes in mental status.

Patients with acute hepatic porphyrias may not have all the manifestations of neurologic dysfunction. Recurrent abdominal pain may be the only symptom. Acute intermittent porphyria is most common in persons of Swedish or English ancestry, is more frequent in women than in men, and is the most frequently noted of the 4 hepatic porphyrias that have abdominal pain as the primary symptom. South Africa has a high incidence of porphyria variegata. The incidence of these acute hepatic porphyrias in North America is not known. Porphyria cutanea tarda (PCT) is the most frequently observed hepatic porphyria in North America; patients with this porphyria have only dermatologic symptoms.

Acquired porphyria and porphyrinuria can occur in poisoning from heavy metals, sedatives, and chemicals such as hexachlorobenzene, benzene, and carbon tetrachloride. Porphyrinuria has also been reported in a variety of medical disorders, particularly liver disease. In acute attacks, the Watson-Schwartz test is a reliable screening method.

Treatment of the acutely ill patient includes carbohydrate loading, correction of associated electrolyte abnormalities, and control of pain. Propranolol may be of help in controlling tachycardia or hypertension. Magnesium sulfate carries the least risk in the management of seizures. The safety of diazepam treatment is controversial, but it should be considered as a second line of therapy.

▶ There is no more wearing patient in all of emergency medicine than the patient admitted to the ED repeatedly with abdominal pain that cannot be specifically diagnosed. Before we label the etiology psychogenic and call for a psychiatric consult, it would be wise to consider the various obscure causes of recurrent abdominal pain: sickle cell crisis (both SS and SC disease), lead poisoning, intermittent obstruction, intestinal volvulus, internal hernia, carcinoid syndrome, and porphyria.

This article is an excellent review of acute porphyria and contains almost everything the emergency physician needs to know about the subject. All 4 of the acute hepatic porphyrias cause abdominal pain and have neurologic findings. These are the ones that should concern the emergency physician most. Porphyria cutaneous tarda PCT, the most common form of porphyria, is a hepatic porphyria, but with PCT, the symptoms are chronic (involving the skin and liver) and not acute.

The authors are to be commended for reminding us about the porphyrias and for rendering a rather complicated subject easier to understand.— H.H. Osborn, M.D.

---

**Dilevalol in Severe Hypertension: A Multicenter Trial of Bolus Intravenous Dosing**
Wallin JD, Cook ME, Fletcher E, Holtzman JL, Winer N, Gavras H, Grim CE, Ramanathan KB, Vidt DG, Johnson BF, Hall D, Stom M, Poland M, Cubbon J (Tulane Univ; VA Med Ctr, Minneapolis; Cleveland Clinic Found; Univ of Missouri; Univ of Massachusetts, et al)
*Arch Intern Med* 149:2655–2661, 1989                                    3–66

---

Dilevalol achieves vasodilation by $\beta_2$-adrenergic stimulation but, unlike labetalol, has no $\alpha$-blocking properties. To study further its ability to lower severe high blood pressure, 101 patients whose supine diastolic blood pressure was greater than 120 mm Hg received in sequence multiple bolus intravenous injections ranging from 10 to 100 mg. Total doses ranged from 35 to 585 mg.

From an initial mean blood pressure of 200/129 mm Hg, a decrease to 149/101 mm Hg was seen. A decrement in supine diastolic blood pressure to less than 100 mm Hg or a 30 mm Hg decrease was achieved by 61% of patients, and a reduction in diastolic blood pressure to 100 mm Hg occurred in another 7%. Black men and patients recently treated with $\beta$-adrenergic blockers had less successful results than the others. Older persons tended to have a better response rate than younger persons. No significant orthostatic hypotension occurred.

Sixty-four patients were then transferred to oral dilevalol therapy plus diuretic. Their blood pressure after 1 month averaged about 160/100 mm Hg.

Intravenous dilevalol appears to be safe and effective in most severely hypertensive patients and can be used in an ED. After intravenous therapy, patients can transfer to oral treatment.

▶ The authors propose a nonselective $\beta$-antagonist with selected $\beta_2$-agonism as an option for intravenous control of urgent hypertension. In addition, conversion to an oral form of the drug is available. True emergent hypertension in the emergency setting probably is still best treated by short-acting vasodilators, which provide precise control in the acutely compromised patient. Much of urgent hypertension can be adequately managed by the oral route when dramatic changes are not indicated or useful. As with most intravenous preparations, concern for orthostatic hypotension remains, although it was not described as a problem by the authors.—D.K. Wagner, M.D.

---

**Salutary Effects of Modest Fluid Replacement in the Treatment of Adults With Diabetic Ketoacidosis: Use in Patients Without Extreme Deficit**
Adrogué HJ, Barrero J, Eknoyan G (VA Med Ctr, Houston; Baylor College of Medicine, Houston)
*JAMA* 262:2108–2113, 1989                                         3–67

---

Fluid administration therapy is a fundamental procedure in the management of diabetic ketoacidosis (DKA), yet the optimal rate of fluid administration to correct the volume deficit remains undefined. Two regimens of fluid therapy that differed exclusively in the rate of fluid infusion were prospectively evaluated in 23 adult patients with DKA. Patients in circulatory shock or with severe renal insufficiency or persistent oliguria were excluded.

In protocol 1, 12 patients received normal saline infusion administered at a rate of 1,000 mL/hr ($\approx$14 mL/kg/hr) in the initial 4 hours and 500 mL/hr ($\approx$7 mL/kg/hr) during the subsequent 4 hours. In protocol 2, 11 patients received normal saline infusion at one half the rates of protocol 1. Insulin therapy and potassium replacement regimens were similar in both groups.

As expected, acid-base parameters showed progressive recovery toward normalcy in both groups. However, the increment in plasma bicarbonate

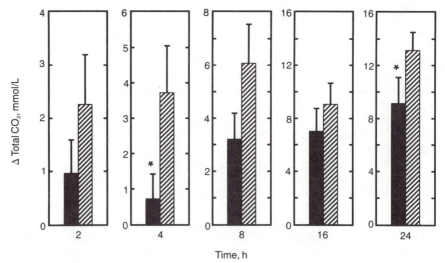

Time, h

Fig 3–6.—Influence of the rate of fluid infusion on speed of recovery, as assessed by the increment in serum total $CO_2$ from the initial value ($\Delta$ total $CO_2$) at different times after admission with protocols 1 *(dark bars)* and 2 *(slashed bars)*. *Asterisk* indicates $P <.05$ vs other protocol at the same time. Note: Scales of the ordinates are not identical in all panels. (Courtesy of Adrogué HJ, Barrero J, Eknoyan G: *JAMA* 262:2108–2113, 1989.)

concentration from admission levels at all points of observation was greater with protocol 2, attaining statistical significance at 4 and 24 hours after admission (Fig 3–6). Patients experienced no untoward side effects with either treatment protocol.

Relatively modest fluid replacement in the treatment of DKA in adult patients without extreme volume deficit results in prompt recovery and a significant reduction in the overall cost of medical care. The slower recovery from DKA with the high infusion rates is most likely caused by the relatively greater acute expansion with a bicarbonate-free solution and a sustained loss of bicarbonate precursors in the urine because of continued volume expansion.

▶ This study suggests that a modest volume of intravenous fluid replacement of approximately one half of current practice for DKA without severe volume depletion achieves a prompt, satisfactory, and safer therapeutic regimen.— G.V. Anderson, M.D.

## Venous and Vascular Emergencies

**Real-Time Ultrasonography for the Diagnosis of Lower Extremity Deep Venous Thrombosis: The Wave of the Future?**
Becker DM, Philbrick JT, Abbitt PL (Univ of Virginia, Charlottesville)
*Arch Intern Med* 149:1731–1734, 1989                                    3–68

Fifteen articles published since 1977 compared real-time ultrasonography with venography in diagnosing deep venous thrombosis (DVT) of the lower extremity. Real-time ultrasonography involves the use of high-resolution real-time (B-mode) transducers to assess the deep venous system for patency, the presence of intraluminal thrombi, vein compressibility, blood flow, and response to hemodynamic maneuvers.

When the studies were evaluated with 8 standards, none of them met all the standards, and only 4 met more than half of them. The mean sensitivity of ultrasonography was 96% and its mean specificity was 99% when thigh and popliteal DVT was considered. Sensitivity and specificity for all DVT were as low as 78%. Four studies found that real-time ultrasonography can help diagnose states mimicking acute DVT such as Baker's cyst and calf hematoma. None of the studies established the reliability of the ultrasonographic method.

Considerable data support the claim that real-time ultrasonography is an accurate means of noninvasively diagnosing DVT in the lower extremity, but clear limitations exist in present knowledge of this method. Clinical limitations also exist. For instance, the study cannot be used to accurately evaluate calf thrombi. Future studies should involve real-time ultrasonography to outline cost-effective strategies for the initial and follow-up evaluation of suspected DVT.

▶ This is a fairly rigid review of 15 articles evaluating the use of real-time ultrasonography for the evaluation of DVTs. Similar to CT scans in trauma, the reliability of this test is dependent on the examiner's experience. Ultrasound is practically limited to evaluating DVTs in the femoral and popliteal distribution, and it cannot visualize the calf and iliac veins. However, the presence of clinically significant DVTs in the calf is nonexistent, and radiologists at this institution believe that their ability to simultaneously visualize a clean inferior vena cava and femoral-popliteal venous system by ultrasound makes it unlikely that a nonvisualized iliac thrombus would be missed. Since clots begin in the popliteal and femoral region and propagate proximally, an isolated iliac thrombus is highly unlikely. If such a clot were present, Doppler studies in the femoral region to evaluate flow augmentation with respiration and leg compression should suggest its presence. Sensitivities and specificities for this diagnostic procedure have been reported to be from 89% to 95% and 97% to 100%, respectively.—H. Unger, M.D.

---

**Use of the Triplex Scanner in Diagnosis of Deep Venous Thrombosis**
Persson AV, Jones C, Zide R, Jewell ER (Lahey Clinic Med Ctr, Burlington, Mass)
*Arch Surg* 124:593–596, 1989                                        3–69

---

Many patients with extensive deep venous thrombosis have few or no symptoms. The invasiveness and expense of venography have prompted efforts to develop reliable noninvasive tests for diagnosing deep venous thrombosis. For 2 years, the authors have used the triplex scanner (Angiodynograph). A total of 264 patients in whom deep venous thrombosis was suspected were examined in a 10-month period. Thirty of them underwent venography as well. Lower limb veins were scanned with a 5- or 7.5-MHz transducer. The vessel lumen was defined by color flow within the gray-scale boundaries.

The results of triplex scanning and venography were in total agreement. Intraluminal clot was documented through changes in venous color-flow patterns and the B-mode image. More recent clots were less echogenic and appeared as black areas in a gray-scale image; older clots were more echogenic. The 2 studies agreed on the anatomic site of thrombosis and also on its extent.

Angiodynography alone can be used to diagnose acute deep venous thrombosis and to rule out the need for treatment. There were no false positive or false negative results in this series. The presence of enlarged venous collateral veins, the absence of color flow, and an inability to compress the veins confirmed the diagnosis of acute deep venous thrombosis.

▶ The triplex scanner is both an expensive and accurate diagnostic tool for evaluating deep vein thrombosis. This study does not make an in-depth comparison between the triplex scanner and the less expensive, but accurate, continuous-wave Doppler ultrasound. This latter imaging device is more rapidly available in most hospitals and takes less time to train operators in its function. However, the triplex scanner may be more sensitive in identifying fresh nonocclusive thrombus and is able to evaluate longer segments of vein in a shorter period of time.— H. Unger, M.D.

**Value of Diagnostic Tests for Deep Venous Thrombosis: A Decision Analysis Model**
Venta LA, Venta ER, Mumford LM (Loyola Univ Med Ctr, Maywood, Ill; Loyola Univ, Chicago; Johns Hopkins Univ)
*Radiology* 174:433–439, 1990                                                          3–70

Diagnosis of deep venous thrombosis (DVT) is still a difficult and complex problem. Four diagnostic procedures are available: Doppler study, plethysmography, iodine 125–fibrinogen scanning, and venography. Clinical diagnosis of DVT has been proved inaccurate when compared with venography.

A number of earlier studies that included more than 12,000 patients were reviewed with evaluation of the prevalence of DVT in symptomatic legs; the sensitivity, specificity, and nondiagnostic rate of different noninvasive tests; and the complication rate of venography. A decision analysis model was based on the information gathered.

The selection of a diagnostic strategy should be based not on the sensitivity or specificity of tests but on the percentages of recovery, morbidity, and mortality. Decision analysis offers certain advantages over clinical tests: (1) most relevant factors are considered in the model so that even infrequent events such as death from DVT are considered, and (2) specific patient circumstances can be estimated with sensitivity analysis or by recalculation of outcome probabilities.

The prevalence of DVT in symptomatic legs is 40%, a value at which venography followed by Doppler ultrasound—in patients with nondiagnostic or unsuccessful venography—is preferred to the sequence of Doppler-plethysmography, provided the sensitivity of the latter is less than 94%. If the prevalence of DVT decreases to 25% or the sensitivity of Doppler is 95% or higher, the sequences of Doppler-plethysmography and venography-Doppler are equal in helping to minimize resultant morbidity and mortality.

The decision analysis reveals that if venography is to be used at all, it is best done before noninvasive tests are performed. Because of the greater clinical significance of proximal (above the knee) DVT, the analysis was modified to reflect changes in prevalence, sensitivity of noninvasive tests, and the rate of pulmonary embolus caused by proximal DVT. In that case, plethysmography is slightly superior to venography, followed by Doppler study or plethysmography.

Because the difference in the total morbidity and mortality rates between the top strategies is small, cost could be a deciding factor.

▶ This is a complex statistical report that emergency physicians should review on their own. Physicians need to plug probability data from their own institution into the decision trees in the paper to arrive at their own conclusions. The results should be discussed with other members of the faculty at the specific institution to arrive at the best branch of the decision tree to follow in each circumstance. The decisions may change as patient populations and equipment accuracy change at any particular institution.

This subject of investigative procedures for DVT remains confusing, but a joint decision by the faculty, after review of this article, and an analysis of the institution's own data could alleviate most of this confusion.— G. Ordog, M.D.

---

### The Limitations of Impedance Plethysmography in the Diagnosis of Acute Deep Venous Thrombosis

Patterson RB, Fowl RJ, Keller JD, Schomaker W, Kempczinski RF (Univ of Cincinnati)

*J Vasc Surg* 9:725–730, 1989                                                           3–71

Despite its known limitations impedance plethysmography (IPG) has been the mainstay for diagnosing acute deep venous thrombosis (DVT) in most vascular laboratories. In a recent 22-month period, 1,776 patients were evaluated for DVT at 1 laboratory. Sixty patients had ascending venography within 48 hours of noninvasive testing. Noninvasive assessment included IPG and real-time B-mode venous imaging.

B-mode scanning correctly identified acute thrombus in 24 of 27 extremities and the absence of thrombus in 34 of 37; thus, the study was 89% sensitive and 92% specific. Fifteen of 20 thrombi were correctly identified with IPG, but results were normal in only 13 of 29 studies in normal extremities. Impedance plethysmography alone was 75% sensitive and 45% specific. Its overall accuracy was 57% compared with 91% for B-mode scanning.

Combined IPG and venous scanning were not significantly more sensi-

---

Diagnostic Accuracy of Impedance Plethysmography Compared With Venography in Selected Series

|  | n | SENS (%) | SPEC (%) | PPV (%) | NPV (%) |
|---|---|---|---|---|---|
| Wheeler et al. | 78 | 80.0 | 60.4 | 48.8 | 86.5 |
| Flanigan et al. | 207 | 90.1 | 75.7 | 66.0 | 93.6 |
| Moser et al. | 42 | 60.9 | 100 | 100 | 67.9 |
| Hume et al. | 32 | 77.3 | 100 | 100 | 66.7 |
| Dmochowski et al. | 43 | 93.8 | 48.1 | 51.7 | 92.9 |
| Sandler et al. | 50 | 63.0 | 67.0 | NA | NA |
| Ramchandani et al. | 100 | 63.0 | 83.0 | NA | 77.0 |
| Meyer et al. | 36 | 42.9 | 59.1 | 40.0 | 62.0 |
| Comerota et al. | 308 | 49.0 | 85.0 | 80.0 | 58.0 |
| Paiment et al. | 937 | 12.3 | 99.1 | 46.7 | 92.4 |
| Present series | 49 | 75.0 | 44.8 | 48.4 | 72.2 |

*(Abbreviations: SENS, sensitivity; SPEC, specificity; PPV, positive predictive value; NPV, negative predictive value.*
(Courtesy of Patterson RB, Fowl RJ, Keller JD, et al: *J Vasc Surg* 9:725–730, 1989.)

tive than scanning alone. Specificity was significantly less when IPG was added to venous scanning.

The accuracy of IPG varies substantially at different institutions (table). If B-mode scanning is available, the rarity of isolated iliac vein thrombosis and the high false positive rate of IPG preclude its continued use. In a high-risk patient strongly suspected of having DVT despite normal findings on a scan, venography is in order before anticoagulation is withheld.

▶ Clearly, better approaches are needed to the stubborn problem of diagnosing DVT. B-mode ultrasound in these authors' hands looks promising. Ultrasound is a technique of wide potential applicability in emergency medicine and lately has been popping up in 1 form or another to address a variety of diagnostic problems (1–3). Its major weakness in this indication seems to be its inability to image the veins proximal to the inguinal ligament, for which IPG may still be the noninvasive diagnostic procedure of choice, although the authors recommend doing a venogram initially in these patients.

I look forward to further reports on this technique and hope particularly that emergency medicine physicians will publish their personal experience with the ultrasound equipment that is currently being marketed specifically for ED use.—J. Schoffstall, M.D.

*References*

1. Sternbach G: *Ann Emerg Med* 15:195, 1986.
2. Puylaert JBCM, et al: *N Engl J Med* 317:666, 1987.
3. Munter DW, et al: *Am J Emerg Med* 7:117, 1989.

# 4 Special Emergencies

## Toxicologic Emergencies/Cocaine Abuse

**"Cotton Fever": A Benign Febrile Syndrome in Intravenous Drug Abusers**
Harrison DW, Walls RM (Vancouver Gen Hosp; Univ of British Columbia, Vancouver)
*J Emerg Med* 8:135–139, 1990                                          4–1

Cotton is a well-recognized pyrogen used in animal models to provoke fever and inflammatory response. It has been implicated as the cause of "cotton fever" in intravenous drug addicts who inject drug suspensions that have been filtered through cotton balls. The condition is a benign and self-limiting syndrome, but it may be confused with sepsis.

Woman, 33, was first seen at an ED with malaise, chills, and pain in the abdomen and legs that had started suddenly soon after intravenous self-administration of a mixture of pentazocine and methylphenidate. She admitted having strained the injected material through a cotton filter. Treatment with intravenous fluids and thiamine was initiated while awaiting laboratory and radiographic results. Two hours later, the patient was still febrile, and her level of consciousness started to deteriorate gradually. After consultation with the internal medicine service she was admitted to the hospital, where her symptoms were resolved spontaneously during 12 hours without specific treatment.

Cotton fever in the context of intravenous drug abuse is resolved spontaneously within 12–24 hours. Symptoms may include headache, malaise, chills and rigors, dyspnea, palpitations, nausea, emesis, abdominal pain, low back pain, myalgias, and arthalgias. Patients typically appear acutely ill, with temperatures ranging from 38.5°C to 40.3°C soon after injection. Tachycardia and tachypnea are common, despite otherwise normal cardiorespiratory examinations and chest radiographs.

Recognition of this clinical syndrome along with a history of filtration of injected substances through cotton should alert an ED physician to the possibility of a more benign diagnosis. Such patients might be appropriate candidates for admission to an ED observation unit. Hospital admission would be indicated only if a patient's status does not improve within 12–24 hours after presentation. Such a practice would represent a significant savings in health care costs because it would decrease the number of admissions for febrile drug users by approximately 12% to 20%.

▶ Patients with cotton fever may look acutely ill, with high fever, leukocytosis, and an altered mental status. It's well known that intravenous drug abusers with high fever cannot be prospectively diagnosed as having a benign (e.g., viral) or serious (e.g., endocarditis) cause for their fever with great accuracy; therefore, those with cotton fever should be treated as sepsis until proved otherwise (1). Given the plethora of infections that can occur in the immunocompromised intravenous drug abuser, it's difficult to handle such patients with prolonged observation in the ED, as the authors suggest, unless you have a bona fide observation unit. Remember that this is a retrospective diagnosis only. Many physicians are unaware of this syndrome, but it's probably on the decline with the rise of crack-cocaine. We will, however, see it again as heroin makes its inevitable comeback.—J.R. Roberts, M.D.

*Reference*

1. Marantz PR, et al: *Ann Intern Med* 106:823, 1987.

---

### Clonidine Poisoning in Young Children
Wiley JF II, Wiley CC, Torrey SB, Henretig FM (Children's Hosp of Philadelphia; St Christopher's Hosp for Children; Delaware Valley Regional Poison Control Ctr, Philadelphia)
*J Pediatr* 116:654–658, 1990                                                                                 4–2

---

Clonidine is an α-adrenergic agonist that is used to treat hypertension, migraine, Tourette's syndrome, opiate withdrawal, nicotine addiction and attention deficit disorder with hyperactivity.

The course of clonidine poisoning was retrospectively examined in 47 consecutive inpatients, aged 9–84 months, seen at 2 hospitals in a 5-year period. Their mean age was 27 months.

The mean dose of clonidine was unknown in 21 and was estimated to be 1.6 mg in 26 patients. All but 3 patients had CNS changes, (mainly lethargy, miosis, and hyporeflexia). Nearly 80% had cardiovascular abnormalities (bradycardia, hypotension). About one third of patients had apnea or depressed respirations. Three fourths of the patients were symptomatic within 1 hour of ingesting clonidine. The remainder were symptomatic within 4 hours of ingestion. Routine toxicologic screening does not detect this drug, but specific serum studies detected clonidine in 4 of 5 patients.

Eighteen patients received syrup of ipecac, and 33 underwent gastric lavage. All but 1 patient received activated charcoal. Six patients needed intubation and ventilation. Seven patients were given atropine for bradycardia. Naloxone was given to 19 patients, but only 3 had definite improvement. The mean duration of symptoms was about 10 hours, and the mean hospital stay was 33 hours.

▶ The clinical course of children after accidental ingestion of clonidine has been well documented previously. The key clinical findings are lethargy, bradycardia, apnea, and hypotension. Treatment is usually symptomatic and supportive. For hypotension, dopamine has the longest track record of safety if fluid boli do not restore the blood pressure. The naloxone issue revolves around the fact that individual case reports have suggested that its use in clonidine over-dose will reverse the clinical findings. In this study, only 3 of 19 patients were believed to have clinically benefitted from naloxone. However, the clinical course of these patients was not altered by the use of naloxone. One of the 19 had hypertension after the administration of naloxone (also previously reported) for which he was given hydralazine. The authors call for a prospective, random-ized nalaxone treatment in clonidine overdose. I suggest that we stop using naloxone as an adjunct for clonidine overdose. Key point: The findings of cloni-dine overdose may mimic those of narcotics. If the history is not suggestive of clonidine, naloxone should be given to all such patients.—S. Wason, M.D.

---

**Quantitative Serum Toxic Screening in the Management of Suspected Drug Overdose**
Mahoney JD, Gross PL, Stern TA, Browne BJ, Pollack MH, Reder V, Mulley AG (Massachusetts Gen Hosp, Boston)
*Am J Emerg Med* 8:16–22, 1990                                                4–3

---

The impact of screening blood, urine, and gastric contents on the diag-nosis and treatment of 176 emergency room patients with suspected drug overdose was analyzed retrospectively. Quantitative serum toxic screens, done in 93% of the cases, disclosed positive results for drug overdose in 81%. Six classes of drugs—ethanol, benzodiazepines, salicylates, acet-aminophen, barbiturates, and tricyclic antidepressants—were responsible for almost 70% of all drug detections and were associated with 80% of all admissions. Drug-specific treatment was prompted by toxic screening results in only 1% of the patients. Substances for which specific treat-ment had already been initiated on clinical grounds were confirmed by toxic screening in 7% of the patients. Results of the screening prompted drug-specific treatments to be discontinued in 2%. Nineteen percent of the patients were admitted to a medical service, but only 4% were admit-ted primarily because of their toxic screening results. The other patients were admitted because of clinical abnormalities requiring inpatient care.

Most drug overdoses result from only a few classes of drugs. Results of the toxic screening rarely change the treatment or disposition of patients suspected of overdose. Decisions about treatments and whether to admit such patients are typically based on clinical parameters.

▶ The role of toxic screens is unclear in the emergency setting. The point to keep in mind is that there is no such entity as a "toxic screen." Each hospital has a toxic screen testing for many similar and many different drugs. My mes-sage is: Tell the laboratory exactly what you are looking for and ask them if they can detect it. Keep in mind those drugs whose quantification may lead to specific therapeutic intervention: acetaminophen (*N*-acetylcysteine), iron (defer-oxamine), lithium (hemodialysis), theophylline (hemoperfusion), ethylene glycol, and methanol (hemodialysis). The problem is that many of these drug inges-tions cannot be suspected on clinical grounds because they produce toxicity relatively late in the course of ingestion (e.g., acetaminophen, ethylene glycol, and methanol).— S. Wason, M.D.

---

**Pralidoxime in the Treatment of Carbamate Intoxication**
Kurtz PH (California Dept of Food and Agriculture, Sacramento)
*Am J Emerg Med* 8:68–70, 1990                                                    4–4

---

Carbamate insecticides inhibit cholinesterase enzymes that are essential for normal nerve function. Intoxication by cholinesterase inhibitors is treated with atropine, which blocks acetylcholine receptors. The use of enzyme reactivators such as pralidoxine in carbamate intoxication is controversial. The source of this concern was examined, and some practical guidelines for the use of pralidoxime were given.

Clinicians have no way to predict whether the toxicity of a specific carbamate compound will be enhanced or antagonized by oxime therapy. With few exceptions, atropine has been superior to oximes in treating carbamate intoxication and therefore the antidote of choice. In some cases, oxime therapy combined with atropine therapy is slightly more effective than atropine alone. The use of pralidoxime as an adjunct to atropine is indicated only in cases in which atropine proves inadequate, in serious poisoning with unknown cholinesterase inhibitors, and in serious mixed poisoning of organophosphorus and carbamate compounds together.

▶ There is still some confusion regarding the appropriate use of pralidoxime in cholinesterase inhibitor poisoning. It is generally believed that pralidoxime is indicated for organophosphates where the inhibition of the enzyme may be alleviated by its use, whereas it is believed that pralidoxime may be harmful if given to patients after carbamate overdose. The authors review the literature but are still unable to make a clear recommendation. In my experience, in addition to atropine, pralidoxime should be given to patients when it is certain that an organophosphate has been taken. In other situations, the treating physician should be aware that the so-called contraindications for pralidoxime are based on scant, generally older evidence. In a life-threatening situation, nobody could object to its use.— S. Wason, M.D.

---

**Myocardial Infarction With Normal Coronary Arteries After Acute Exposure to Carbon Monoxide**
Marius-Nunez AL (Edgewater Med Ctr, Chicago)
*Chest* 97:491–494, 1990                                                    4–5

---

Because myocardial ischemia may occur after carbon monoxide poisoning, ECG is a useful screening test in such cases.

Man, 46, was found unconscious after carbon monoxide exposure. Myocardial infarction was demonstrated by ECG and serum enzymes. The coronary angiogram done 1 week after hospitalization did not show evidence of coronary obstructive lesions. The patient's medical profile was negative for risk factors for coronary heart disease.

During carbon monoxide exposure, myocardial damage may occur from (1) a decreased oxygen transport capacity of the blood leading to a reduced amount of oxygen available to tissues, and (2) an impaired mitochondrial function resulting from a reversible inhibition of the intracellular respiration by the formation of cytochrome $a$, $a_3$-CO ligand.

▶ The author does not report novel findings. The take-home message from this report is this: always look for evidence of myocardial infarction in patients who are resuscitated from fires. Infarcts are not limited to the infirm, elderly, or those with risk factors.— S. Wason, M.D.

---

**Use of Diphenhydramine for Local Anesthesia in "Caine"-Sensitive Patients**
Pollack CV Jr, Swindle GM (Univ of Mississippi, Jackson; US Naval Hosp, San Diego)
*J Emerg Med* 7:611–614, 1989                                          4–6

---

The patient with a laceration requiring sutures who reports being allergic to the "caine," local anesthetics (e.g., lidocaine and procaine) poses a problem for the emergency physician. The history often is difficult to interpret, but true hypersensitivity to local anesthetics does occur. Diphenhydramine hydrochloride may be a useful substitute in this situation.

Three patients with lacerations and a history of allergy to the caines were successfully treated using a 1% solution of diphenhydramine for anesthesia. None had adverse effects. Diphenhydramine hydrochloride is a suitable substitute for caine anesthetics in patients who report sensitivity. Infiltration with 1.5–5 mL of 1% solution is recommended; epinephrine in a 1:100,000 dilution may be added. Allergic reactions to diphenhydramine are rare, but local hypersensitivity may develop after repeated doses even if low concentrations are used.

▶ This is a very useful report for emergency physicians indicating that 1% diphenhydramine is a useful alternative to the caines. Although most ED physicians are aware of the topical anesthetic effects of diphenhydramine, this report reminds us of the earlier literature attesting to its parenteral properties. Now we need a comparative study of diphenhydramine infiltration vs. topical application to lacerations vis-à-vis a solution of tetracaine, epinephrine, and cocaine.— S. Wason, M.D.

---

**Rhabdomyolysis: Need for High Index of Suspicion**
Reha WC, Mangano FA, Zeman RK, Pahira JJ (Georgetown Univ Hosp)
*Urology* 34:292–296, 1989                                          4–7

---

Rhabdomyolysis is classically defined as the triad of traumatic skeletal muscle injury, pigmented urine, and acute renal failure. Nontraumatic rhabdomyolysis associated with a more subtle form of myoglobinuria and acute renal failure has also been reported.

Nontraumatic rhabdomyolysis may be more difficult to diagnose than traumatic rhabdomyolysis, and a high index of suspicion is required. A history for certain risk factors, such as jogging, infections, metabolic derangements, seizures, diuretics, alcohol, or drug use, should be sought. Physical examination may show only mild muscle weakness and swelling. Rhabdomyolysis may also occur as a result of prolonged immobilization during surgery

The diagnosis of rhabdomyolysis is confirmed by laboratory studies. Marked elevation of creatinine kinase without associated cardiac or brain injury is a distinguishing diagnostic feature. A disproportionate elevation of serum creatinine to blood urea nitrogen values may also be noted. Routine urinary assays for myoglobin are unreliable, but the presence of pigmented granular casts, consisting of myoglobin and sloughed tubular cells, is suggestive. Radiologic tests with contrast enhancement are contraindicated. If radiography is performed, bilateral dense striated nephrograms are suggestive of the diagnosis, but they may also be secondary to a number of other conditions.

Adequate hydration to maintain a brisk diuresis is the cornerstone of therapy. Mannitol can be used to bring about osmotic diuresis, and furosemide can be given for additional diuresis. The addition of bicarbonate or calcium supplementation remains controversial. Dialysis is indicated for life-threatening hyperkalemia, oliguric or anuric renal failure, uremic pericarditis, or uremic encephalitis. Excellent prognosis is achieved with early diagnosis and prompt treatment.

▶ The authors point out the need to maintain early recognition of rhabdomyolosis if favorable outcome is to be evoked. Further, it should be remembered that the orthotoluidine test (Hema-test) of the urine is unreliable in that it does not differentiate between myoglobin and hemoglobin. Consequently, as the authors point out, the diagnosis rests on a marked elevation of creatine kinase levels in the absence of brain or myocardial injury or causation. Although the orthotoluidine test, as noted, is unreliable, evaluation of the urine sediment for pigmented granular cells may be helpful to evoke the diagnosis.—D.K. Wagner, M.D.

## Organophosphate Poisoning From Wearing a Laundered Uniform Previously Contaminated With Parathion

Clifford NJ, Nies AS (Univ of Colorado, Denver)
JAMA 262:3035–3036, 1989

4–8

The index case spilled a 76% parathion solution on his work uniform contaminating the inguinal area. He apparently showered immediately and changed his clothes and boots. He failed to report the incident to anyone until 2 days later when he developed nausea, vomiting, weakness, and sweating. Plasma cholinesterase level was 340 units/L (nL > 7,000).

One week or so later another worker in the same plant developed nausea, vomiting, and weakness. When seen in an ED, he had a seizure and became apneic. His plasma cholinesterase level was 410 units/L.

A third worker developed nausea, vomiting, miosis, and diaphoresis at an unknown time after the second patient became symptomatic. His cholinesterase level was 500 units/L.

All 3 patients recovered.

Because no cases of organophosphate poisoning were seen in this manufacturing plant for several years before this clustering of cases, the safety officer was able to trace a single uniform that all 3 men had worn. Although it had been laundered several times, analysis revealed 70,000 ppm of parathion.

▶ This report is a timely reminder that clothing contaminated with organophosphates continues to be a potential hazard despite repeated laundering.

The vigilant safety officer should be congratulated for his efforts. One point of curiosity: One would have expected the first patient to be the most seriously sick. Although he had the lowest cholinesterase activity, he was not as sick as the second patient, who had a presumably lower exposure approximately 1 week later. Was this overzealous detective work?—S. Wason, M.D.

---

### The Metabolic Effects of Fatal Cyanide Poisoning

Singh BM, Coles N, Lewis P, Braithwaite RA, Nattrass M, FitzGerald MG (Gen Hosp; Dudley Road Hosp, Birmingham, England)
*Postgrad Med J* 65:923–925, 1989                                                    4–9

---

Detailed toxicologic and metabolic studies were possible in a case of fatal cyanide poisoning.

Man, 24, previously well, was found unconscious after working alone in a silver plating tank removing residue of silver cyanide sludge without protective clothing or a respirator. The air in the tank contained 200 ppm of hydrogen cyanide. Brick-red cyanide burns were present on exposed skin, and there was a strong odor of bitter almonds. The patient was apneic and had a faint pulse of 120 beats/minute but no recordable blood pressure. The pupils were fixed and dilated. Intubation was carried out, and cobalt edetate and 50% dextrose were given. Breathing returned only transiently. The skin was washed and gastric lavage performed. Anuria was followed by a phase of gross polyuria. Acidosis resolved within 24 hours, and blood pressure and urine output were stable at this time, but an electroencephalogram showed no cerebral activity. Brain stem activity was absent 3 days after admission, and ventilation was discontinued.

This patient exhibited lactic acidosis and severe insulin resistance, which persisted despite early detoxification, intensive supportive treatment, and insulin infusion. Acidosis resulted from excess lactate produced by anaerobic glucose metabolism.

► The authors provide data regarding the metabolic defects of fatal cyanide poisoning. Although the presence of lactic acidosis has been recognized, its production pathways have been less well understood. The authors provide plausible explanations. The refractive nature of the condition mandates protective and preventive workplace measures.—D.K. Wagner, M.D.

---

## Superwarfarin Poisoning

Katona B, Wason S (Francis Scott Key Med Ctr, Baltimore; Children's Hosp Med Ctr, Cincinnati; Univ of Cincinnati)
*J Emerg Med* 7:627–631, 1989                                                    4–10

---

Newly synthesized compounds called superwarfarins are currently in use as anticoagulant rodenticides (ACRs). Because the management of patients who have ingested superwarfarins is unclear, the clinical effects were studied in 143 patients in 3 series.

Superwarfarins are more potent than warfarin with longer anticoagulant activity. Their pharmacokinetics in human beings are unknown. Monitoring of the same laboratory parameters should be performed as would be indicated after warfarin ingestion. Prothrombin time (PT) can become prolonged 24–36 hours after ingestion.

Individual case reports from the literature have described patients who had deliberately ingested superwarfarin and probably involved single acute ingestions in most cases. Only 1 of these patients had life-threatening hemorrhage. All patients had prolonged PTs, which were not correctable by menadione (vitamin $K_3$).

In 1 series of 8 children who had ingested variable quantities of ACRs, 2 had normal PTs and none required treatment. In a series of 110 children who had also ingested variable amounts of ACRs, 8 had abnormal PTs. One patient became symptomatic with diarrhea that was fecal occult blood positive. Among 25 children with accidental ingestion of ACR in another series, 16 had normal PTs and none had complications.

Accidental childhood ingestion of ACRs does not generally cause bleeding problems. No treatment should be necessary for children who have ingested 1 or 2 grains of rodent bait. For larger amounts, emesis should be instituted within 30 minutes if possible. If not possible, activated charcoal should be administered. Because deliberate ingestion usually involves large amounts of ACRs, gastric emptying, activated charcoal, and vigilant follow-up, including PT determination over several days, are recommended. Vitamin $K_1$ is the compound of choice in such circumstances.

► If a child ingests standard warfarin sodium (Coumadin)–based rat poison, treatment is not required as long as you can identify the specific product as not being one of the newer, more potent compounds. (It's best to touch base with the regional poison center.) Children who are found playing with superwarfarin compounds can be followed as outpatients by checking PT in 36–48 hours. Those with suicidal ingestions should be admitted. I advise not prescribing routine vitamin K (you should use vitamin K₁ [Aquamephyton], but rather to follow the patient. The vitamin may delay the coagulopathy, making it difficult to know when to stop the follow-up. Clotting defects develop gradually, so it's safe to be conservative. If no coagulopathy is present at 48 hours, you're home free. Superwarfarins demand respect, since significant, prolonged toxicity has occurred.—J.R. Roberts, M.D.

---

**Repeated Acetaminophen Overdosing: Causing Hepatotoxicity in Children**

Henretig FM, Selbst SM, Forrest C, Kearney TK, Orel H, Werner S, Williams TA (The Children's Hosp of Philadelphia; Univ of Pennsylvania; Delaware Valley Regional Poison Control Program, Philadelphia)
*Clin Pediatr* 28:525–528, 1989                                    4–11

---

Data on 2 young children who had hepatotoxicity caused by repeated acetaminophen overdosing were compared with data on similar patients. Hepatic failure developed in both children, aged 11 and 22 months, after receiving acetaminophen suppositories for 8 doses of 60 mg/kg over 32 hours (400 mg/kg/day) and 10 doses of 52 mg/kg over 72 hours (174 mg/kg/day), respectively. An acetaminophen level of 240 mg/mL at 11 hours and 32 mg/L at 24 hours after the last reported dose were in the highly toxic range, even in the context of a single, acute overdose. The overdosage was the result of documented prescription errors. The second child also had renal failure and hypoglycemia. Both patients responded to supportive care.

The similarity of clinical course and laboratory abnormalities in these children to those previously reported in the literature provides support for the causal association between long-term repeated acetaminophen overdosing and significant hepatotoxicity. In light of studies published on acute acetaminophen overdose in children, clinicians should be aware that merely doubling the recommended therapeutic dose of acetaminophen for several days would put children at risk of severe hepatotoxicity.

▶ Most commonly, persistent fever in the child is caused by inadequate or inappropriate dosage with acetaminophen. However, the authors identify 2 situations in which we see repeated acetaminophen administration result in hepatotoxicity. It is important to remember that repeated, inadvertent or deliberate dosing of 1.5 times the recommended therapeutic dosage will rapidly produce toxic levels in the child. Acetaminophen suppositories occur in 120-, 325-, and 650-mg sizes. Their use in the vomiting child should probably be limited to the emergency setting and rarely recommended for home usage.—D.K. Wagner, M.D.

## Pharmacokinetics and Toxic Effects of Diltiazem in Massive Overdose

Ferner RE, Odemuyiwa O, Field AB, Walker S, Volans GN, Bateman DN (Freeman Hosp, Newcastle upon Tyne, England; New Cross Hosp, London)
*Hum Toxicol* 8:497−499, 1989                                              4−12

Little is known of the pharmacokinetics of diltiazem overdose. One patient had drug levels of more than 30 times the estimated maximum therapeutic concentration.

Man, 50, had angina and known stenosis of the anterior descending branch of the left coronary artery. He had taken 98 (60-mg) diltiazem tablets with beer and was hypotensive on arrival at the hospital, with a junctional escape rhythm and nonspecific ST-segment changes. The systolic blood pressure was 55 mm Hg. A 6-second period of ventricular asystole was noted. The patient vomited a dose of activated charcoal with residues of many tablets. A transvenous pacing electrode was placed after 2 intravenous injections of calcium gluconate were ineffective. His blood pressure rose as dopamine was infused, and sinus rhythm returned. Digoxin was given when fast atrial fibrillation appeared. The serum level of diltiazem 4 hours after admission was 6,090 µg/L.

An attempt should be made to remove diltiazem from the gut, because absorption may be greatly prolonged. Patients with severe bradycardia require temporary pacing, whether or not a conduction abnormality is present. Dopamine effectively restores blood pressure. The prognosis would seem to be good if adequate cardiovascular support is provided, even if levels of diltiazem are many times the maximum therapeutic concentration.

▶ This paper reviews the clinical course of a massive diltiazem overdose in a man. Clinical details of overdose with this category of calcium channel blockers are scarce. The paper also reviews some of the suggested management for these agents, including assurance of the ability to insert a pacemaker, the use of calcium salts, and the use of pressor agents. Some authors cite the value of hypertonic saline infusion when combined with calcium salts to convert arrhythmias and restore blood pressure (1). Anecdotally, some authorities have also suggested attempting to utilize glucagon as a last resort for both calcium channel blocker and β-blocker toxicity when massive overdoses of these agents are encountered.—F. Henretig, M.D.

*Reference*

1. Ramoska EA, et al: *Ann Emerg Med* 19:649, 1990.

## Drug- and Toxin-Induced Rhabdomyolysis

Curry SC, Chang D, Connor D (Good Samaritan Med Ctr, Phoenix)
*Ann Emerg Med* 18:1068−1084, 1989                                    4−13

Numerous causes have been identified in rhabdomyolysis, a condition in which injury to skeletal muscle results in the leakage of intracellular contents from myocytes into the plasma. Prompt treatment can prevent complications, but this potentially fatal disease can be difficult to diagnose. Researchers reviewed English literature in the field to define the pathophysiology, etiologic agents, clinical presentation, diagnosis, and treatment of drug- and toxin-induced rhabdomyolysis.

Rhabdomyolysis can result from any process that impairs the production or use of adenosine triphosphate (ATP) by skeletal muscle or causes energy requirements to exceed ATP production. Drugs or toxins that interfere with the production or use of ATP can damage skeletal muscle. Among those substances are agents that deplete the body of potassium, chlorphenoxy herbicides, drugs used to treat hypercholesterolemia, plants, bites or stings of venomous animals, ethanol, heroin, and corticosteroids.

Although pain or weakness from muscle damage would be anticipated, at least 50% of patients with rhabdomyolysis in 1 study did not have such symptoms at admission. And symptoms such as grossly red urine, fever, and leukocytosis may be mistaken for signs of other illnesses. Clinical presentation varies considerably. Patients who have had seizures, fight restraints, and have an altered mental status or serious fluid and electrolyte disorders should be suspected of having rhabdomyolysis, as should all patients who are symptomatic from metabolic poisons. Myoglobinuria and renal failure are major complications of the disease. Other conditions that may accompany rhabdomyolysis include hyperkalemia, hyperuricemia, hypocalcemia, hypercalcemia, disseminated intravascular coagulation, metabolic acidosis, acute cardiomyopathy, respiratory failure, compartment syndromes, and peripheral neuropathies.

The most sensitive indicator of muscle damage is elevated serum creatine phosphokinase levels. The urine dipstick test for blood is not sensitive for rhabdomyolysis. Areas of soft tissue involved in the disease have been identified by bone scans with technetium 99m phosphorus compounds, sonograms, and CT and gallium scans.

Treatment should begin with the halting of further muscle destruction. The patient may have to be controlled with sedatives or even pharmacologic paralysis. Hyperthermia is then treated in the same way as heat stroke. The patient should be examined regularly for compartment syndrome. Renal failure can be minimized by the coadministration of mannitol and saline and urinary alkalinization. With accurate diagnosis and treatment of the various complications, most patients will recover from rhabdomyolysis without permanent disability.

▶ This extraordinary review article is far and away the most comprehensive discussion of rhabdomyolysis that I have ever seen and should be part of every emergency physician's and toxicologist's files. It includes an exhaustive survey of the literature regarding drugs and toxins known to have caused this syndrome, as well as an excellent review of basic muscle physiology and mechanisms of toxicity and a rational discussion of the approach to clinical diagnosis and management. There is a cogent description of the details involved in interpreting urine and blood tests for myoglobinemia, myoglobinuria, and hemoglobinuria. (See also Abstract 4–7.)—F. Henretig, M.D.

---

### Chloroquine Poisoning in a Child

Kelly JC, Wasserman GS, Bernard WD, Schultz C, Knapp JF (Children's Mercy Hosp; Univ of Missouri, Kansas City)
*Ann Emerg Med* 19:47–50, 1990                                                    4–14

---

The toxic effects and lethality of chloroquine in children are widely known. An infant died after receiving a dose of only 300 mg.

Girl, 12 months, was seen in the ED about 30 minutes after sucking on 12 chloroquine tablets and perhaps eating 1. She exhibited apnea, no blood pressure, and a pulse rate of 20. After resuscitation was begun, an ECG showed ventricular bradycardia and wide QRS complexes, which were converted to normal by an isoproterenol drip (Fig 4–1). Gastric lavage was performed, and activated charcoal was given. She was then taken to another hospital. The infant had continuous seizures and a Glasgow Coma Scale score of 3. Seven hours after ingestion of the chloroquine, serum level was 4.4 mg/L. Hypokalemia was present, but after

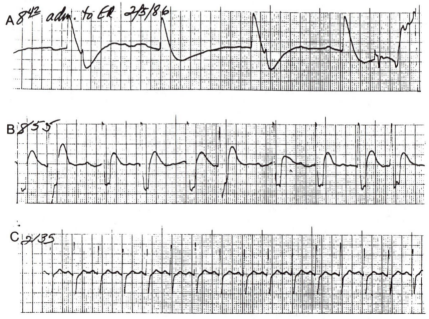

Fig 4–1.—ECG recorded at 8:42 PM, 2 minutes after infant's admission to emergency department, shows idioventricular rhythm with ventricular bradycardia of 33 after chloroquine ingestion; **B,** isoproterenol given at 8:50 PM—ECG recording at 8:55 PM shows progressive recovery with ventricular rate of 56 and atrial rate of 75; **C,** ECG recording at 9:35 PM shows normal sinus rhythm with rate of 115. (Courtesy of Kelly JC, Wasserman GS, Bernard WD, et al: *Ann Emerg Med* 19:47–50, 1990.)

intravenous injection of maintenance levels of potassium, the potassium level rose to 7.3 mEq/L at 24 hours. Urine output became low. She was treated with phenytoin, polystyrene sulfonate, furosemide, restricted fluids, mannitol, dexamethasone, and hyperventilation, but she continued to deteriorate. Eventually life support was discontinued.

This case demonstrates the extreme sensitivity of children to chloroquine and establishes a new minimum lethal dose and serum level. Because supportive treatment in cases such as this is futile, further study to find better treatment for children is needed. Use of the bitter-tasting generic form of the drug might decrease the amount children ingest.

▶ Chloroquine is one of those drugs that can kill quickly, especially in the pediatric patient. A relatively small number of milligrams per kilogram can be rapidly fatal in the small child. I don't think that people respect the potential danger of chloroquine as much as they should. The major problem with chloroquine is that it has a quinidine-like activity on the cardiovascular system and is very rapidly absorbed from the stomach. One should still attempt gastric decontamination and administration of activated charcoal but realize that there is little response to the usual decontamination procedures. It is then important to provide hemodynamic monitoring to observe for quinidine effects.

Several articles cited in the literature suggest intravenous diazepam (Valium) used early in the treatment plan may prevent the patient from having seizures and complete cardiovascular collapse. Although the mechanism is not fully understood, the pediatric dosages include a loading dose of 1 mg/kg, followed by a continuous infusion of 0.25–0.40 mg/kg/hour for approximately 48 hours if cardiac symptoms occur or if the dose of chloroquine exceeds 30 mg/kg of body weight. Patients should be admitted to an intensive care unit, and one should be prepared to intubate and provide ventilatory support. Prevention of this tragedy is obviously the only safe alternative. Chloroquine should be prescribed in its bitter generic form with childproof caps and labeling that lets the parent or patient know that this medication is potentially fatal if ingested by a child.—R.W. Schafermeyer, M.D.

---

**Acute Iron Poisoning: Rescue With Macromolecular Chelators**
Mahoney JR Jr, Hallaway PE, Hedlund BE, Eaton JW (Univ of Minnesota, Biomedical Frontiers, Inc, Minneapolis)
*J Clin Invest* 84:1362–1366, 1989                                     4–15

---

Acute iron intoxication is an important cause of life-threatening accidental poisoning in children. Deferoxamine (DFO), a potent iron chelator, is the drug of choice for treatment of acute iron poisoning, but its effectivity is limited by its adverse effects on blood pressure. To obviate this problem, a new class of iron chelators comprised of DFO covalently attached to high molecular weight carbohydrate polymers, such as dextran and hydroethyl starch, was developed. These macrolecular chelators do not cause detectable hypotension in experimental animals, even when administered intravenously in very large doses; they are less toxic and persist in the circulation much longer than the unconjugated chelator.

The efficacy of these new macromolecular chelators in alleviating the effects of acute iron poisoning was studied in an animal model. Intraperitoneal or oral administration of the conjugated DFO completely prevented the mortality associated with lethal doses of iron. In contrast, treatment with polymers alone or a combination of free DFO and polymers did not significantly improve survival. The high molecular weight iron chelators also abrogated the iron-mediated hepatotoxicity, suppressing the release of alanine aminotransferase. Delayed administration of the DFO conjugate 1 hour after giving iron intraperitoneally was also associated with a significant improvement in survival.

Macromolecular DFO conjugates hold promise for the effective treatment of acute iron intoxication. High molecular weight DFO conjugates may also be useful in other clinical conditions in which control of free, reactive iron is therapeutically desirable.

▶ This paper presents an interesting approach to the development of a new antidote and examines the role of deferoxamine covalently attached to high molecular weight polymers to develop a macromolecular chelating agent that the authors suggest may be preferable to the currently available deferoxamine in the treatment of acute iron poisoning. The results are convincing and their discussion suggests that there may certainly be a future potential for these agents, but in my clinical experience, their implication that the efficacy of deferoxamine is significantly limited by its adverse effects on blood pressure has not proved to be true. In fact, the majority of children and adults who are iron poisoned require no chelation therapy, and in those who do, the current regimens of deferoxamine, which are routinely recommended, seem quite well tolerated. For patients with life-threatening toxicity, the deferoxamine infusion should be given at a maximum rate of 15/mg/kg/hour. Using lower doses is probably sufficient for moderate intoxications. The frequently cited problem of hypotension when deferoxamine is given intravenously has, in fact, never been experienced in my own practice, even in the critically ill, acidotic children with serum iron levels of nearly 7,000 µg/dL (1). One does well with the currently available form of deferoxamine as long as the currently recommended regimens are followed.—F. Henretig, M.D.

*Reference*

1. Henretig FM, et al: *Ann Emerg Med* 12:306, 1983.

---

**A Toxicity Study of Parenteral Thiamine Hydrochloride**
Wrenn KD, Murphy F, Slovis CM (Grady Mem Hosp; Emory Univ, Atlanta)
*Ann Emerg Med* 18:867–870, 1989                                            4–16

---

Overt thiamine deficiency syndromes, such as Wernicke-Korsakoff encephalopathy or beriberi, may require rapid parenteral repletion. However, because of previously reported serious and sometimes fatal reactions to parenterally administered thiamine, physicians are reluctant to administer thiamine hydrochloride intravenously. In a prospective study designed to assess the safety of large doses of intravenously administered thiamine hydrochloride, 989 consecutive patients, aged 16–80 years, were given a 100-mg bolus of thiamine hydrochloride intravenously. Alcoholism was the most common reason (80%) for administration of thiamine.

A total of 1,070 doses of thiamine hydrochloride were given. Adverse reactions were observed in 12 patients (1.1%). Minor reactions consisting of transient localized burning were observed in 11 patients (1.02%). A major reaction consisting of generalized pruritus was observed in 1 patient (0.093%).

Thiamine hydrocholoride may be administered intravenously without undue concern in patients at significant risk for thiamine deficiency. Intradermal tests before administration may not be warranted except in patients with previous allergic reactions.

▶ This report demonstrates quite adequately that intravenous thiamine administration is a safe procedure. The number of reactions, most of which could have occurred if intravenous saline was injected too rapidly, was very small. Their "major reaction," which consisted of mild and apparently self-limited pruritus, was not described as requiring any intervention whatsoever. This incidence of side effects occurring in approximately 1,000 doses of a parenterally administered drug could easily have occurred had a placebo been given, and I would consider this study to prove conclusively that parenteral thiamine may be given safely by the intravenous route.—F. Henretig, M.D.

## Severe Metabolic Acidosis After Acute Naproxen Sodium Ingestion
Martinez R, Smith DW, Frankel LR (Stanford Univ)
*Ann Emerg Med* 18:1102–1104, 1989                                      4–17

The propionic acids are the least toxic class of nonsteroidal anti-inflammatory drugs (NSAIDs), but reports of adverse side effects, such as acidosis, continue to accumulate. Severe metabolic acidosis developed in a patient after acute overdosage of naproxen sodium, a propionic acid derivative.

Girl, 15 years, ingested 50 275-mg tablets of naproxen sodium. Profound metabolic acidosis, obtundation, and generalized seizures rapidly followed naproxen ingestion. With supportive care, serum bicarbonate levels returned to normal 12 hours after admission, correlating with the known pharmacokinetics of naproxen. There were no long-term sequelae from the overdose.

Careful examination of the acid-base status should be performed in patients with overdose of NSAIDs. Because both naproxen and its metabolites are acids, the acidosis may be related to the large amounts of naproxen and its metabolites in the serum. Treatment is directed toward limiting drug absorption and supportive care. Hospital observation is recommended for patients with intentional overdose and those who are symptomatic or have impaired liver and kidney functions.

▶ This case report of a severe overdose of naproxen in a teenage girl simply proves the old truth that if you take too much of anything, bad consequences may result. On the whole, overdoses with propionic acid derivatives of NSAIDs tend to be fairly benign; however, reports of significant effects, including seizures and metabolic acidosis, are accumulating even with this category of agents. The bottom line is that patients who overdose on these agents and have any significant symptomatology should probably be admitted to a hospital at least overnight for observation on seizure precautions and should be followed for impaired hepatic or renal function, as well as monitored for their acid-base status.—F. Henretig, M.D.

### Absorption of Lidocaine and Prilocaine After Application of a Eutectic Mixture of Local Anesthetics (EMLA) on Normal and Diseased Skin

Juhlin L, Hägglund G, Evers H (Univ Hosp, Uppsala, Sweden; Astra Pain Control, Södertälje, Sweden)

*Acta Derm Venereol (Stockh)* 69:18–22, 1989 4–18

A eutectic mixture of 5% lidocaine and prilocaine (EMLA) is used topically under occlusion to produce anesthesia for superficial surgery. This material was applied for 1–2 hours to 25–100 cm$^2$ of skin of healthy subjects. In addition, 4–6 g of EMLA was applied for 1 hour to normal and diseased skin in a 25-cm$^2$ area on the forearm.

When applied to normal skin EMLA was absorbed more rapidly from the face than from the forearm. Absorption from diseased skin was faster than from normal skin, and higher plasma levels were reached. The anesthetic effect occurred more rapidly but lasted a shorter time. Plasma levels in the general circulation were 100 times lower than those associated with toxicity. Levels of prilocaine were 200%–300% lower than those of lidocaine in the general circulation.

Care must be taken in applying EMLA when large areas of diseased skin are treated. The finding that analgesic and vascular effects on lesional skin begin sooner and disappear faster than on normal skin should be kept in mind when superficial surgery is carried out.

▶ This report once again serves to remind us that topical anesthetic agents may have the potential for causing systemic toxicity, although the particular findings of this study are offered as reassurance that when used appropriately, this particular combination of anesthetics is presumably unlikely to reach toxic level in the systemic circulation. However, it is well to remember that in pediatric practice it is commonly suggested that topical mixtures of lidocaine gel, aluminum and magnesium hydroxide (Maalox), and diphenhydramine hydro chloride (Benadryl) be applied to oral mucous membranes for the treatment of viral stomatitis and that there have been now several reports of serious and potentially life-threatening toxicity resulting from ingestions of viscous lidocaine. My own inclination is to avoid the use of topical lidocaine anesthetics as much as possible in average emergency center practice, particularly in terms of medications to be prescribed for at-home use.—F. Henretig, M.D.

---

**Whole-Bowel Irrigation Versus Activated Charcoal in Sorbitol for the Ingestion of Modified-Release Pharmaceuticals**
Kirshenbaum LA, Mathews SC, Sitar DS, Tenebein M (Univ of Manitoba; Manitoba Poison Control Ctr, Winnipeg)
*Clin Pharmacol Ther* 46:264–271, 1989                                                          4–19

---

Whole-bowel irrigation is a routine colonoscopy preparative procedure that involves rapid enteral administration of large volumes of polyethylene glycol electrolyte lavage solution to irrigate the gastrointestinal tract. The efficacy of whole-bowel irrigation as a potential decontamination strategy after overdose with modified-release pharmaceuticals was compared with administration of activated charcoal in sorbitol. In this 3-phase, randomized crossover protocol, 10 adult volunteers ingested 9 325-mg doses of enteric coated acetylsalicylic acid on 3 occasions with at least 1 week between each administration period.

Compared with control, both whole-bowel irrigation and activated charcoal in sorbitol decreased peak salicylic acid concentration, time-to-zero salicylic acid concentration, and area under the serum salicylic acid concentration vs. time curves. However, whole-bowel irrigation was significantly superior to activated charcoal in sorbitol in all 3 criteria (Fig

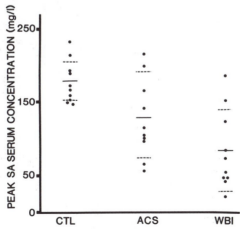

Fig 4–2.—Peak serum salicylic acid *(SA)* concentrations for control *(CTL)*, activated charcoal in sorbitol *(ACS)*, and whole-bowel irrigation *(WBI)* phases after ingestion of 2,925 mg (16.25 mmol) of enteric-coated acetylsalicylic acid. Individual data are reported as mean values *(solid line)* ± SD *(dashed line)*. A treatment effect was demonstrated ($P < .01$), and treatments differed from each other ($P < .05$). (Courtesy of Kirshenbaum LA, Mathews SC, Sitar DS, et al: *Clin Pharmacol Ther* 46:264–271, 1989.)

4–2). Adverse effects were fewer and less severe during whole-bowel irrigation, and 9 persons preferred whole-bowel irrigation over activate charcoal in sorbitol.

Whole-bowel irrigation should be considered for the treatment of overdose with other modified-release pharmaceuticals. Because modified-release pharmaceuticals can persist for several hours within the small intestine, at which time administration of syrup of ipecac, gastric lavage, and activated charcoal would be ineffective, whole-bowel irrigation may be an effective intervention.

▶ This is another application for whole-bowel irrigation that has been brought to prominence for us by Dr. Tennenbein and his colleagues from Winnipeg. This group has been touting the benefits of using a polyethylene glycol electrolyte lavage solution to irrigate the contents of the bowel in the toxicologic context for several years now, beginning with its use in pediatric elemental iron intoxications, an area for which gastric emptying procedures and the use of activated charcoal have been of relatively low value. Subsequently, whole-bowel irrigation has been adopted by the toxicologic community as potentially beneficial in a variety of situations, including patients admitted with late symptoms from massive overdoses, ingestions with iron and other heavy metals that are not bound to activated charcoal, and the ingestion of packets or vials of foreign materials such as crack-cocaine. Now in the context of delayed-release pharmaceutical products, there is yet another role for whole-bowel irrigation. In my own experience, this technique has proved to be very efficacious with minimal side effects even in young pediatric patients such as toddlers who have consumed massive amounts of their parents' iron pills and for whom initial attempts at gastric evacuation have been followed by abdominal films that still visualize radioopaque matter. Patients tolerate whole-bowel irrigation without obvious significant accumulation of fluid or alteration in their electrolyte status, and I expect to see this technique being used more and more in these slightly unusual poisoning cases where routine efforts at gastric evacuation or the use of activated charcoal might have suboptimal effects.—F. Henretig, M.D.

**Charcoal Lung: Bronchiolitis Obliterans After Aspiration of Activated Charcoal**
Elliott CG, Colby TV, Kelly TM, Hicks HG (Univ of Utah; Mayo Clinic and Found, Rochester, Minn)
*Chest* 96:672–674, 1989                                          4–20

Suicide attempts involving ingestion of an overdose of sedatives or tricyclics are routinely treated by stomach lavage or induced emesis, followed by instillation of activated charcoal. Bronchiolitis obliterans accompanied by hypoxemia and hypercapnia has been associated with aspiration of gastric contents containing food particles but not with aspiration of gastric contents and activated charcoal. Obliterative bronchiolitis developed in a girl after she aspirated activated charcoal.

Girl, 16 years, was brought to the ED of a local hospital after ingestion of 60 nortriptyline tablets. The stomach was lavaged until clear of pill fragments, followed by lavage with activated charcoal. The patient had a grand mal seizure accompanied by cardiac arrest 10 minutes later. After successful resuscitation, she was transferred comatose to the University of Utah hospital. Chest radiography revealed bilateral alveolar infiltration and a right subpulmonic pneumothorax. Fiberoptic bronchoscopy showed extensive charcoal staining of both main stem bronchi but no signs of tracheal laceration. A total of 33 mL of thin gray sputum was suctioned during the next 24 hours. Over the next few days, her arterial blood gas values improved to a pH of 7.46, and the coma resolved. The patient underwent extubation on day 15 after admission and discharged 4 days later. She was readmitted 6 days later, complaining of fever, cough, dyspnea, and headaches. The sternum moved paradoxically and she had late inspiratory rales over both lower lobes. She slowly deteriorated to where she required reinstitution of mechanical ventilation. The patient died 10 weeks after readmission and 14 weeks after the suicide attempt.

Postmortem examination revealed extensive charcoal deposition along the airways in all regions of the lung. Histologic staining visualized scarring and fibrous obliteration of the bronchioles associated with a prominent foreign body giant cell reaction. There was no evidence of food aspiration or pneumonia at the time of death. The final diagnosis was extensive bronchiolitis obliterans and progressive respiratory failure associated with massive aspiration of activated charcoal. Chest radiography failed to identify the large amount of charcoal aspirated during lavage.

▶ This paper describes the occurrence of a bronchiolitis obliterans syndrome after massive aspiration of activated charcoal in the context of a severe tricyclic antidepressant overdose. This girl, who was 16 years old, was described as being combative at the time of her admission to the hospital. There is little detail offered about additional clinical findings on her arrival, but she underwent gastric lavage and activated charcoal administration. Ten minutes later, a grand mal seizure occurred, which was accompanied by cardiac arrest. The primary subject matter of this report is the documentation of a pulmonary complication following aspiration of activated charcoal; that it's not great to aspirate a lot of charcoal into the tracheobronchial tree is not particularly surprising. In fact, as the authors acknowledge, similar cases have been noted previously. The traditional dogma has been that aspirating charcoal is no worse than aspirating stomach contents, but I doubt that it has any protective effects in this context. What impressed me most about this paper is the reminder that patients who take massive overdoses of tricyclic antidepressants are walking time bombs. I think the take-home message of this case is that before you try to put a lavage tube down a struggling 16-year-old girl who has just taken 60 nortriptyline tablets and follow it with a belly full of charcoal, you should probably do a careful and controlled elective tracheal intubation.—F. Henretig, M.D.

### Efficacy of Charcoal Cathartic Versus Ipecac in Reducing Serum Acetaminophen in a Simulated Overdose

McNamara RM, Aaron CK, Gemborys M, Davidheiser S (Med College of Pennsylvania, Philadelphia; New York City Poison Control Ctr; McNeil Pharmaceuticals, Fort Washington, Pa)

*Ann Emerg Med* 18:934–938, 1989                                     4–21

The role of gastric emptying as the initial step in the management of poisoned patients has been questioned. Some physicians have advocated immediate activated charcoal administration. In patients with acetaminophen overdose, ipecac-induced emesis might interfere with subsequent

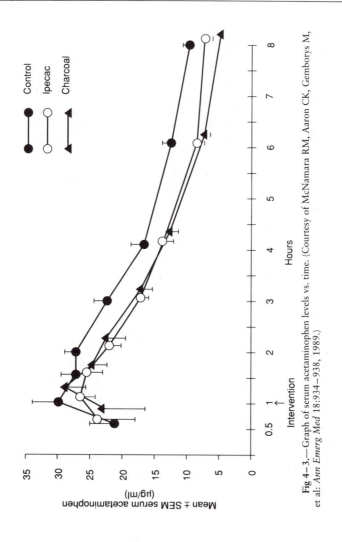

Fig 4–3.—Graph of serum acetaminophen levels vs. time. (Courtesy of McNamara RM, Aaron CK, Gemborys M, et al: *Ann Emerg Med* 18:934–938, 1989.)

oral antidotal treatment. Therefore the efficacy of initial therapy with ipecac was compared with activated charcoal-cathartic in a simulated acetaminophen overdose.

Ten healthy volunteers participated. After taking 3 g of acetaminophen, they were given no treatment, 30 mL of ipecac, or 50 g of activated charcoal-sorbitol solution at 1 hour. Serial acetaminophen levels were determined at intervals for 8 hours. Both treatments significantly decreased the area under the curve compared with no treatment. No significant differences were found between ipecac and activated charcoal-cathartic (Fig 4–3).

Both ipecac-induced emesis and activated charcoal-cathartic were effective in reducing total drug absorption. When emesis is contraindicated or when prolonged emesis might interfere with the timely administration of *N*-acetylcysteine (NAC), physicians should consider using activated charcoal-cathartic alone as initial treatment.

---

### Large Surface Area Activated Charcoal and the Inhibition of Aspirin Absorption

Dillon EC Jr, Wilton JH, Barlow JC, Watson WA (Univ of British Columbia, Vancouver; Royal Columbian Hosp, New Westminister, BC; Millard Fillmore Hosp, Buffalo; Univ of Missouri, Kansas City)
*Ann Emerg Med* 18:547–552, 1989                                               4–22

---

Studies suggest that although the surface area of an activated charcoal preparation is important in determining its adsorptive ability in binding drugs in the gastrointestinal tract, other factors may have an important impact on the net effect of the preparation on drug absorption. The abilities of 2 activated charcoal preparations to inhibit gastrointestinal absorption of aspirin in humans were compared.

Actidose-Aqua, 1,500 $m^2/g$, and Super Char, 3,000 $m^2/g$, were compared in 12 healthy men. The men fasted for 8 hours before and 4 hours after taking an oral dose of 20 mg of aspirin/kg. One hour after taking the aspirin, each man received no charcoal, 25 g of Actidose-Aqua, or 25 g of Super Char in a randomized crossover design. Total urine volumes were collected over 12-hour intervals from 12 hours before the aspirin was taken to 72 hours after the aspirin dose. The fractions of aspirin dose recovered in urine were 0.96, 0.78, and 0.5 for the control, Actidose-Aqua, and Super Char treatment phases, respectively. In vitro, Super Char bound more salicylic acid than Actidose-Aqua at pH 8.1.

Both activated charcoal preparations were effective adsorbents, reducing the gastrointestinal absorption of aspirin when given 1 hour after aspirin dosing. Super Char, the larger-surfaced area preparation, was 2.6-fold more effective than Actidose-Aqua in decreasing the gastrointestinal absorption of aspirin. The relationship between surface area and the clinical effectiveness of activated charcoals in inhibiting drug absorption is supported.

▶ This simple, yet elegant, study supports many others that have demonstrated the superiority of superactivated charcoal over regular-activated charcoal. Two points: First, it has never been demonstrated that this difference affects clinical outcome. Second, as of this writing, Super Char is not available in the United States because its only manufacturer has stopped production as a result of technical problems.— S. Wason, M.D.

---

**Potentiation of Cocaine Toxicity With Calcium Channel Blockers**
Derlet RW, Albertson TE (Univ of California, Davis Med Ctr, Sacramento)
*Am J Emerg Med* 7:464–468, 1989                                        4–23

---

Treatment modalities for cocaine intoxication have been empirically selected to antagonize cocaine-induced signs and symptoms and include treatment with calcium channel blockers. An animal model of cocaine intoxication was used to assess the efficacy of 3 calcium channel blockers in preventing cocaine-induced seizures and death. Rats were pretreated with normal saline (control), diltiazem, nifedipine, or verapamil 30 minutes before being challenged with cocaine hydrochloride, 70 mg/kg, intraperitoneally.

In control animals, seizures occurred within 6 minutes, followed by death within 10 minutes. Cocaine-induced seizures and death occurred more rapidly in animals pretreated with diltiazem, nifedipine, or verapamil than in controls, and at specific doses, death rate was higher in all pretreated animals than in controls. When lower doses of cocaine were used after pretreatment with nifedipine, 2 mg/kg, significant augmentation of the incidence of seizures and death were observed.

Clinically, available calcium channel blockers fail to protect against the toxic effects of cocaine and, in fact, many augment cocaine-induced seizures and death in rats. Calcium channel blockers may enhance uptake of cocaine and the cerebral delivery of cocaine through peripheral peritoneal or cerebral vasodilation. In addition, these agents may induce pump failure to the adrenergic crisis incited by cocaine. Calcium channel blockers also may augment cocaine intoxicity by interacting at selected sites in the CNS.

▶ The search for a cocaine antidote continues. Absence of demonstated cocaine receptors, a plethora of adverse clinical effects, and the inconsistency of animal studies all have been obstacles to defining the best clinical approach to serious cocaine toxicity. Even β-blockers have recently been incriminated. Although used for years to combat tachycardia, propranolol has been demonstrated to augment cocaine-induced coronary artery vasospasm (1).

There is evidence to support the use of calcium channel blockers for the treatment of severe cocaine-induced hypertension or coronary constriction, but their parameters were not evaluated in this study. Unfortunately, the authors looked at only the effect of pretreatment on death by seizures. Benzodiazepines, in high enough doses to be effective, still remain the first-line choice for cocaine neurotoxicity. Based on this study, it would be premature to label calcium channel blockers as worthless, or even dangerous, therapy for cocaine toxicity.—J.R. Roberts, M.D. ·

*Reference*

1. Lange RA, et al: *Ann Intern Med* 112:897, 1990.

---

**Acute Cocaine Abuse Associated With Cerebral Infarction**
Seaman ME (Valley Med Ctr, Fresno, Calif)
*Ann Emerg Med* 19:34–37, 1990                                          4–24

---

Ischemic cerebral infarction temporally associated with cocaine abuse has been reported. Among the possible mechanisms by which infarction may occur are promotion of thrombogenesis, vasospasm, impaired cerebral vascular autoregulation, and adverse affects on cerebral metabolism.

Woman, 29, smoked 1 g of crack-cocaine in about 1 hour, then suffered a tonic-clonic seizure lasting 1 minute. An initial noncontrast CT scan of the brain was normal, showing no signs of cerebral infarction or hemorrhage. Further work-up on the second day of her hospitalization included an echocardiogram, which demonstrated no valvular vegetations or thrombus. On the third day, Holter monitoring showed rare premature ventricular contractions and several short runs of ventricular tachycardia. On the fifth day, a repeat noncontrast CT scan of the brain demonstrated a cerebral infarction in the right basal ganglion. The patient was hospitalized for 3 weeks, during which she had improvement in left leg strength but not in the left arm motor deficit.

This case stresses that neurologic deficits after cocaine abuse may result not only from intracranial bleeding or subarachnoid hemorrhage but also from cerebral infarction.

▶ The patient in this report had a seventh cranial nerve deficit as well as a paralyzed left arm, so this disturbing report does not suggest that patients with cocaine-induced seizures should be hospitalized for delayed development of cerebral pathology. Usually, if the initial CT and results of the cervical puncture are normal, the diagnosis of stroke is not pursued unless other findings crop up. A high percentage of patients with cocaine-induced stroke have an underlying cerebral aneurysm or arteriovenous malformation, but this report links the infarction to thrombosis or vasospasm instead of hemorrhage. Cocaine-induced cerebral vasculitis, which can mimic stroke, can be diagnosed only by arteriogram (1).—J.R. Roberts, M.D.

*Reference*

1. Kaye BR, Fainstat M: *JAMA* 258:2104, 1987.

---

**Neonatal Cocaine-Related Seizures**
Kramer LD, Locke GE, Ogunyemi A, Nelson L (King–Drew Med Ctr, Los Angeles)
*J Child Neurol* 5:60–64, 1990                                                    4–25

Cocaine abuse is associated with a variety of severe acute neurologic complications in the abuser, including ischemic stroke, subarachnoid and intraparenchymal hemorrhage, headaches, syncope, seizures, and death. Sixteen children with presumed cocaine-related seizures caused by maternal consumption were observed.

The children's ages ranged from 16 hours to 8 years at the time of the examination. All were assessed only because of requests for neurologic consultation. The mothers' pregnancy histories were similar. The children uniformly exhibited postdelivery tremulousness, irritability, and excessive startle responses. Shortly after birth, each child had stereotypic episodes with ictal electroencephalographic confirmation in 7 cases. Eight neonates continued to have seizures after the first month of life.

Several mechanisms may be involved in a child with cocaine-related seizures. Transient neurochemical changes in the neonatal period may be precursors of long-term changes and epilepsy. Case-control studies are needed to determine the degree of long-term potential for the induction of epilepsy by cocaine.

▶ This scenario is probably of more relevance to the neonatologist faced with a seizing newborn, but infants recently discharged home are also at risk for cocaine-related seizure if the mother still uses the drug. Cocaine is excreted in breast milk, and the baby who breathes sidestream or exhales crack smoke can become cocaine toxic. Other obstetric sequelae of cocaine use include spontaneous abortion and abruptio placentae. A transient decrease in cardiac output at birth has been reported in infants of cocaine-using mothers (1).—J.R. Roberts, M.D.

*Reference*

1. van de Bor M, et al: *Pediatrics* 85:30, 1990.

---

**Reversible Cardiomyopathy Associated With Cocaine Intoxication**
Chokshi SK, Moore R, Pandian NG, Isner JM (Tufts Univ, Boston)
*Ann Intern Med* 111:1039–1040, 1989                                              4–26

Cocaine intoxication may produce cardiovascular complications including acute infarction. Dilated cardiomyopathy rarely is described.

Acutely dilated cardiomyopathy in temporal relation to smoking crack-cocaine was observed.

Woman, 35, was admitted with seizures after daylong smoking of crack. Hypotension was treated with intravenous fluids and dopamine, and because of severe hypoxemia, intubation and mechanical ventilation were initiated. An ECG showed only sinus tachycardia. Echography showed left ventricular dilation with severe, global ventricular hypokinesis; the estimated left ventricular ejection fraction was 10%. Inotropic agents and diuretic therapy were given, but an intra-aortic balloon assist device was placed because intracardiac filling pressures remained elevated. Results of endomyocardial biopsy were normal. The patient required no pressor agents after the first week. Repeat echocardiography showed a nondilated left ventricle with a left ventricular ejection fraction of 45%.

The patient's course resembled those reported in patients with pheochromocytoma and associated catecholamine cardiomyopathy. Reversible depression of myocardial contractility has been ascribed to a direct effect of high levels of circulating catecholamines on cardiac myocytes. Acutely depressed ventricular function is a potential sequel of cocaine abuse. Aggressive treatment is indicated.

▶ Fortunately, the cardiomyopathy in this report was reversible and responded to standard therapy for congestive heart failure. Contraction band necrosis and infiltrative myocarditis have been associated with both chronic cocaine use and pheochromocytoma (1), so there may be a common pathophysiology. Other causes of dyspnea in the cocaine user are noncardiogenic pulmonary edema, cocaine-induced myocardial infarction, pulmonary hemorrhage, pneumonia, or pneumothorax. Of course, an alcoholic cardiomyopathy may coexist. As with the seizure work-up in a child, it appears that a drug screen may uncover an unexpected toxic cause for what seems like straightforward congestive heart failure.—J.R. Roberts, M.D.

*Reference*

1. Virmani R, et al: *Am Heart J* 115:1068, 1988.

---

**Migrainelike Headache and Cocaine Use**
Satel SL, Gawin FH (Yale Univ; West Haven Veterans Hosp, West Haven, Conn)
*JAMA* 261:2995–2996, 1989                                                      4–27

---

Three patients had new-onset migraine-like headaches that were temporally associated with cocaine use. They had no history of trauma, illness, or major medical problems associated with using cocaine. None was dependent on alcohol or opiates. No patient had a family history of migraine.

Man, 27, had used 5–8 g of cocaine/week for 1 year, both by smoking and intravenous administration. For 1 month he had smoked 3 g of cocaine/day. Throbbing headaches had developed behind the right eye 5 days before admission, associated with sensitivity to light and noise. The pain responded rapidly to cocaine administration, but recurrent pain after 90 minutes prompted the serial readministration of cocaine. There were no neurologic abnormalities, and meningeal signs were absent. Lumbar puncture was refused. The headache responded to some degree to oral ibuprofen, and subsequently headaches were aborted by sublingual ergotamine tartrate. After 2 months the patient was abstinent from cocaine and had had no further headaches.

Headache in cocaine users is ascribed to the aftereffects of cocaine binging. There is evidence relating migraine to serotonin dysregulation, and cocaine influences serotonergic function. The time course of the headaches is consistent with the rapid response of migraine to serotonin-enhancing agents such as ergot.

▶ It's tempting to attribute headache during a cocaine binge to this migraine variant, but life is not so simple. Cocaine can cause stroke (via cerebral infarct, subarachnoid hemorrhage, intracerebral hemorrhage) or cerebral vasculitis (1–2). Clinically it's probably impossible to differentiate these entities, so most patients will require lumbar puncture and CT. Vasculitis is diagnosed only with an arteriogram. Also, headache can be related to head trauma during a cocaine-induced seizure or a blow to the head from a drug deal gone bad. Subdural or epidural hematoma or skull fracture is in the differential. If the drug is used intravenously or the patient has AIDS, headache can also be caused by CNS infection, often by exotic organisms.—J.R. Roberts, M.D.

*References*

1. Klonoff DC, et al: *Arch Neurol* 46:989, 1989.
2. Kaye BR, Fainstat M: *JAMA* 258:2104, 1987.

---

**The Effect of Haloperidol in Cocaine and Amphetamine Intoxication**
Derlet RW, Albertson TE, Rice P (Univ of California, Davis)
*J Emerg Med* 7:633–637, 1989                                    4–28

---

The number of patients admitted to EDs with stimulant intoxication from cocaine or amphetamine overdoses has been increasing. There is anecdotal evidence that haloperidol antagonizes the CNS in stimulant-intoxicated patients. However, there are no clinical studies and only a few animal studies available that prove the efficacy of haloperidol against either seizures or death resulting from amphetamine or cocaine exposure. The protective effect of haloperidol pretreatment against amphetamine- or cocaine-induced seizures and death was evaluated in a rat model of stimulant intoxication.

Toxic effects were induced in Sprague-Dawley rats by intraperitoneal injection of either amphetamine (75 mg/kg) or cocaine (70 mg/kg) doses, which provide a reasonable time of observation before death. Animals were pretreated with either dimethyl sulfoxide (DMSO) or haloperidol dissolved in DMSO, given 30 minutes before amphetamine or cocaine administration in doses ranging from 0.5 to 20 mg/kg. All animals were observed for 3 hours and reexamined 24 and 48 hours later. Animals that died after the initial 3-hour observation period were reported as late deaths.

All DMSO-pretreated amphetamine controls and 82% of the DMSO-pretreated cocaine controls died. Haloperidol failed to significantly protect against amphetamine-induced seizures at all doses tested but did lower the mortality rate at most doses tested. In contrast, haloperidol decreased the incidence of cocaine-induced seizures at the 2 highest doses but did not lower the mortality rate at any dose. These findings suggest a protective role for haloperidol against death from high-dose amphetamine exposure and against seizures from high-dose cocaine exposure.

▶ Haloperidol or phenothiazines are probably safe to use to treat the severe anxiety or agitation of cocaine poisoning, but the issue of whether or not these drugs lower the seizure threshold in human beings has never been definitely answered. Animal studies are always difficult to extrapolate to human beings, especially the cardiovascular pathophysiology, so this study does not settle the issue. Death by seizure is the norm for cocaine toxicity, so why haloperidol reduced seizures yet failed to influence mortality is confusing.

A possible disadvantage of haloperidol is that it may precipitate acute dysuria or the neuroleptic malignant syndrome. Since it's clinically impossible to differentiate amphetamine from cocaine toxicity, I firmly believe that benzodiazepines are still the initial drugs of choice, because they control agitation, have no significant cardiovascular downside, and clearly are protective against cocaine-induced seizures.—J.R. Roberts, M.D.

---

**Generalized Seizures in an Infant Due to Environmentally Acquired Cocaine**
Rivkin M, Gilmore HE (The Floating Hosp for Infants and Children, Boston)
*Pediatrics* 84:1100–1102, 1989                                              4–29

The adverse neurologic consequences of cocaine ingestion in adults and adolescents have been well documented. A few reports have described the neurologic effects of cocaine in infants who acquired the drug from the maternal circulation during gestation from breast-feeding, or through the consumption of breast milk. Cocaine ingestion by infants without maternal involvement has not been reported until now.

Female infant, 9 months, was brought to the hospital for evaluation of new-onset generalized tonic-clonic seizures. Both alcohol and cocaine powder had been used during a party on the previous evening. The next morning the parents found the infant playing with the uncleared remains of foods and beverage.

Shortly thereafter, the infant experienced jerking movements of all 4 extremities, shallow breathing, and duskiness. She was taken to a local hospital, where she continued to have prolonged generalized tonic-clonic seizures that abated only after intravenous administration of diazepam, phenobarbital, and phenytoin. The infant underwent intubation and was transferred to a second institution, where her course was uneventful. Cocaine was detected in a subsequent toxicology screen.

Drug availability in the parents' home should be considered when infants with new-onset seizures are evaluated. Younger children undergoing the adverse effects of cocaine ingestion may need a longer course of hospital observation than is needed by older patients.

▶ No doubt, most physicians presented with a seizing infant would make the diagnosis of a benign, febrile seizure if the CT and ultrasound were normal and the seizure stopped spontaneously. Finding cocaine-induced fever and a mild leukocytosis would erroneously clinch the missed diagnosis. The route of exposure was unknown in this report, but it could be sidestream smoke from a crack-smoking patient, accidental oral ingestion of a drug stash found by an inquisitive toddler, or even as a result of intentional overdose by a parent bent on child abuse. Others have reported similar cases (1), so unfortunately it's time to add a routine urine drug screen to the diagnostic work-up of a seizure disorder. The fact that multiple drugs and intubation were required to terminate status epilepticus attests to the severe neurotoxicity of cocaine. It would have been interesting to see if the infant had a low serum pseudocholinesterase level (the enzyme that helps metabolic cocaine) as a risk factor for prolonged seizures.—J.R. Roberts, M.D.

*Reference*

1. Ernst AA: *Ann Emerg Med* 18:774, 1989.

---

### Cocaine-Induced Coronary-Artery Vasoconstriction

Lange RA, Cigarroa RG, Yancy CW Jr, Willard JE, Popma JJ, Sills MN, McBride W, Kim AS, Hillis LD (Univ of Texas, Dallas)
*N Engl J Med* 321:1557–1562, 1989                    4–30

Because recreational cocaine use in high doses has been related to chest pain and myocardial infarction, the wide use of intranasally administered cocaine for local anesthesia during rhinolaryngologic surgery is of concern. The effects of 10% intranasally administered cocaine, 2 mg/kg, on coronary blood flow and coronary artery dimensions was investigated in 45 patients undergoing cardiac catheterization for chest pain. The left coronary artery was measured by quantitative angiography before and 15 minutes after intranasal administration of saline or cocaine. Of the patients, 21 had single-vessel coronary disease and 13 had multivessel disease.

Heart rate, arterial pressure, and the rate-pressure product increased after cocaine administration. Myocardial oxygen demand increased, but coronary sinus blood flow decreased. All patients had an increase in coronary vascular resistance. Diffuse constriction of the left anterior descending and circumflex coronary arteries was noted. No patient had chest pain or ECG evidence of ischemia. The hemodynamic and angiographic sequelae of cocaine were reversed by intracoronary phentolamine, but not by saline infusion.

Cocaine administered intranasally in doses close to those used for topical anesthesia can constrict the coronary arteries and reduce coronary blood flow. These effects appear to be mediated by α-adrenergic stimulation. The changes are probably more marked with the much higher doses of cocaine that are abused.

▶ This is the first study to confirm the long-held belief that cocaine precipitates coronary artery spasm. Of concern is that it does so in the presence of perfectly normal coronary arteries and at such low doses. This study is also important since it suggests that phentolamine (Regitine), a drug used to treat acute adrenergic-induced hypertension, may be the drug of choice for reversing cocaine-induced myocardial ischemia. Patients in this study were asymptomatic, and the effect was mild, so the clinical consequences of using cocaine to pack a nose are unclear. It will be prudent, however, to eschew this commonly used ear, nose, and throat drug in the elderly or those with known coronary artery disease and to keep the dose to a minimum (1 mg/kg). It's advisable to use the equally effective 4% solution (40 mg/mL) instead of the 10% formulation. Myocardial infarction has been attributed to the topical use of cocaine for nasal surgery (1).—J.R. Roberts, M.D.

*Reference*

1. Chiu YC, et al: *Arch Otolaryngol Head Neck Surg* 112:988, 1986.

---

### Acute Non-Q Wave Cocaine-Related Myocardial Infarction
Kossowsky WA, Lyon AF, Chou S-Y (Brookdale Hosp Med Ctr, Brooklyn; State Univ of New York, Brooklyn)
*Chest* 96:617–621, 1989                                                    4–31

---

Cocaine can produce myocardial ischemia and infarction in patients with or without preexisting coronary disease. An initial report in 1984 showed 6 patients with acute myocardial infarction temporally related to cocaine use. Data on 19 other patients, with an average age of 31 years, in whom ischemic chest pain syndromes occurred after cocaine use were reviewed.

Non–Q wave infarction developed in 17 patients (89%) and Q-wave infarction developed in 2 patients after intranasal or intravenous use of cocaine or after smoking of cocaine. Angina with marked ST-segment elevation and associated ventricular tachycardia was present in 1 patient.

None of the patients had diabetes mellitus or hypertension, and all but 1 were cigarette smokers. The mean serum cholesterol level was 162 mg/ dL. Of 5 patients who consented to undergo coronary angiographic studies, 4 had normal coronary arteries, and 1 had proximal stenosis of the right coronary artery. None of 7 patients who underwent the cold pressor test had angina or ECG changes induced by cold stimulation. There were no deaths. Cocaine-induced non−Q wave infarction may be more prevalent than previously appreciated. Its pathogenesis may involve that of cocaine-induced coronary vasospasm.

▶ Cocaine, even in relatively small doses, can produce coronary vasospasm and even precipitate acute myocardial infarction in patients with absolutely normal coronary arteries (1). Cocaine also commonly elicits serum creatine phosphokinase (CPK) levels (but not MB fraction), and young cocaine users frequently exhibit nondiagnostic abnormalities or J-point elevation as normal variants on the ECG. Therefore, one is left with nonspecific clinical and laboratory data and a patient with chest pain and cocaine use. Currently, there is no definitive way to rule in or rule out myocardial ischemia in the ED, so some patients are admitted. However, the majority do rule out or leave against medical advice before the answer is known. One yet-to-be-proved approach used by many physicians is to observe all patients with nondiagnosed chest pain for 6 hours in the ED and discharge those who have a normal CPK-MB value and a persistently normal ECG (see Abstract 3–23). This study suggests that any patient with ST-T wave changes should be admitted. It has been suggested that cocaine-induced chest wall rhabdomyolysis may masquerade ischemia (2).—J.R. Roberts, M.D.

*References*

1. Lange RA, et al: *N Engl J Med* 321:1557, 1989.
2. Rubin RB, Neugarten J: *Am J Med* 86:551, 1989.

## Barotrauma, Environmental, and Allergic Emergencies

### Hypoxic Hazards of Traditional Paper Bag Rebreathing in Hyperventilating Patients

Callaham M (Univ of California, San Francisco)
*Ann Emerg Med* 18:622–628, 1989                                    4–32

Acute hyperventilation as the result of anxiety traditionally is managed by having the patient rebreathe into a paper bag. In 3 patients who were hypoxemic or had myocardial ischemia, this measure resulted in death. These deaths prompted a study of the effects of rebreathing in healthy adult volunteers. Twenty persons with an average age of 36 years hyperventilated to an average end-tidal $CO_2$ of 21.6 mm Hg and then continued hyperventilating into a paper bag containing sensors for a capnograph and an oxygen monitor.

The mean change in oxygen from room air was −16 after 30 seconds of rebreathing and −20.5 after 60 seconds. At 3 minutes the mean change was −27. A few subjects achieved a $CO_2$ level as high as 50, but many could not reach a value of 40. When 3 subjects rebreathed into a plastic bag filled with 100% oxygen, $CO_2$ values rapidly exceeded 40, but oxygen levels were less than 10% at 15 minutes.

Bag rebreathing is potentially very hazardous and should never be instituted unless myocardial ischemia can be excluded and the patient's oxygenation is immediately assessable, conditions that are not feasible outside a hospital. It is far better to use oxygen supplementation and other measures that do not alter the inspired gas concentration.

▶ This is a must-read paper. Dr. Callaham points out the dangers of bag rebreathing in hyperventilating patients. The ED physician is compelled to discover the etiology of the hyperventilation, focusing especially on pulmonary embolus, angina, metabolic acidosis, toxic inhalation, or cocaine toxicity. He presents evidence for using supplemental oxygen in all of these patients, independent of the etiology of the hyperventilation and especially when bag breathing is employed. What this paper does not do is give a clear treatment protocol for those patients who are hyperventilating because of anxiety. Because of the hypoventilation and hypoxemia stage that occur after periods of hyperventilation, use of sedating agents may be unwise. Since this paper was published, we no longer administer diazepam to the anxious hyperventilator. Hydroxyzine (25 mg given intramuscularly), cupped-hand breathing, and reassurance work well.—E.J. Reisdorff, M.D.

---

**Patent Foramen Ovale and Decompression Sickness in Divers**
Moon RE, Camporesi EM, Kisslo JA (Duke Univ)
*Lancet* 1:513–514, 1989                                          4–33

The search continues for individual risk factors associated with neurologic damage caused by decompression sickness. A patent foramen ovale may be a risk factor by allowing the passage of venous gas emboli into the systemic circulation. Thirty sports scuba and professional divers with a history of decompression sickness were examined for the presence of patent foramen ovale by bubble-contrast, 2-dimensional echocardiography, and color-flow Doppler imaging.

During bubble-contrast echocardiography, 11 patients (37%) had right-to-left shunting through a patent foramen ovale during spontaneous breathing. Eleven of 18 patients (61%) with serious signs and symptoms of decompression sickness had shunting. In contrast, none of the 12 patients with mild symptoms and only 9 of 176 healthy controls (5%) had shunting. None of the patients with decompression sickness had detectable shunting with color-flow Doppler imaging.

The presence of patent foramen ovale is a risk factor for the development of decompression sickness in divers. Bubble-contrast echocardiography appears to be a sensitive method for detecting patent foramen ovale in these patients.

▶ It is difficult to place this article in practical context. Certainly, it would be difficult to screen all scuba divers with bubble-contrast echocardiography. However, for the emergency physician involved in hyperbaric medicine or environ-mental medicine, the concept is important. Certainly, it would seem that all pa-tients suffering from decompression sickness with neurologic symptoms would be candidates for this evaluation, especially if they intend to continue to dive in the future.—J.T. Amsterdam, M.D.

---

**Exercise-Associated Collapse in Endurance Events: A Classification System**
Roberts WO (MinnHealth PA, White Bear Lake, Minn)
*Phys Sports Med* 17:49–55, 1989                                                        4–34

---

Exercise-associated collapse (EAC) may develop during or after 2–6 hours of endurance sports, such as marathons. Based on observation of casualties at 6 Twin Cities Marathons in 1982–1987, a clinical classifi-cation system for EAC was developed to be used by physicians who cover endurance events and promote a scientific approach to the pathogenesis of EAC. This classification system can be used to classify casualties of en-durance events lasting 2–24 hours.

The major diagnostic criteria of EAC are body temperature and mental status. The syndrome consists of abnormal body temperature, altered mental status, muscle spasms, and inability to walk unassisted. The 3 classes of EAC are hyperthermic (≥39.5°C), normothermic (36.7°C–38.9°C), and hypothermic (≤36.1°C). Each class is further subdivided as mild, moderate, or severe. Mild EAC includes any of the symptoms and ability to walk with or without assistance. Moderate EAC is character-ized by extra fluid loss from diarrhea or vomiting, inability to walk, se-vere muscle spasms, and abnormal body temperature. Severe cases show changes in mental status, such as delirum, confusion, or unconsciousness, and extreme body temperatures.

Management involves fluid and fuel replacements. Treatment of warm runners includes application of ice bags wrapped with wet towels to ma-jor areas of heat loss (neck, axilla, and groin) to lower core body temper-atures. Treatment of cool runners involves removing wet clothing, drying the skin, and insulating with wool blankets.

▶ This article reviews the pathophysiology and treatment of heat exhaustion. It proposes a 9-category clinical classification system to evaluate athletes who collapse at endurance events. Although the classification system is somewhat confusing, it may provide a better tool for the evaluation of the exercise-asso-ciated collapse.—E.J. Reisdorff, M.D.

---

**Exercise-Induced Angioedema and Asthma**
Leung AKC, Hegde HR (Univ of Calgary; Alberta Children's Hosp, Calgary)
*Am J Sports Med* 17:442–443, 1989                                                     4–35

---

Occasionally exertion is complicated by urticaria, angioedema, asth-matic attacks, laryngospasm, cardiac arrhythmias, and vascular collapse.

In 1 patient angioedema and asthmatic attacks developed on more than 6 occasions after physical exertion.

Boy, 15 years, was seen at the ED with sudden onset of painless facial and periorbital swelling and breathing difficulties after playing basketball for 30 minutes. He had no itchiness or rash and there was no urticaria. He described similar episodes that had occurred 6 times within 6 months, usually after 20–30 minutes of exercise in the gymnasium. He had not taken any medication. On previous occasions physical examination confirmed angioedema and wheezing. Neither hot baths nor nervousness brought on periorbital edema or asthmatic attacks, and his family history was negative for angioneurotic edema. Results of laboratory tests were within normal limits. His bronchospasm was relieved promptly with 0.3 mL of 1:1,000 epinephrine subcutaneously and salbutamol by inhalation. He was given 25 mg of diphenhydramine every 4 hours. His periorbital and facial edema resolved within 2 days. Cimetidine prophylaxis (300 mg twice daily) reduced the frequency and severity of these attacks.

Angioedema is a nonitchy swelling in the deep dermis or subcutaneous tissue with a predilection for the face and oral soft tissues. The nonpruritic nature of the lesion is explained by the paucity of sensory nerve endings in affected areas. Cimetidine is a useful prophylactic in this condition.

▶ The authors report a case of exercise-induced angioedema. Two thirds of children with asthma will have an exercise-induced component. This case was treated immediately with an $H_1$ blocker; an $H_2$ blocker was an effective prophylactic agent. In cases of exercise-induced angioedema and asthma, both $H_1$ and $H_2$ blockade are effective treatment. Among $H_1$ blockers, hydroxyzine (25 mg) causes less drowsiness.—E.J. Reisdorff, M.D.

---

**Neuropsychological Consequences of Circulatory Arrest With Hypothermia: A Case Report**
Newman S, Pugsley W, Klinger L, Harrison M, Aveling W, Treasure T (Univ of London)
*J Clin Exp Neuropsychol* 11:529–538, 1989                                    4–36

---

The actual value of the measures intended to protect against cerebral ischemia during circulatory arrest has been difficult to determine because much of the research in this area has involved infants and children whose brains are functionally so plastic they may possibly mask cerebral damage. The effects of circulatory arrest with cooling and barbiturate "protection" were studied in 1 adult patient.

Woman, 66, had been hypertensive for many years. Aortic incompetence and later ascending aortic dissection were diagnosed. Cardiopulmonary bypass was instituted as the core temperature was lowered to 18°C. The patient received 2 g of thiopentone. The initial course after aortic graft placement was quite uneventful, but the patient remained drowsy for some time. "Soft" neurologic signs were present 24 hours after operation, but these were absent on day 8. Performance on tests of attention and concentration resembled that seen in coronary artery bypass patients, with initial decline and later restoration of function. Perceptuomotor performance did not improve to the preoperative level. Memory function was poorest at 8 days; by 8 weeks performance was similar to that of patients who have coronary artery bypass surgery.

In general the neuropsychologic tests showed considerable preservation of function in this patient, especially considering that circulatory arrest lasted 24 minutes and that electroencephalographic activity was absent for some time after injection of thiopentone. It appears that the combination of hypothermia and barbiturates conferred protection.

▶ Although the intraoperative situation this case report addresses is not really within the scope of emergency medicine physicians, the problem of cerebral preservation in the face of ischemia caused by cardiac arrest is of great interest to us and is the focus of much ongoing research. Barbiturates alone, once thought promising, have since proved worthless. There is currently much interest in hypothermia. Even mild degrees of hypothermia, 34°C–36°C, can produce substantial improvements in neurologic outcome in dogs (1). Research protocols to use head cooling in human cardiac arrest patients are being developed.—J. Schoffstall, M.D.

*Reference*

1. Lenov Y, et al: *J Cereb Blood Flow Metab* 10:57, 1990.

---

**Closed Thoracic Cavity Lavage in the Treatment of Severe Hypothermia in Human Beings**
Hall KN, Syverud SA (Univ of Cincinnati)
*Ann Emerg Med* 19:204–206, 1990                                      4–37

---

Partial cardiopulmonary bypass is the treatment of choice for severe hypothermia complicated by cardiac arrest, but this treatment modality is not readily available in many settings. Alternate treatments include closed- or open-chest cardiac compression for circulatory support and active core rewarming with peritoneal lavage, open or closed pleural lavage, heated aerosol inhalation, or gastric lavage. Closed thoracic cavity lavage (CTCL) has been evaluated in animal studies, but the technique has not previously been used in human beings. In 2 cases, CTCL was used to rewarm cardiac arrest victims with severe hypothermia for whom cardiopulmonary bypass was not available.

*Case 1.*—Man, 72, was found unconscious at home with profound bradycardia and a rectal temperature of 23.9°C. On arrival in the ED, he was given intravenous bretylium tosylate. After oral intubation, he was treated with heated aerosol inhalation by endotracheal tube, warmed intravenous fluids, and gastric lavage with warmed saline. His rectal temperature increased during the next 2 hours to 26.7°C. After 2 hours in the ED, spontaneous movement on the cardiac monitor suddenly ceased, and there was a loss of pulse and blood pressure. Closed thoracic cavity lavage was initiated, and 40 L of warming fluid was instilled over 20 minutes, after which the patient's esophageal temperature increased to 32.8°C. The advanced cardiac life support protocol was followed during the rewarming period, but there was no resolution of his asystole. Autopsy showed deep vein thrombosis and massive pulmonary embolus.

*Case 2.*—Woman, 36, was found in her automobile without pulse or respiration. The cardiac monitor showed asystole. On arrival at the ED, her rectal temperature was 25°C. Closed thoracic cavity lavage was initiated, and after 20 minutes of rewarming, the patient's esophageal temperature had increased to 32.4°C. Advanced cardiac life support was not successful. Toxic screen at autopsy confirmed tricyclic overdose.

Although both patients died, the use of CTCL resulted in a rapid elevation of core temperature in both patients. The true efficacy of CTCL can be assessed only when it can be attempted in patients suffering from pure environmentally induced hypothermia not complicated by other conditions.

▶ In cases of severe hypothermia, slow core warming (1°C–2°C/hour) is advocated. Rapid core warming is usually used when the patient has cardiopulmonary arrest. Rapid core warming can have many detrimental effects when compared with slow core warming. Practically, rapid core warming eliminates the need to do prolonged cardiopulmonary resuscitation (often 10–15 hours) until one elevates the core temperature to 37°C to legally pronounce the patient dead. Unfortunately, whether or not this procedure improves outcome was not shown in this paper.—G. Ordog, M.D.

---

**Emergency Treatment of Exertional Heatstroke and Comparison of Whole Body Cooling Techniques**
Costrini A (Savannah, Ga)
*Med Sci Sports Exerc* 22:15–18, 1990                                    4–38

---

Exertional heatstroke is a serious and potentially fatal disease. Its treatment relies on prompt recognition of symptoms and early institution of appropriate therapy. A comparison of whole-body cooling techniques for exertional heatstroke was presented.

The use of cold water immersion with skin massage has been successful in rapidly lowering body temperatures and in avoiding severe complications or death. In a study of young soldiers with heatstroke, rectal temperatures dropped from 41.1°C–43.1°C to 39°C at a rate of 0.15°C/minute during a 10- to 40-minute immersion in ice water (mean time 19.2 minutes) and vigorous skin massage. No cases of seizures or of renal or other organ failure were observed. There were no deaths.

Recently, alternatives to water immersion have emerged. They include the use of warm air spray, helicopter downdraft, and pharmacologic agents. Although those methods were effective and resulted in faster cooling rates, none proved to be more effective than cold water immersion in preventing death.

All treatment centers should establish a heatstroke therapy protocol using ice water immersion. If other methods of cooling are used initially, the ice water bath should be used if body temperature is not reduced to 38.9°C within 30 minutes. Treatment should begin at the point of collapse, because the number and severity of complications are directly related to delays in instituting vigorous cooling therapy.

▶ The single, best treatment for cooling a hyperthermic patient is immersion, which also complicates monitoring. Whoever rubs the victim with ice, winds up with stiff, painful hands. We keep in the ED a homemade mesh stretcher top like the King Saud University cooling bed mentioned here.—T. Stair, M.D.

---

**Radio Frequency (13.56 MHz) Energy Enhances Recovery From Mild Hypothermia**
Hesslink RL Jr, Pepper S, Olsen RG, Lewis SB, Homer LD (Naval Med Research Inst, Bethesda, Md; Naval Aerospace Med Research Lab, Pensacola, Fla)
*J Appl Physiol* 67:1208–1212, 1989                                      4–39

---

The rate of warming after hypothermia depends on what is used as a rewarming source. Hot water immersion is a standard method for actively rewarming hypothermic individuals, but this method has limited application for field use. Insulated sleeping bags, which are currently used to rewarm victims of hypothermia, require the individual's own limited body heat for rewarming. Recent advances in radio frequency (RF) energy (13.56-MHz) delivery systems have shown great promise in animal studies. The effectiveness of RF energy as a rewarming source was assessed in 6 healthy male volunteers using the illustrated RF rewarming coil system (Fig 4–4).

After fasting overnight, 6 men with a median age of 25 years wearing bathing trunks were instrumented with esophageal, rectal, and surface skin temperature probes. Each study participant was immersed to nipple level in a well-stirred cold water tank until his rectal temperature had dropped by 0.5°C. The man was then removed from the tank, lightly towel dried, and rewarmed for 60 minutes using either RF energy, immersion in hot water at 41°C, or wrapping in an insulated cocoon (IC). Blood samples were collected 30 minutes after insertion of an indwelling catheter into the antecubital vein, just before removal from cold water, and at 5, 10, 30, and 60 minutes into the rewarming period. Each man served as his own control for 3 rewarming trials, which were also recorded on video cassette for the determination of a shivering response.

Radio frequency warmed the thoracic cavity faster than either hot wa-

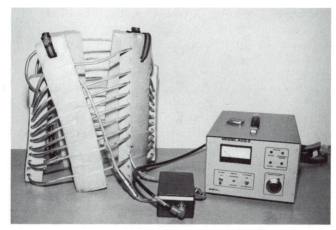

**Fig 4–4.**—Radio frequency rewarming coil system and commercial frequency generator. (Courtesy of Hesslink RL Jr, Pepper S, Olsen RG, et al: *J Appl Physiol* 67:1208–1212, 1989.)

ter or an IC. Thus, the potential for cardiac arrhythmias associated with low core temperature may be diminished when RF rewarming is used after hypothermia. Rectal temperatures did not increase as rapidly as did esophageal temperatures. Each man immediately stopped shivering on entry into the hot water tank. When RF warming was used, moderate intermittent shivering was observed during the first 30 minutes but not during the last 30 minutes of the rewarming period. With use of the IC, all men were observed to shiver throughout the entire 60-minute rewarming period.

Radio frequency rewarming is a new and promising alternative for rewarming victims of hypothermia in the field. Radio frequency energy reheated the thoracic region more rapidly than did either immersion in hot water or wrapping in an IC.

▶ The number of noninvasive methods for active rewarming of the hypothermic patient are limited. This paper describes a new RF rewarming coil that exceeds the rate of rewarming achieved with either warm water immersion or placement with an insulated cocoon. Unfortunately, the experimental design limits its application to mildly hypothermic patients (core temperature decrease of 0.5°C). Clinically, these patients do not require active rewarming, and it is only an assumption that in the profoundly hypothermic patient its superior effect will persist. Intuitively, this hypothesis seems reasonable, but further studies with lower core temperatures are necessary. A major drawback to this experimental device is the inability to obtain ECG data in close proximity to RF energy. Most patients who require rewarming are at risk for cardiac arrhythmias and consequently require cardiac monitoring. In addition, nonmetallic thermocouples that might require the purchase of specialized equipment by the ED must be used. The effect of RF energy on implanted metals (e.g., surgical staples, pacemakers) that might limit patient use is not mentioned.—H. Unger, M.D.

## Anaphylactic Shock Occurring Outside Hospitals

Sørensen HT, Nielsen B, Nielsen JØ (Thisted Hosp; Aalborg Hosp North; Aarhus Amtssygehus; Aalborg Hosp South, Denmark)
*Allergy* 44:288–290, 1989                                          4–40

Anaphylactic shock (AS) is the result of either acute hypersensitivity or non-IgE-mediated mast cell mediator liberation. Both mechanisms produce the same clinical result, which includes anxiety, palpitations, urticaria, respiratory distress, and cardiovascular collapse. All cases of AS occurring in a hospital catchment area from 1973 to 1985 were reviewed. Twenty patients (13 men and 7 women, average age 49 years) with AS were recorded, giving an incidence of 3.2 cases per 100,000 inhabitants per year. There was 1 death.

The precipitating agents were penicillin in 7, aspirin in 3, food in 2, and bee or wasp stings in 8. In 2 of the 3 cases attributed to aspirin, there was doubt as to whether aspirin was the precipitating agent because aspirin was administered in conjunction with other drugs. In all instances, the drugs were given orally. Ingestion of celery and shrimp resulted in 2 cases of food-induced AS. A bee sting was the cause of the single death.

Admission records on the frequency of AS-related symptoms and signs revealed that in 11 patients the first symptoms occurred within 5 minutes of exposure, in 2 between 5 and 15 minutes after exposure, and in 4 more than 15 minutes later, with a maximal time from exposure to occurrence of symptoms of 2 hours. Time of onset was not recorded for the other 3 patients. Only 1 patient reported a history of atopic disease, whereas 15 had previously been in contact with the precipitating agent. Three of the 15 had had 1 or more anaphylactic reactions to the precipitating agent (1 each to aspirin, shrimp, and bee sting). No history was available for the patient who died.

Anaphylactic shock rarely occurs outside the hospital; however, orally administered penicillin is a more important cause than was previously considered. Because hypersensitivity tests for both penicillin and *Hymenoptera* venoms are available and desensitization to the latter is possible, it would appear that recurrent episodes of AS are preventable; however, prevention of initial episodes does not seem possible.

► The authors of this paper on anaphylactic shock outside the hospital demonstrate that this disease is underreported and often misdiagnosed, at least in Denmark, anyway. The same is probably true in this country.

On a more disturbing note, only 1 of the 20 patients described had an atopic history, and only 3 had had a previous anaphylactic reaction. The authors make no mention of family history. Thus, few of these reactions could have been predicted in advance.

However, for those who have experienced anaphylactic reactions, a careful history should be obtained, and the patient should be warned against further exposure to offending agents. For those who are sensitive to *Hymenoptera* venom, desensitization should be strongly recommended. Immunotherapy has something to offer to this limited but important group of patients.—H.H. Osborn, M.D.

---

### Comparison of Cimetidine and Diphenhydramine in the Treatment of Acute Urticaria

Moscati RM, Moore GP (Darnall Army Community Hosp, Fort Hood, Tex; Maricopa Med Ctr, Phoenix)
*Ann Emerg Med* 19:12–15, 1990                                                    4–41

---

It is traditionally accepted that $H_2$ receptors have a very limited role in the pathogenesis of acute urticaria. At the cellular level, $H_2$ blockade increases local histamine release by interruption of feedback inhibition and thus may even exacerbate symptoms. However, cimetidine, an $H_2$ blocker, has been used effectively to treat chronic and recalcitrant acute urticaria. To investigate further, the efficacy of cimetidine in acute urticaria was compared with that of diphenhydramine, an $H_1$ blocker, in a prospective double-blind study. Ninety-three patients with acute urticaria were randomly treated with either 50 mg of diphenhydramine or 300 mg of cimetidine intramuscularly. A numeric scale was used to quantitate itching, sedation, wheal intensity, wheal extent, and overall improvement.

Both diphenhydramine and cimetidine significantly improved itching and wheal intensity. Both drugs caused significant sedation, but diphenhydramine caused significantly more sedation than cimetidine. Overall improvement was perceived by 87% of cimetidine-treated patients compared with 76% of diphenhydramine-treated patients. None of the patients in either groups reported worsening of symptoms.

Cimetidine is effective in the treatment of acute urticaria with less sedative effects. Cimetidine should be recommended as the initial treatment of acute urticaria.

▶ This excellent, prospective, randomized, and double-blind study compares 2 histamine antagonists, an $H_1$ and an $H_2$ blocker, in the treatment of acute urticaria. In so doing, it offers us a new, and from all appearances, effective therapy and casts serious doubt on our understanding of the pathophysiology of this disorder.

The relatively short observation period and the lack of any placebo control are significant limitations in this otherwise well-designed and executed study. Cimetidine proved to be just as effective in the relief of symptoms as diphenhydramine. The authors are not justified in claiming that the perception of overall improvement was greater with cimetidine since the numerical advantage they report is not statistically significant.

Further studies will no doubt increase our understanding of the role of histamine receptors in mediating acute allergic reactions as well as the place of cimetidine (and other $H_2$ blockers) in treating them.

In the meantime, cimetidine should be considered a first-line agent in the treatment of acute urticaria. Consideration of side effects (e.g., sedation), cost, and possible drug interactions should inform the decision to use any 1 particular agent.— H.H. Osborn, M.D.

▶ This paper once again demonstrates that activated charcoal may prevent the absorption of an ingested toxin as well as any of the commonly used methods of gastric emptying. The authors go on to comment on the advisability of using activated charcoal in the particular context of acetaminophen overdose, a subject that has been widely discussed among toxicologists. In former times, we believed that activated charcoal is contraindicated in this context because of the possibility of interference of NAC absorption by the administered activated charcoal. But as the authors point out in their discussion, most studies have found little in vivo effect on the absorption of NAC. However, one paper published in 1987 described an approximately 40% reduction in NAC absorption when 100 g of activated charcoal was given 30 minutes after the administered dose of NAC. My own belief about this is based not so much on controlled studies but a kind of common-sense approach based on what I perceive to be the relative risk/benefit ratios of various interventions. For the patient admitted within the first 2–3 hours after an overdose and in a setting where a rapid turnaround time for acetaminophen levels is feasible, drug levels can dictate therapy. There is no question that giving activated charcoal within the first few hours after an acetaminophen overdose will help prevent the development of a toxic acetaminophen level. On the other hand, if the patient is seen more than 4 hours after the overdose, the likelihood that the charcoal will significantly reduce absorption is fairly slim, and there is the potential complication of a modest reduction in NAC absorption. Further, in this context, it is probably desirable to administer the loading dose of NAC immediately without waiting for the results of the acetaminophen level. It has been shown by the Rocky Mountain Poison Control Center Group that the maximum efficacy of NAC is probably achieved if the antidote can be administered within the first 8 hours after acetaminophen ingestion (1).— F. Henretig, M.D.

*Reference*

1. Smilkstein MJ, et al: *N Engl J Med* 319:1557, 1989.

---

**Loxosceles reclusa Envenomation**
Gendron BP (Madigan Army Med Ctr, Tacoma, Wash)
*Am J Emerg Med* 8:51–54, 1990                                        4–42

---

Spiders of the genus *Loxosceles* are widely distributed; the most common species in the United States is *Loxosceles reclusa,* or brown recluse. The incidence of *Loxosceles* spider bites is unknown. The pathophysiology of the brown recluse venom may be related to the sphingomyelinase D component of the venom.

The clinical spectrum of loxoscelism range from a very mild local reaction to systemic involvement. The spider bite may manifest as a nonspecific small erythematous papule or often as a slow-healing necrotic lesion.

Systemic involvement develops at 24–48 hours after the bite, particularly among children. Diffuse intravascular coagulation and renal failure may occur. Systemic symptoms are directly related to the amount of envenomation but not the severity of skin lesion.

Diagnosis is often difficult and is usually based on a clinically consistent lesion and the known presence of the spider in the area. Treatment consists of local conservative care. When started within 12 hours of the bite, dapsone may prove beneficial in some patients. Specific antivenom may minimize sequelae. Surgery should be considered only for necrotic ulcers greater than 1–2 cm in diameter and only after the borders of the lesions are well established. Spider bites can be avoided by staying away from the spider's habitat.

▶ Except in rare cases, the diagnosis of a *Loxosceles* bite is clinical. Following a relatively painless bite, the lesion begins as a small, erythematous papule and progresses to a blister that quickly becomes a necrotic ulcer. No doubt, the spider can wreak havoc, but fortunately most envenomations are limited to soft-tissue injury. Antivenom is not currently available. Corticosteroids and early bite excision are best avoided. The safety of dapsone (100 mg twice daily) for such bites is unproved, but short-term use is probably safe (5–7 days); thus, it's reasonable to start it empirically. The drug is approved only for dermatitis herpetiformis and leprosy, and it can cause aplastic anemia, hemolysis in glucose-6-phosphate dehydrogenase deficiency and methemoglobinemia. Early hyperbaric oxygen treatment has also been advocated, but the benefit is unproved.—J.R. Roberts, M.D.

### A Comparative Double Blind Study of Amoxycillin/Clavulanate *vs* Placebo in the Prevention of Infection After Animal Bites
Brakenbury PH, Muwanga C (Middlesbrough Gen Hosp, Middlesbrough, England)
*Arch Emerg Med* 6:251–256, 1989                                      4–43

Preventing wound infection is the main objective in the management of patients with animal bites. The value of prophylactic antibiotics has not been established. A prospective double-blind study of 185 consecutively enrolled patients compared a broad-spectrum antibiotic with placebo in the treatment of full-thickness animal bite wounds.

Initial wound treatment involved thorough wound cleansing, débridement, and irrigation. The patients were then assigned to either treatment or placebo groups. Patients, aged 6–12 years, were given 125 mg of amoxycillin and 62 mg of clavulanic acid or placebo. Patients older than age 12 years were given 250 mg of amoxycillin and 125 mg of clavulanic acid or placebo. The antibiotic produced no significant benefit when the wounds were less than 9 hours old. However, in patients seeking medical attention 9–24 hours after the injury, antibiotic treatment significantly reduced the rate of infection. Prophylactic broad-spectrum antibiotic treatment should be considered when bone, joint, and tendon involvement is suspected.

▶ This is yet another study that demonstrates the uselessness of routine prophylactic antibiotics following soft-tissue injuries.

An exception to this scenario is a cat bite—a condition where it's impossible to properly clean tiny puncture wounds. When a feline is the culprit, most physicians prescribe a penicillin or tetracycline to thwart *Pasteurella multocida* infections. Antibiotics given 9 hours after a bite are more therapeutic than prophylaxis, and this may account for a clinical response in "old" wounds. It's a cliché but still true that no amount of expensive antibiotics will substitute for early, proper wound cleansing.—J.R. Roberts, M.D.

---

**Clinical and Immunologic Features and Subsequent Course of Patients With Severe Insect-Sting Anaphylaxis**
Lantner R, Reisman RE (State Univ of New York at Buffalo)
*J Allergy Clin Immunol* 84:900–906, 1989                                    4–44

---

A better understanding of the natural history of insect sting anaphylaxis is needed. One hundred fifty-eight patients ranging from 3 to 80 years of age (mean age 29.7 years) with severe life-threatening anaphylactic reactions were evaluated. Thirty-three patients were younger than age 10 years.

Symptoms included potentially fatal venom anaphylaxis—hypotension, loss of consciousness, throat or laryngeal edema, or marked respiratory distress. The incidence of atopy was 20%. One hundred twenty-seven patients had been stung previously, 27 of whom had prior systemic reactions. Almost all patients had venom-specific IgE, with a wide range of radioallergosorbent test titers. The 45 patients who lost consciousness were older, had an increased incidence of cardiac disease and β-blocker use, and had stings in the head area. Also in this group, resting reactions occurred in patients who did not receive venom immunotherapy (VIT). In the 37 patients receiving VIT, 106 restings occurred with no systemic reactions. Thirty-eight restings occurred in 18 patients who refused VIT, producing 14 systemic reactions in 11 of them.

There are no characteristics, including age, that would distinguish patients who are susceptible to severe venom anaphylaxis from those who are not. Venom immunotherapy proved to be an effective prophylaxis in this series.

▶ There's no question that an insect sting may be fatal, and rarely is the patient aware of his or her hypersensitivity before the anaphylaxis occurs. This impressive review underscores the value of venom immunotherapy, so it's important to refer seriously affected patients to an allergist. In the meantime, a self-injecting epinephrine kit may be lifesaving. It's interesting that severe anaphylaxis occurred frequently in young children, but it was impossible to prospectively identify patients at high risk. Many patients with anaphylaxis to an initial sting are restung without any serious sequelae or tolerate a number of prior stings before anaphylaxis ensues. Patients taking β-blockers may be more susceptible to cardiovascular collapse and more refractory to therapy. In such cases, glucagon, calcium, or both may be of help if traditional therapy with epinephrine is not effective. Even in the healthy patients with anaphylaxis, it's dangerous to use bolus alliquots of intravenous epinephrine. It's more prudent to titrate a continuous infusion (1–2 mg in 1 L).—J.R. Roberts, M.D.

## Infant and Childhood Emergencies

### Patterns of Injury in Children

Peclet MH, Newman KD, Eichelberger MR, Gotschall CS, Guzzetta PC, Anderson KD, Garcia VF, Randolph JG, Bowman LM (Children's Natl Med Ctr, Washington, DC)
*J Pediatr Surg* 25:85–91, 1990                                    4–45

Injuries killed more than 8,000 children in the United States in 1985, and more than 100,000 children were permanently disabled. Trauma is the chief cause of death of children aged more than 1 year. Injury patterns therefore were studied in 3,472 children admitted in a 3-year period to a regional pediatric trauma center.

The mean age was 5.5 years; boys accounted for 64% of admissions. The mortality was 2.2%, and most deaths occurred within 48 hours of initial resuscitation (Fig 4–5). Head injuries were most frequent among victims of child abuse, crashes, and falls. Thoracic and abdominal injuries occurred mainly in children with stab and gunshot wounds. Limb injuries predominated in cyclists and pedestrians. Mechanisms of injury correlated with age and mortality.

Occupants in motor vehicle crashes were younger than victims of other

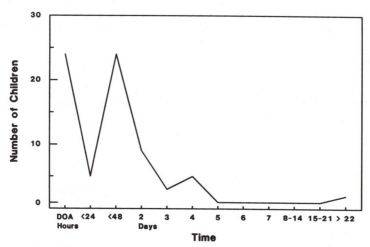

**Fig 4–5.**—Time between resuscitation and death of children treated at a pediatric trauma center. (Courtesy of Peclet MH, Newman KD, Eichelberger MR, et al: *J Pediatr Surg* 25:85–91, 1990.)

traffic-related trauma and were more severely injured. Victims of falls were the least severely injured children with blunt trauma. Children with burn injury or smoke inhalation were among the youngest in the series. Victims of child abuse were the youngest of all and had the most severe injuries.

Nearly three fourths of admissions to this urban pediatric trauma center were for traffic-related injury, falls, and burn injury. Overall mortality was low, but a disproportionately large number of the deaths resulted from child abuse, drowning, and penetrating trauma.

▶ Pediatric trauma is still the leading killer and disabler of our children. This article really does not add any new information as to the epidemiology of the causes of pediatric trauma but does stress that prevention is a must and identifies an overall mortality rate that other institutions can use to monitor their effectiveness in managing pediatric trauma.

The motor vehicle is definitely not a child's friend; it is the leading cause of death and disability for childhood trauma. Urban teenagers with their gang and drug activities have markedly increased the amount of penetrating trauma that inner-city hospitals manage.

Our EDs and prehospital care providers have learned how to better manage pediatric trauma over the past 10 years, but we will not make a significant dent in the morbidity until we convince parents and children to make injury prevention a permanent part of their life-style. This past weekend brought home this point to me. Once again, there was another bad auto wreck with 1 dead child at the scene, another child arresting en route to the hospital, and 2 children with injuries severe enough to necessitate a laparotomy shortly after arrival in the hospital. That same day on my way home, I saw at least 20 children riding bicycles, and not 1 was wearing a safety helmet.

The emergency physician must also consider that child abuse or neglect may have been the cause of this child's injury, and it may be a matter of life and death for us to identify early that this child is abused and report the case to the appropriate authorities. We must raise the public's awareness of how to identify and report child abuse and how to promote injury prevention.—J.W. Schafermeyer, M.D.

---

**Ingestion of Prescription Drugs by Children: An Epidemiologic Study**
King WD, Palmisano PA (Children's Hosp of Alabama, Birmingham; Univ of Alabama, Birmingham)
*South Med J* 82:1468–1471, 1989                                          4–46

---

The Poison Prevention Packaging Act (PPPA) of 1970, which mandates child-resistant packaging of hazardous household products and prescription drugs, has resulted in a 65% decline in ingestions of products packaged in child-resistant containers. Ingestion of aspirin alone has declined by more than 75%. However, ingestion of prescription drugs by children has declined by only 36%. During the past 5 years, ingestion of prescription drugs accounted for 62% of ingestion-related hospitalizations at 1 institution. The records of 849 children younger than 6 years who ingested prescription drugs were reviewed.

Of the 849 children, 205 (24%) were 12–23 months old, and 456 (54%) were 24–35 months old. The peak hour of the day for these ingestions was between 6 and 7 P.M. More than 75% involved tablets or capsules in non-child-resistant packages or loose pills in no container at all. The leading solid prescription drugs that resulted in hospitalization when ingested were ferrous sulfate, clonidine, lorazepam, digoxin, diphenoxylate-atropine, amitriptyline, and oxycodone-acetaminophen. Although the parents' prescriptions accounted for 54% of the ingestions, nearly 30% involved grandparents' medication.

These findings suggest that the original intent of the PPPA has not been achieved fully with regard to prescription drugs. Children still are being exposed to many dangerous drugs, resulting in too many unnecessary hospitalizations or emergency department visits. Unit-dose packaging, at least of those prescription drugs that are most toxic to children, might be a viable option for lowering the incidence of prescription drug ingestions by children.

▶ This survey of ingestion of prescription drugs by children reported to a poison control center reviews some important facts for the emergency physician: Most ingestions are by toddlers or 2-year-olds and occur around dinner time when there is more activity and less supervision by adults. In any child for whom an ingestion is suspected, one must find out what medications the parents, grandparents, and family members are taking. The authors review which are the most toxic and common prescription drugs that require hospitalization in children. Perhaps as emergency physicians, we should be ordering child-proof packaging on all prescriptions written for these more toxic drugs and warning the patients of their toxicity if ingested by children or grandchildren.—K.N. Shaw, M.D.

## Injuries Among 4- to 9-Year-Old Restrained Motor Vehicle Occupants by Seat Location and Crash Impact Site

Agran P, Winn D, Dunkle D (Univ of California, Irvine)
*Am J Dis Child* 14:1317–1321, 1989                                    4–47

Children aged 4–9 years appear to be less protected by selt belts and child safety seats than younger children and adults. Children in this age group are placed in seat belt systems designed for adults, although their weight, height, and center of gravity differ markedly from that of older passengers. The patterns of injury in restrained 4- to 9-year-olds were examined by seat location and crash impact site in 131 children involved in a crash between 2 passenger vehicles with a single impact site.

Most serious injuries occurred with children seated on the side of the impact during lateral collisions; 41% of these children had injuries with a Maximum Abbreviated Injury Score (MAIS) of 2 or greater. Children seated on the side opposite the impact had only minor injuries. Of the children in the front passenger seat, 20% sustained an injury with an MAIS of 2 or greater in frontal impacts. In children restrained in the back seat, injuries of this severity occurred in 10% during frontal impacts and in 7% during rear impacts. Injuries to the head or face were sustained by 70% of the children, primarily the result of frontal images. Only 6% of the children had upper-torso injuries. Lower-torso injuries were more common (18%), especially in frontal impacts. Spinal injuries were generally minor and occurred most often to children in the front seat during a rear impact.

Until improvements in vehicle design are made, the middle rear seat appears to offer children the greatest safety in a lateral impact. Until special safety seats are available for children aged 4−9 years, the front seat should be moved as far back from the dashboard as possible to lower the risk of head and face injures.

▶ This study makes several practical points: (1) the safest place to seat your child is in the middle of the back seat (if you have only 1 child); (2) it is better to have a car with solid, impact-absorbing doors; and (3) lap-shoulder belts may prevent significant head injuries by preventing hyperextension of the upper torso, which can occur in children wearing just a lap belt.

Once a child has outgrown the infant car seats (18 kg or 102 cm), 3 options are currently available for restraint in motor vehicles: lap belt, lap-shoulder belt, or booster seat in conjunction with a lap-shoulder belt. All 3 methods are better than no restraining device but have potential problems. The National Highway Traffic Safety Administration states that the shoulder portion should not be used if it crosses the neck or face, whereas the National Transportation Safety Board states that the shoulder strap should always be used regardless of its position on the child. This study supports the latter opinion. Although the number of children in lap-shoulder restraints is small, there were no seat-shoulder belt-related injuries and also no significant head trauma. However, if the shoulder portion of the belt is not used, it should never be placed under the arm of either children or adults, because severe internal injuries may occur from rib fractures and puncture in the event of a significant impact (place the shoulder belt behind the child). This study does not evaluate booster seats, which should also prevent hyperextension and significant head injury. Controversy exists as to whether the minishield pressure against the abdomen may cause internal injuries at crash forces. This is an area that needs further research.— K.H. Shaw, M.D.

---

**Self-Administered Nitrous Oxide for Fracture Reduction in Children in an Emergency Room Setting**
Wattenmaker I, Kasser JR, McGravey A (Children's Hosp, Boston)
*J Orthop Trauma* 4:35–38, 1990                                          4–48

---

Traditional ways of achieving analgesia for fracture reduction in children may be difficult, anxiety producing, and time consuming. The use of self-administered 50:50 nitrous oxide−oxygen gas in 22 children requiring closed reduction of fractures in the emergency room was evaluated. Most patients had forearm fractures. The Nitronox Scavenger system was used by the patient as the fracture was reduced and the cast applied, and oxygen then was administered for several minutes. The patients were at least 4 years old (average age, 10 years).

No other form of analgesia was used except for a hematoma block in 1 patient and a digital block in another. In all patients, a single maneuver without fluoroscopy was considered likely to succeed. Closed reduction during nitrous oxide analgesia administration succeeded in all but 2 patients. The average time of nitrous oxide administration was 16 minutes. None of the patients had severe pain, and most had no more than minimal pain at any time. No complications related to nitrous ocide use occurred.

Self-administered 50% nitrous oxide is a safe and effective analgesic for fracture reduction in the emergency room setting. This approach is recommended if a single maneuver not requiring muscle relaxation is considered extremely likely to succeed.

▶ Conscious sedation of the pediatric patient has always been a difficult issue for the practitioner. The choices for conscious sedation include the age-old cocktail of meperidine (Demerol), promethazine (Phenergan), and chlorpromazine (Thorazine) or some similar mixture of medications. This mixture did not work in every patient and occasionally caused agitations, seizures, or a cardiopulmonary arrest.

Some clinicians used sedative hypnotic agents but noted that they worked only for nonpainful procedures, such as CT scanning or electroencephalograms. One could use local infiltrative anesthesia for fracture reductions, but the clinician had to pay close attention to the total amount of anesthetic agent injected, because, again, some children had an adverse outcome from excessive dosage of the anesthetic agent.

The bottom line is safety and efficacy in the care of the small child. We should get away from the turf battles and false issues surrounding the use of nitrous oxide. This article points out that self-administered nitrous oxide was an ideal agent for the management of painful pediatric procedures. Nitrous oxide would be an ideal agent for debridement of burns or abrasions, reduction of dislocations, and fracture pin placement in trauma patients.

There are several important issues if one is to institute the use of nitrous oxide: (1) use appropriate cardiopulmonary monitoring of the patient, (2) use a 50:50 mix of nitrous oxide and oxygen, and (3) be sure that the agent is self-administered to avoid an overdose of nitrous oxide. Thus, the age and intelligence level of the child will be limiting factors in the use of nitrous oxide. In setting up nitrous oxide in your department, you will also need to have a scavenger device so that nitrous oxide fumes do not escape into the environment.

Conscious sedation of the pediatric patient has always been a controversial and unsatisfactory component of caring for children. As reflected in the article by Hawk et al. (1), a significant number of physicians are dissatisfied with the method or methods that they select. I believe that the use of self-administered nitrous oxide might change their opinion.— R.W. Schafermeyer, M.D.

*Reference*

1. Hawk W, et al: *Pediatr Emerg Care* 6:84, 1990.

---

**Efficacy of Sponging vs Acetaminophen for Reduction of Fever**
Friedman AD, Barton LL, Sponging Study Group (St Louis Univ)
*Pediatr Emerg Med* 6:6–7, 1990                                                    4–49

---

Three common methods of fever control were compared in 73 children with acute febrile illness. The children, aged 4 months–4 years, were randomly assigned to treatment with acetaminophen (n = 26), acetaminophen and sponging (n = 28), or sponging alone (n = 19).

All groups showed temperature reduction at 1 hour after the initial temperature reading. The greatest temperature reduction was achieved with acetaminophen plus sponging. The least effective method was sponging alone.

The routine use of sponging alone in febrile infants and children should be reassessed. In addition to its being less effective than acetaminophen alone or in combination with sponging in reducing fever, sponging alone is time consuming and inconvenient to the child and may result in accidental drowning.

▶ Some practitioners still advocate fever reduction only for hyperpyrexia, usually temperature more than 40°C, arguing that there are beneficial physiologic effects of elevated body temperature. As a practicing pediatrician and a parent, I have no doubt that fever reduction improves the comfort level of ill children. Many previously irritable children become alert and playful after their temperature is brought toward normal. Keep in mind that the response of the fever to antipyretic therapy does not predict the seriousness of the underlying illness (1).

Friedman and Barton address the issue of the most effective therapy for fever reduction. The results of this study are similar to a study of almost 20 years ago (2). In both studies, patients were randomized to sponging alone, acetaminophen alone, or a combination of acetaminophen with sponging. Hunter also included a placebo group and a group treated with aspirin. In both studies, acetaminophen-treated patients fared better than sponging alone (and the no therapy group included by Hunter). The combined therapy patients exhibited minimal improvement in fever reduction compared with patients given only acetaminophen. Several other studies have also reached the same conclusions; Steele (3) noted that bathing caused an extra dimension of discomfort to the child. The time and staff required as well as the discomfort to the patient may not make the addition of the sponging worthwhile. For a busy ED, acetaminophen alone would be the preferred initial therapy until an examination room is available.

For those interested in further reading on the subject, Martin Lorin produced an elegant short book covering all aspects of fever in children (4). The section on bacteremia is somewhat dated now, but the chapters on the mechanisms of temperature regulation and the pathophysiology of fever are complete and well written. Lorin points out that based on the mechanisms of fever production in infections, an upward resetting of the hypothalamic temperature control center, antipyretic medication is the rational therapy of choice.— R.M. Rutstein, M.D.

*References*

1. Baker MD, et al: *Pediatrics* 80:315, 1987.
2. Hunter J: *Arch Dis Child* 48:313, 1973.
3. Steele RW, et al: *J Pediatr* 77:824, 1970.
4. Lorin M: *The Febrile Child*. New York, John Wiley & Sons, 1982.

**Tape Measure to Aid Prescription in Paediatric Resuscitation**
Hughes G, Spoudeas H, Kovar IZ, Millington HT (Charing Cross Hosp, London)
*Arch Emerg Med* 7:21–27, 1990                                              4–50

The United Kingdom has only a few dedicated children's hospitals and even fewer specialized pediatric EDs. Consequently, emergencies among children are treated most often in adult ED settings by staff not trained in the emergency treatment of children. Prescription of drugs and fluids for rehydration in children is based largely on body weight and surface area parameters. However, true weights are usually unobtainable in emergencies, and drug and fluid therapy doses are estimated. To reduce the potential for error in determining drug and fluid replacement doses for children, a simple and rapid tape measure method that enables an accurate estimate of body weight in children was developed.

In a test of reliability, pediatric nurses measured 61 children aged 6 weeks–10 years during routine visits to a pediatric outpatient clinic, experienced ED nursing staff measured 78 children aged 9 days–10 years who were brought to an ED, and junior emergency medicine physicians measured 24 children aged 1 month–9 years who also were brought to the ED. Twenty-eight of the 61 children seen in the pediatric outpatient clinic also were assessed by a junior pediatrician.

The body weights estimated with the tape measure method clearly were correlated with the true body weights for all 139 children. This study confirmed that the tape is a reliable tool for estimating body weight in children, even in inexperienced hands. The use of this tape would reduce significantly the margin of error in calculating drug and fluid requirements for severely ill or injured children brought to an ED where trained pediatric emergency staff is not available.

▶ This is the British documentation of an idea developed in North Carolina by Jim Broselow, M.D. All who have used the tape system find it to be a handy reference guide. The system is not 100% accurate. Its use takes some thought and looking at the patient's body habitus. For those not used to working with children and even for those who are, it is more accurate than taking a guess at the child's weight. I highly recommend the use of the Broselow tape.— S. Ludwig, M.D.

### Pediatric Procedures: Do Parents Want to Watch?

Bauchner H, Vinci R, Waring C (Boston Univ)
*Pediatrics* 84:907–909, 1989                                      4–51

Basic invasive medical procedures such as performing venipuncture or obtaining intravenous access are frightening and painful experiences for acutely ill young children and their parents. Many pediatricians do not want parents to be present for these procedures, but parental preference under these circumstances has never been surveyed. A study was conducted to determine whether parents prefer to watch or leave when their children undergo venipuncture or intravenous catheter placement.

During a 2-month period, parents who brought a child to the ED for an acute, noncritical illness were asked to complete a questionnaire that asked whether they would want to watch while their child had blood drawn or an intravenous catheter started, why they would want or not want to watch, and whether an explanation of the procedure would be helpful if they chose not to watch.

Of 253 eligible parents, 250 completed the study. Of the 250 parents, most (88%) were mothers, most (54%) were black, and most (94%) had completed at least some high school. The mean age of the parents was 30 years, and the mean age of the children was 4.5 years. Reasons for coming to the ED included fever (18%), upper respiratory tract infection (10%), vomiting or diarrhea (7%), earache (10%), laceration (14%), and other (41%).

Analysis of the data showed that 196 (78%) of the 250 parents would want to watch if their child would need to have blood drawn or an intravenous catheter started. Of those who would want to watch, 80% said it would make them feel better, 91% believed it would make the child feel better, and 73% believed it would help the physicians. Of the 54 parents who did not wish to watch, 4 did not understand the procedures involved, 29 were scared, 22 believed it would hurt their child, and 2 believed that an explanation of the procedure would be helpful.

Parents who wished to watch were significantly more likely to have had other children who underwent procedures, be black rather than Hispanic or white, and have completed more school than those who did not want to watch. Age, gender of the child or parent, number of children in the family, marital status, type of health insurance, or reason for the visit did not influence the choice of whether or not to watch.

Most parents prefer to be present when their children undergo basic procedures such as venipuncture or placement of an intravenous catheter. Physicians should be encouraged to allow parents to be present when their children undergo these basic procedures, because most children will be helped by their parents' presence.

▶ This article documents what most parents know: they want to be present to comfort and protect their children as much as possible. Although some physicians are uncomfortable with parents observing, for nonacute procedures this is a reasonable request. In our pediatric ED, we assume parents will be present for intravenous placement and blood drawing. The issue of parental presence is often an issue when the procedures perceived are more invasive but not life-threatening, such as most lumbar punctures and urethral catheterizations. It would be interesting to confirm these findings for other procedures and in other populations.— K.N. Shaw, M.D.

---

**Use of Cyanoacrylate Tissue Adhesive for Closing Facial Lacerations in Children**
Watson DP (Guy's Hosp, London)
*BMJ* 299:1014, 1989                                           4–52

---

The value of cyanoacrylate tissue adhesive for closure of facial lacerations was prospectively assessed in 50 children aged younger than 14 years. A new method of applying the glue by means of capillary tubing was also assessed.

The skin edges were held together and glue dabbed along the wound with glass capillary tubing. The wound was then held together until the glue polymerized and became opaque. Of the 50 children, 45 returned at 2 weeks, 40 returned at 3 months, and 21 returned at 6 months for follow-up. Cosmetic results were generally excellent, with only 5 complications; 2 wounds became infected, 1 had hypertrophic scarring, 1 patient picked the wound open, and 1 patient had an inclusion body type reaction along the wound scar.

Cyanoacrylate tissue adhesive is fast, atraumatic, and cost effective and gives excellent cosmetic results. Because there are no stitches to remove, a return visit is not necessary.

▶ I am not aware of this product currently being used in the United States. The lacerations in this study were all less than 3 cm, straight, nonhemorrhagic, and not on the eyelids or mucocutaneous junctions of the mouth. I question whether Steri-Strips might not give the same results in these situations, especially when applied with benzoin to a dry surface. Steri-Strips have the same advantages over suturing that are mentioned in this brief report. The 1 complication of a foreign body reaction is worrisome.— K.N. Shaw, M.D.

---

**Comparison of Topical Tetracaine, Adrenaline, and Cocaine Anesthesia With Lidocaine Infiltration for Repair of Lacerations in Children**
Hegenbarth MA, Altieri MF, Hawk WH, Greene A, Ochsenschlager DW, O'Donnell R (Children's Hosp Natl Med Ctr, Washington, DC; Fairfax Hosp, Falls Church, Va)
*Ann Emerg Med* 19:63–67, 1990                                4–53

---

Lidocaine infiltration for laceration repair is safe, but its use in children is often painful and frightening. A topically applied solution of 0.5% tetracaine, 1:2,000 adrenaline (epinephrine), and 11.8% cocaine (TAC) appears to provide effective anesthesia for laceration repair in children and adults. However, the efficacy and safety of TAC is still being questioned. This prospective, randomized, unblinded study was done to compare TAC with lidocaine for local anesthesia of superficial lacerations in children.

The study population comprised 467 children, aged 7 months–18 years (mean 6.3 years), of whom 262 received topical TAC and 205 received lidocaine infiltration. Of 262 TAC-treated children, 218 had facial or scalp wounds, and 44 had extremity or trunk wounds. Of 205 lidocaine-treated children, 158 had facial or scalp wounds, and 47 had extremity or trunk wounds. The 2 groups were well matched for age, gender, and race. However, children with extremity or trunk lacerations were significantly older than those with facial or scalp lacerations.

Adequate anesthesia of facial and scalp wounds was achieved for 81% of the TAC-treated wounds and 87% of the lidocaine-treated wounds. Effective anesthesia of extremity wounds was achieved for only 43% of the TAC-treated wounds compared with 89% of the lidocaine-treated wounds. No systemic side effects were seen in any patients. The incidence of wound infection was 2.2% for both TAC and lidocaine. Wound dehiscence of facial or scalp wounds occurred in 7 TAC-treated patients and 2 lidocaine-treated patients. Wound dehiscence also occurred in 5 TAC-treated and 4 lidocaine-treated extremity wounds. The differences were statistically not significant. Wound erythema was seen slightly more often in TAC-treated patients than in lidocaine-treated patients, but the difference was also not significant.

The solution of TAC was well accepted by patients and parents, particularly when used on facial and scalp lacerations. Parents of children with TAC-treated extremity or trunk wounds were significantly less satisfied with the anesthesia. The use of TAC is a more humane alternative to lidocaine infiltration for anesthetizing superficial facial and scalp lacerations in children. It is less useful for anesthetizing extremity wounds.

▶ Topical TAC has been around for many years and is advocated for use on small, superficial lacerations.

If one chooses to use topical analgesia, there are 2 other tricks that I have used over the years. One is to adjust the pH of lidocaine by placing 1 mL of sodium bicarbonate with 10 mL of lidocaine. For patients with abrasions that need cleaning or removal of road tars, I have used the 2% or 4% lidocaine (Xylocaine) jelly. Because each of these has a higher amount of lidocaine per milliliter than TAC, one needs to pay particular attention to the total volume used. Do not exceed a dose of 3 mg of lidocaine/kg.

Conscious sedation is another means to approach lacerations in children.—R.W. Schafermeyer, M.D.

---

**Intramuscular Meperidine, Promethazine, and Chlorpromazine: Analysis of Use and Complications in 487 Pediatric Emergency Department Patients**

Terndrup TE, Cantor RM, Madden CM (State Univ of New York, Syracuse)
*Ann Emerg Med* 18:528–533, 1989                                    4–54

The use of DPT, a mixture of merperidine (Demerol), promethazine (Phenergan), and chlorpromazine (Thorazine), has been accepted to some degree by the pediatric community, but recommendations for its use still differ. Patterns of DPT use were examined in a review of nearly 500 pediatric patients seen in an ED in a 2-year period. The mixture was given to 1.7% of all pediatric patients seen in the ED this time.

The mean age of patients given DPT was 2.7 years. Only 9% of the patients had evidence of chronic illness; lung disease and chronic neurologic disease were most frequent. Therapy with DPT was most often used in cases of repair of a laceration or fracture reduction; the former indication was present in 69% of cases. Lacerations most commonly involved the face, and they were considered to be complex in a clear majority of cases. Eight patients required repeat sedation. Two patients had respiratory depression after receiving DPT, and 1 had an apneic episode.

The use of DPT appears to be relatively effective and safe for sedation of selected pediatric patients in the ED. Resuscitation equipment should be at hand when DPT is administered, and it should be used cautiously, if at all, in patients with neurologic illness or abnormal mental status.

▶ The concensus of the Emergency Medicine Interest Group's workshop in sedation and analgesia in the pediatric outpatient setting at the national meeting of the Ambulatory Pediatric Association in May 1990 was that the use of intramuscular DPT results in unpredictable timing, degree, and duration of sedation and analgesia. The complications of oversedation, prolonged sedation, respiratory depression of arrest, and cardiovascular instability are unacceptable. The titration of individual, shorter-acting drugs to a desired sedative or analgesic effect is safer and would produce the desired outcome more consistently.

I would interpret these study results differently than the authors. Use of potentially life-threatening medications that resulted in 8 serious complications over a 2-year period for the repair of lacerations that were predominantly of the face and finger is needless, especially when a topical anesthetic agent or digital block could be used instead. One should be extremely reluctant to sedate any child with altered mental status and should never use DPT with its prolonged effect and difficulty in reversal in this situation. If DPT is used, one must provide prolonged monitoring of the patient, which few EDs have the time or facilities to do. (See also Abstract 5–19.)—K.N. Shaw, M.D.

---

## Utility of the Cervical Spine Radiograph in Pediatric Trauma

Lally KP, Senac M, Hardin WD Jr, Haftel A, Kaehler M, Hossein Mahour G (Univ of Southern California, Los Angeles)
*Am J Surg* 158:540–542, 1989                                                     4–55

---

Current guidelines for the initial evaluation of trauma patients include obtaining a routine cervical spine radiograph. However, injured children have a much lower incidence of cervical spine injuries than adults, and the level of cervical injury in children differs from that in adults. The utility of obtaining routine cervical spine radiographs in pediatric trauma patients was determined in 187 children aged 1 month–18 years who had radiographs during a 2.5-year period. The children's mean age was 6.6 years. The number of vertebrae visualized and the quality of the radiographs were determined by a single radiologist.

All 7 cervical vertebrae were seen in only 57% of the initial radiographs. A second study visualized all 7 cervical vertebrae in 38 patients, and a third study was required in another 8 patients. Complete visualization of all 7 vertebrae was never achieved in 48 patients, 34 of whom did not have repeat study. Only 1 nondisplaced fracture of the body of C7 was seen in an 11-year-old child, who had fallen from 1.8 m.

A review of the medical records of all children admitted during a 20-year period revealed that 16 children had been admitted with a diagnosis of cervical spine injury. Only 3 of those 16 children had injuries below C4, and all were more than 8 years of age. All patients with cervical spine fracture and dislocation were symptomatic with neck pain or a neurologic deficit, or were comatose on admission. The routine cervical spine radiograph in the pediatric trauma setting is therefore a very low-yield test.

▶ Cervical spine injuries are uncommon in children and increase with age. To reduce costs and radiation exposure, investigators have attempted to define when cervical spine radiography should be performed in traumatized children. Jaffe et al. (1) developed a clinical algorithm based on the presence of 1 of 8 variables (neck pain, neck tenderness, limitation of mobility, trauma to the neck, and abnormalities of strength, reflexes, sensation, or mental status) that identified 58 of 59 children with cervical spine injuries. They recommended validation trials.

This is one of several small studies of cervical spine injuries in children. The authors reviewed all pediatric cervical radiographs done over 2 years to determine the number of vertebrae visualized and the quality of the films. It appears from their study that a significant number of children required repeat films to adequately visualize C7, and in 26%, C7 was never visualized.

They also reviewed 16 children with cervical spine injuries. Following previous trends, upper cervical spine injury was more common, and all children were symptomatic with neck pain or neurologic deficits or were comatose on arrival. These findings reflect similar studies and should prompt future prospective, large multicenter trials of clinical markers to predict cervical spine injuries in children. (See also Abstracts 2–18 and 2–8.)—J.M. Mitchell, M.D.

*Reference*

1. Jaffe DM, et al: *Ann Emerg Med* 16:1270, 1987.

---

**Emergency Endotracheal Intubation in Pediatric Trauma**
Nakayama DK, Gardner MJ, Rowe MI (Children's Hosp of Pittsburgh; Univ of Pittsburgh)
*Ann Surg* 211:218–223, 1990 4–56

---

Timely endotracheal intubation in trauma care provides a therapeutic margin that may ensure survival under critical circumstances. Many authorities recommend that patients with severe head injuries also undergo early endotracheal intubation, because it assures optimal gas exchange and allows controlled hyperventilation to decrease intracranial pressure through cerebral vasoconstriction. Despite compelling arguments in favor of early endotracheal intubation, the efficacy of early airway management protocols is as yet unknown. The effectiveness and associated problems of emergency intubation were evaluated in 605 head-injured children, 63 of whom underwent endotracheal intubation either at the scene of injury, at a referring hospital, or in the ED. Of the 63 children, 90.4% had head injuries and 39.7% had multiple injuries. Indications for intubation included coma (74.6%), shock (28.6%), apnea (22.2%), and airway obstruction (3.2%). When intubations at the scene of injury were successful, they more often required more than 1 attempt compared with those performed at the referring hospital or at the ED. Of 14 intubations attempted at the scene, 6 were unsuccessful, 4 of which were subsequently successful at the referring hospital or at the ED. The other 2 children who also underwent unsuccessful cricothyroidotomy died of their injuries before ventilation was established.

Airway-related complications occurred in 16 patients and were immediately life threatening in 13. Complications included 5 main stem intubations, 2 massive barotraumas, 2 failures of adequate preoxygenation, 1 esophageal intubation, 1 attempt at nasotracheal intubation in an open facial fracture, and 1 extubation during transport. There were 3 late complications, including 2 patients with vocal cord paresis and 1 with subglottic stenosis. There were 4 complication-associated fatalities, all at the scene. Problems in respiratory management occurred in 28 (44.4%) of the children after arrival at the ED, including major airway complications, hypoxemia, or hypercarbia. These factors were significantly more common in scene intubations. Despite endotracheal intubation, head-injured children remain at considerable risk for secondary brain injury from hypoxia and intracranial hypertension.

▶ The first thing we learn in our emergency medicine residency is the "ABCs." Airway control is the most important principle and technique we learn as residents. The emergency physician must be able to approach control of the airway in every possible situation. He or she represents the only specialist with an unprejudiced approach to total airway evaluation and control (i.e., endotracheal intubation, upper airway bypass, or lower airway chest decompression). All physicians understanding emergent airway control will occasionally have difficulties and failures. Appropriate training and skill maintenance will keep these to an acceptable minimum. (See also Abstract 6–13.)—D.K. Wagner, M.D.

---

**Epiglottitis: Comparison of Signs and Symptoms in Children Less Than 2 Years Old and Older**
Losek JD, Dewitz-Zink BA, Melzer-Lange M, Havens PL (Med College of Wisconsin, Milwaukee)
*Ann Emerg Med* 19:55–58, 1990                                    4–57

Epiglottitis is a life-threatening infectious disorder that is characterized by acute onset of fever, sore throat, dysphagia, drooling, muffled voice, preference for upright position, and breathing difficulties. Although it commonly occurs in children aged 3–7 years, it also occurs in infants and adults. Recent reports suggest that children aged younger than 2 years have different manifestations of epiglottitis than older children. The signs and symptoms of epiglottitis in children of these 2 age groups were retrospectively compared. During a 20-year period, 236 children were treated for epiglottitis; 58 children were aged younger than 2 years, and 178 were aged 2 years or older. To assess the association of age with clinical manifestation and diagnosis, the frequency of 21 signs and symptoms was determined for each age group.

The 5 most common characteristics for children aged younger than 2 years were fever, difficulty breathing, irritability, change in voice, and not sleeping. The 3 most common findings on physical examination were stridor, retractions, and fever. The 5 most common characteristics for children aged 2 years or older were fever, change in voice, sore throat, difficulty breathing, and irritability. The 3 most common findings on physical examination were identical to those in the younger age group. Sore throat was significantly more common in older children with epiglottitis and was the only characteristic that was statistically significantly different between the 2 age groups. Pneumonia was the most common extrasupraglottic infection. The diagnosis initially was missed in 11 children (19%) aged younger than 2 years and in 49 children (28%) aged 2 years or older. One of the younger children and 6 of the older children died. Blood cultures were positive for *Hemophilus influenzae* in 128 children (54%). The signs and symptoms of epiglottitis in children aged younger than 2 years are similar to those seen in children aged 2 years and older.

▶ Epiglottitis is a disease that is well respected and feared by the emergency physician. The following trends are occurring: First, its incidence in infants and children is decreasing. This may serve to wrongly lower one's threshold for concern and diagnosis. Second, its incidence in adolescents and adults is increasing. This may serve to wrongly lower one's concern for possible mortality. Third, the rapidity of clinical symptoms is inversely proportional to age and size of airway. Finally, the availability and use of bedside fiberoptic nasopharyngoscopy can help to ameliorate the first 3 concerns. (See also Abstract 3–3.)— D.K. Wagner, M.D.

---

**Circumstances Surrounding the Deaths of Children Due to Asthma: A Case-Control Study**
Miller BD, Strunk RC (Univ of Colorado, Denver; Washington Univ, St Louis)
*Am J Dis Child* 143:1294–1299, 1989                                4–58

---

Many studies have investigated the circumstances surrounding deaths caused by asthma, but none has been case controlled. The life circumstances and course of events in 12 children aged 10–18 years who died of an acute asthma episode were compared with those in 12 control children aged 11–17 years who suffered a life-threatening asthma attack but survived.

Information obtained by structured interviews with families and physicians and from medical records was used to characterize the patient and his or her family, to define the severity and treatment of asthma during the 6 months before the attack, and to describe the medical circumstances and patient characteristics on the day of and during the acute episode. The 12 case patients were carefully matched to their controls for similar use of long-term medication and overall ratings of disease severity.

Analysis of the variables pertaining to the 6-month period preceding the attacks showed that case patients had a greater frequency of respiratory failure requiring intubation, a decrease in steroid use in the month before the attack, a history of family disturbance, and an abnormal reaction to separation or loss and had expressed hopelessness and despair.

Analysis of the variables pertaining to the medical circumstances and patient characteristics on the day of the attack showed that case patients more often had attacks started during sleep but less frequently experienced vomiting during the course of the attacks. Treatment of the attack by the parents was poor in 7 of the 12 children who died, but poor treatment was also a factor in 6 of the 12 children who survived. None of the many other variables analyzed for this study discriminated between case patients and controls.

Although the data suggest that certain characteristics of asthmatic children may place them at greater risk for death from an acute asthma attack, there may be as yet unidentified inherent differences in the mechanisms of the acute attacks between children who died and those who survived.

▶ Although this is a matched case-control study, there are several areas of potential bias: interviewer, recall, and selection bias. Much of the information was obtained during an interview by the investigators with parents. However, it is certainly important to obtain a previous history of severity of illness, including episodes of respiratory failure, medication usage with attention to decreased steroid use, and precipitating or exacerbating situations in the evaluation of children with asthma in the ED. This study stresses the role of the emergency physician in recognizing risk factors for serious morbidity and mortality in evaluating children with chronic disease. (See also Abstract 3–7.)—K.N. Shaw, M.D.

---

**Pulse Oximetry to Identify a High-Risk Group of Children With Wheezing**
Rosen LM, Yamamoto LG, Wiebe RA (Univ of Hawaii, Kapiolan, Med Ctr for Women and Children, Honolulu)
*Am J Emerg Med* 7:567–570, 1989                                    4–59

---

To investigate the value of pulse oximetry in treating children who are brought to the ED with wheezing-associated respiratory illnesses, the initial oxygen saturations (OSATs) were measured in 1,235 patients younger than age 19 years seen over a 5-month period with a wide range of wheezing-associated respiratory illnesses. A total of 1,101 initial OSATs with the patients breathing room air were recorded. The saturations were not recorded if the patient was too uncooperative or fussy to enable a steady-state reading. Initial OSATs were also measured on 138 control pediatric patients who had no evidence of respiratory illness.

The mean OSATs were 95.4% for wheezing children and 98.7% for controls. An initial OSAT of 95% or more indicated a low need for hospitalization, whereas an initial OSAT of less than 85% indicated a high need for hospitalization.

Pulse oximetry is a reliable, noninvasive procedure that is easy to perform, even in children. Initial OSAT measurements in the early phase of an ED encounter may identify which wheezing children are at high risk so that aggressive therapy may be initiated without delay.

▶ The clinician is always looking for a way to identify the asthmatic patient who needs admission or who may be at risk of arresting in the department. In the past, the seriously ill child was placed on oxygen therapy, hopefully a cardiac monitor, and then would have to undergo the process of obtaining arterial blood gases. Not only is the procedure painful, but it can worsen the agitation of the patient. At last there is a simple noninvasive piece of technology that allows us to monitor the asthmatic patient. Pulse oximetry is simple and easy to use, and for the pediatric patient, one can use the ear probe, finger, or toe probe.

An OSAT less than 85% places the child in acute respiratory failure, and that child deserves aggressive airway support and management. That child most likely will need to be admitted to an intensive care unit if he or she does not rapidly respond to oxygenation and adrenergic inhalation therapy.—R.W. Schafermeyer, M.D.

---

**The Child With Simultaneous Stridor and Wheezing**
Poole SR, Mauro RD, Fan LL, Brooks J (Univ of Colorado, Denver; Children's Hosp of Denver; Univ of Rochester, Rochester, NY)
*Pediatr Emerg Care* 6:33–37, 1990                                          4–60

---

Stridor in children usually occurs during inspiration and usually is produced by obstruction to airflow in the extrathoracic airway. Wheezing occurs primarily during expiration and usually is produced by obstruction to airflow in the intrathoracic airway. A child with simultaneous stridor and wheezing may thus have 2 pathologic processes at different levels of the airway or 1 process in either the extrathoracic or intrathoracic airway. The case histories of 25 children with simultaneous stridor and wheezing were reviewed.

Twelve patients with simultaneous stridor and wheezing had treatment at the ED of 1 institution within 2 years. Another 13 cases were found in medical articles. The distinction between stridor and wheezing during physical examination was based on the particular pitch and quality of airway noise as subjectively determined by an examiner. The age at onset ranged from birth to 17 years. The median age at onset was 6 months, with 22 of the 25 children aged 2 years or less when symptoms began. Six patients had 2 separate foci of obstruction causing the stridor and wheezing, of whom 3 had croup and bronchiolitis, 1 had croup and asthma, 1 had epiglottitis and asthma, and 1 had thyroglossal duct cyst and bronchiolitis. The other 19 patients had a single etiology, of whom 8 had congenital airway obstructing lesions, 9 had foreign bodies in their airways or esophaguses, and 2 older children had acquired lesions obstructing their airways. All 8 patients with congenital lesions had symptoms by 4 months of age, all 9 patients with foreign bodies had symptoms between 5 and 30 months of age, and the patients with single lesions were aged 16 and 17 years.

For 18 of the 25 patients, the lesion site was accurately identified with a combination of history, physical examination, and 4 plain radiographs, including lateral neck, posteroanterior chest, lateral chest, and forced expiratory chest. Barium swallow was used in 2 patients with vascular rings. Endoscopy was used to identify accurately the sites of lesions in 3 children with congenital lesions and in 1 child with a bronchial foreign body.

Single, congenital lesions in young infants first seen with simultaneous stridor and wheezing should be highly suspected, whereas foreign bodies are the more likely cause in older infants and toddlers. Single acquired lesions of the airway should be considered for children of all ages but may be more common in older children.

▶ As our skill in saving small, premature infants improves, we are likely to note an increase in the number of children with compromised airways. The report of children with simultaneous stridor and wheezing is documentation of that occurrence. Foreign body in the airway is also a well-documented cause of this symptom complex. The authors note several other rarer causes. Six children had more than 1 apparent cause. All that wheezes is not asthma. All that is stridor is not croup or epiglottitis.—S. Ludwig, M.D.

---

**Serious Respiratory Consequences of Detergent Ingestions in Children**
Einhorn A, Horton L, Altieri M, Ochsenschlager D, Klein B (Children's Hosp Natl Med Ctr, Washington, DC)
*Pediatrics* 84:472–474, 1989 4–61

---

Phosphate detergents have been replaced by nonphosphate detergents containing sodium carbonate and sodium silicate. Eight children aged 1–2.5 years were admitted to a hospital after ingesting or inhaling laundry detergent powder containing sodium carbonate.

Symptoms of airway compromise appeared 1–2 hours after ingestion or immediately after inhalation of small amounts of the detergent. One patient had symptoms 5 hours after ingestion but had damage only to the lips and buccal mucosa. The most frequent symptoms were stridor, drooling, and respiratory distress. Five patients vomited, and 1 had eye injury. All but 1 patient underwent endoscopy of the airway and esophagus. Five were admitted to the intensive care unit, and all but 1 of the 4 children who underwent intubation had edema of the epiglottis. Regardless of type of therapy, all patients had improvement within 12 hours of admission and all were asymptomatic at 72 hours.

Ingestion or inhalation of sodium carbonate or silicate detergent powders can cause severe upper airway compromise. Manifestations of airway compromise appear within 1−2 hours but can develop as late as 5 hours after ingestion. Corneal injury should be ruled out. Therapy consists of supportive control of the airway. There are no consistent indications for either endoscopy or intubation.

▶ Nonphosphorus-containing detergents are toxic and caustic because their pH level is typically greater than 10.0. It is especially toxic to the oropharynx and gastrointestinal tract. It can be irritating to the respiratory tract system if the powders are inhaled into the tracheobronchial tree.

Almost every ED physician who has access to a poison control center or Poisondex knows the proper management for the nonphosphate detergent ingestions. The majority of these children will be placed in the hospital for endoscopy or followed very closely by a pediatric surgeon or general surgeon. It is rare for the detergent to be inhaled into the respiratory tract system. This article, however, relates that it may not be so rare as I thought, and respiratory tract symptoms can appear as late as 5 hours after ingestion. Most of these children had signs of respiratory obstruction or distress, such as stridor, drooling, tachypnea, and wheezing. The child deserves appropriate aggressive airway support and endoscopy to evaluate the tracheobronchial tree. If there are no signs or symptoms of respiratory distress or upper airway obstruction, the child should be watched for 6 hours.—R.W. Schafermeyer, M.D.

---

**Childhood Near-Drowning: Is Cardiopulmonary Resuscitation Always Indicated?**

Nichter MA, Everett PB (Univ of South Florida; All Children's Hosp, St Petersburg)
Crit Care Med 17:993−995, 1989                          4−62

---

There are increasing reports of pediatric near-drowning victims who recover after arriving at the ED in a comatose state. Data on 93 pediatric near-drowning victims were reviewed to evaluate variables that might predict outcome in patients admitted to emergency care with significant physiologic impairment.

Of the 93 near-drowning pediatric patients, 67 survived intact, 7 survived with severe brain damage, and 19 died. Spastic quadraplegia developed in the 7 patients who survived with severe brain damage, and 4 subsequently died. Age, sex, and length of submersion were not reliable predictors of outcome.

Forty-eight intact survivors and 5 impaired survivors received cardio-pulmonary resuscitation (CPR) on the scene. On arrival at the hospital, 17 patients had no perfusing cardiac rhythm; 14 died and 3 survivied impaired. There were no intact survivors in this group. Cardiotonic medication was required by 23 patients; 16 died and 7 survived impaired; no patients in this group survived intact. All intact survivors had pupillary light reactivity on initial admission. On arrival, 23 patients were apneic; 17 died, 5 survived impaired, and 1 survived intact. No response to pain was found in 27 patients; 19 died, 6 survived impaired, and 2 survived intact.

Pediatric near-drowning victims appear to benefit from on-scene CPR; those who require CPR in the emergency room do not have a good prognosis. The need for cardiotonic medication was an absolute predictor of poor outcome in these patients. The decision to use cardiotonic medication on a pediatric near-drowning victim should take into consideration the patient's chances of surviving neurologically intact.

▶ This retrospective review is entirely descriptive without any statistical analysis of the data they review. The authors suggest that the emergency physician should consider not resuscitating warm water, near-drowning victims if they arrive without a perfusing cardiac rhythm or require cardiotonic medications. This conclusion is based on 17 and 23 patients, respectively. When one calculates the 95% confidence intervals on this small number of cases, the true incidence of intact survival in the general population of near-drowning victims is estimated to be up to 15%–20%. This is consistent with the findings of other investigators who report up to a 24% intact neurologic survival in patients requiring CPR in the ED (1).

Although requirement for CPR or cardiotonic medications and lack of pupillary response in the ED are indicators of a low chance of intact neurologic recovery, the ED physician cannot predict absolute poor outcome if these signs are present. Initial resuscitation should be performed in all cases of warm water near-drowning and should be continued in cases of cold water near-drowning until the core temperature is greater than 32°C.—K.N. Shaw, M.D.

*Reference*

1. Allman FD, et al: *Am J Dis Child* 140:571, 1986.

---

**Syncope in Children and Adolescents**
Pratt JL, Fleisher GR (Miami Children's Hosp)
*Pediatr Emerg Care* 5:80–82, 1989                                    4–63

---

The causes of syncope, its frequency, and the best methods for its evaluation are not well studied for children and adolescents. Emergency department records of 77 such patients whose chief complaint was fainting were examined retrospectively.

Careful study indicated that 20 patients did not have a syncopal or near-syncopal episode. Syncope was experienced by 40, and near-syncope occurred in 17 patients. In patients with syncope, the diagnoses included vasovagal syncope in 50%; orthostatic hypotension in 20% because of dehydration or, in a few cases, anemia; atypical seizure in 7.5%; minor head trauma in 5%; and migraine headache in 5%. In the near-syncope group, final diagnoses were lightheadedness in 29%, seizure in 18%, tension headache in 12%, and migraine in 6%.

Abnormalities were found in 17.5% of those with syncope, involving orthostatic blood pressure, heart rate, hematocrit and glucose levels, and ECG tracings. Those with near-syncope had no abnormalities.

Initial evaluation should include history, physical examination, determinations of orthostatic blood pressure and hematocrit and glucose values, and 12-lead ECG. Prospective studies showing outcome over time should be performed to identify the best initial evaluation and explore prognostic implications. Meanwhile, the physician should follow up to see if the clinical situation warrants more invasive testing.

▶ This retrospective study points out that syncope in children is usually benign and vasovagal in origin but suffers from small numbers and incomplete information on each patient. Only 12 patients actually had orthostatic vital signs done, 165 had hematocrit values determined, 14 had ECGs done, and 15 had glucose levels checked. It is difficult to make final determination of diagnoses and predictions with this information.

The most important part of an evaluation for syncope is a complete history and physical examination, which dictate which laboratory studies to obtain. The authors make an important point that the examination should include orthostatic vital signs. In pediatrics, the Dextrostick is usually considered part of the preliminary evaluation. One should consider obtaining ECG readings and hematocrit values if anemia or a cardiac etiology are possible etiologies consistent with the history. Conversely, the history and examination indicate the need for an electroencephalogram, Haltor monitor, or pregnancy test. Follow-up is very important.— K.N. Shaw, M.D.

### Children With Abdominal Pain: Evaluation in the Pediatric Emergency Department
Reynolds SL, Jaffe DM (Northwestern Univ; Children's Mem Hosp, Chicago)
*Pediatr Emerg Care* 6:8–12, 1990                                    4–64

Abdominal pain is a common complaint of children seen in a pediatric ED. However, because the range and frequency of diagnoses for such children have not been assessed previously, the medical records of 371 children seen in a pediatric ED with abdominal pain during 4 seasonally diverse months were reviewed.

Of 197 boys and 174 girls, 182 were aged 2–6 years, 118 were aged 7–11 years, and 71 were aged 12–16 years. Children aged 2–6 years had the highest relative incidence of fever, vomiting, and ill appearance. Teenage patients had the highest percentage of tenderness and guarding.

Ten Most Common Diagnoses in Patients
With Abdominal Pain

|  | No. | % |
|---|---|---|
| Gastroenteritis | 98 | 26 |
| Nonspecific abdominal pain | 98 | 26 |
| Viral illness | 24 | 6 |
| Constipation | 18 | 5 |
| Urinary tract infection | 18 | 5 |
| Pharyngitis | 17 | 5 |
| Appendicitis | 13 | 4 |
| Asthma | 8 | 2 |
| Otitis | 7 | 2 |
| Pneumonia | 7 | 2 |

(Courtesy of Reynolds SL, Jaffe DM: *Pediatr Emerg Care* 6:8–12, 1990.)

Forty-eight different diagnoses were made, but 10 diagnoses accounted for 83% of the patients (table). Gastroenteritis and nonspecific abdominal pain accounted for 59% of the children seen in the ED. Respiratory illnesses were diagnosed for 12%. Thirteen children had appendicitis, representing the only surgical problem occurring in more than 1% of the patients. Most diagnoses (64.4%) were classified as medical, 6.5% as surgical, and 29.1% as nonspecific. Eighteen percent of the teenage patients had surgical diagnoses.

Statistical analysis showed that age, general appearance, presence or absence of vomiting, guarding, and abdominal tenderness were associated significantly with diagnosis type. Guarding and abdominal tenderness were associated most strongly with a surgical diagnosis, whereas decreased appetite, diarrhea, dysuria, location of abdominal pain, and duration of pain before the ED visit were not significantly associated with a surgical diagnosis.

The high percentage of nonspecific diagnoses in children with abdominal pain seen at an ED of a large pediatric teaching hospital illustrates the difficulty of diagnosing abdominal pain in children.

▶ This report by Reynolds and Jaffe presents an interesting, retrospective, epidemiologic profile of the complaint of abdominal pain in children. Because the sample size is small and the study retrospective, it is hard to fully accept the data relating signs and symptoms to final diagnosis. Nonetheless, there are interesting trends that must be substantiated by a more tightly controlled prospective study. The most important take-home message comes in the list of all of the final diagnoses. It teaches us to approach the child with abdominal pain with healthy respect and an open mind to all sorts of problems. The finding that most causes are medical is also important. Only 6.5% of the cases were surgical, but the authors do not provide us with an equally important statistic, the rate of surgical consultation. The diagnosis of appendicitis continues to be a difficult one. There are so many variations in its manifestation. It behooves the ED physician to be liberal in the use of pediatric surgical consultation. (See also Abstracts 2–42 and 2–43.)—S. Ludwig, M.D.

### Emergency Department Thoracotomy in Children—A Critical Analysis

Rothenberg SS, Moore EE, Moore FA, Baxter BT, Moore JB, Cleveland HC (Denver Gen Hosp; Univ of Colorado)
*J Trauma* 29:1322–1325, 1989                    4–65

The use of ED thoracotomy in critically injured pediatric patients has not been adequately evaluated. In an effort to establish guidelines for performing ED thoracotomy in children, results of ED thoracotomies in 83 children treated at level I trauma centers over an 11-year period were reviewed.

Pediatric patients ranged in age from 13 months to 18 years and represented 12% of the 689 ED thoracotomies performed. Causes of injury included blunt trauma (57%), gunshot wound (30%), and stab wound (13%). On arrival at ED, patients were classified as having no signs of life (group 1), waning signs of life without vital signs (group 2), or vital signs present (group 3).

Sixty of these 83 pediatric patients died in the ED. Twenty-three were able to be transferred to the operating room, but only 3 survived surgery. All 3 of these patients eventually had full recovery; 1 was from group 1 and 2 were from group 3. Survival by type of injury was 9% for stab wound, 4% for gunshot wound, and 2% for blunt trauma. Although more than 90% of pediatric fatalities are caused by blunt trauma, such injury mechanism has the poorest outcome. Thus thoracotomy appears unwarranted in blunt trauma victims with no signs of life at ED admission.

The outcome of ED thoracotomy in children is similar to that reported for adults. Both injury mechanism and physiological status on ED admission should be considered in the decision to perform the procedure. Children with penetrating wounds and those with a detectable pulse are likely to benefit but not those arriving lifeless after blunt trauma.

▶ The value of emergency thoracotomy is a topic with a long history of deep controversy and debate. At last, the pediatric patient has been brought into the fray. The findings of this report will hopefully obviate further conflict. My reading of the report is that emergency thoracotomy continues to be a generally unrewarding procedure. It may have value in the rare circumstance of a patient with penetrating thoracic trauma who is brought directly to a level I pediatric trauma center. For the majority of patients with absent vital signs, it is an exercise in futility, a waste of resources, and a possible health risk to those at the bedside.—S. Ludwig, M.D.

### Cardiac Contusion in Pediatric Patients With Blunt Thoracic Trauma

Ildstad ST, Tollerud DJ, Weiss RG, Cox JA, Martin LW (Children's Hosp Med Ctr, Cincinnati)
*J Pediatr Surg* 25:287–289, 1990                    4–66

Cardiac contusion is more frequent than previously recognized in adults sustaining blunt thoracic trauma. Its prevalence in pediatric trauma patients was examined in a review of 7 patients seen in 8 months with significant blunt thoracic trauma that produced rib fracture or pulmonary contusion. The age range was 2.5–18 years.

All of the patients had injury to at least 1 other major organ system. Four patients had bone injury, and 4 had closed head injury. Three patients had cardiac contusion identified by multigated acquisition cardiac scanning. Cardiac enzyme and isoenzyme estimates confirmed myocardial damage in all cases. Ventricular wall motion was abnormal, but no ECG abnormality or ventricular ectopy was noted in these patients. Two patients with cardiac contusion had emergency surgery and tolerated it well. One had a repeat scan 3 weeks after injury, which showed normal myocardial function.

Cardiac contusion may be relatively common in children sustaining severe thoracic injury. The presence of pulmonary contusion, especially with rib fractures, should suggest the possibility of occult myocardial damage.

▶ Although the patient numbers are small, the report by Ildstad and colleagues is important in that it alerts us to a problem that often goes unrecognized in the ED. Children so rarely have cardiac complications to their illnesses that we tend to overlook that system so central to adult pathology. Even when thoracic trauma is the central complaint, cardiac trauma is not considered. At many trauma centers, the consideration of cardiac trauma would be evaluated by an ECG. If the ECG were normal, further studies might not be undertaken. This report gives us pause and indicates that the diagnosis of cardiac contusion needs to be pursued more vigorously. The authors promise a second report in which they will indicate the clinical relevance of their findings. So stay tuned. (See also Abstracts 2–30 and 2–31.)—S. Ludwig, M.D.

---

## The Use of an Insulin Bolus in Low-Dose Insulin Infusion for Pediatric Diabetic Ketoacidosis

Lindsay R, Bolte RG (Univ of Utah, Salt Lake City)
*Pediatr Emerg* 5:77–79, 1989                    4–67

---

To determine if a priming bolus of insulin is necessary before starting low-dose insulin infusion in pediatric diabetic ketoacidosis (DKA), 56 episodes of DKA in 38 children were studied during therapy with an intravenous bolus of insulin (0.1 units/kg), followed by continuous low-dose insulin infusion (0.1 units/kg) (n = 24), or a similar insulin infusion without a prior insulin bolus (n = 32).

Regardless of the degree of acidosis, the decline in serum glucose level and changes in serum osmolality after the first hour of insulin therapy were virtually similar in both the bolus and nonbolus groups. The time required to reach a serum glucose level of less than 250 mg/dL and the total duration of insulin infusion were also similar in both groups. These data show that the use of a bolus insulin before low-dose insulin infusion in pediatric DKA appears unnecessary.

▶ This report by Lindsay and Bolte indicates that it is not necessary to use bolus administration of insulin before starting an intravenous insulin infusion. This is nicely documented in a study of 56 episodes of DKA. This study comes at a time when we have seen the effects of too vigorous therapy in a few patients. One must be careful to weigh the patient properly, make accurate calculations of insulin and fluids, and continue to monitor the patient and his or her laboratory values closely. The rate of glucose fall should be watched and should not exceed 100 mg%/hr. (See also Abstract 3–67.)—S. Ludwig, M.D.

---

**Severe Hypoglycemia in Children With Insulin-Dependent Diabetes Mellitus: Frequency and Predisposing Factors**
Daneman D, Frank M, Perlman K, Tamm J, Ehrlich R (Univ of Toronto; The Hosp for Sick Children, Toronto)
*J Pediatr* 115:681–685, 1989                                                    4–68

---

Children with insulin-dependent diabetes mellitus (IDDM) are at constant risk for hypoglycemia. Several studies have assessed the incidence of severe hypoglycemic episodes among adult patients with IDDM but not among children with IDDM. To define the frequency of hypoglycemic episodes in children with IDDM and to identify any factors associated with the occurrence of severe hypoglycemia, 311 children with a mean age of 11.6 years and a mean duration of IDDM of 4.6 years were surveyed during a 3-month period.

A questionnaire was given to each child and his or her parent to be completed during their visit to a diabetes clinic. Each episode of hypoglycemia was confirmed either by a long concentration of blood glucose measured at home or in an emergency room or by a prompt response to administration of glucagon or glucose. Only severe hypoglycemic episodes confirmed by chart review were included in the analysis. Severe hypoglycemia was defined by the occurrence of coma, convulsion, or both. Moderate hypoglycemia was defined by the occurrence of confusion requiring assistance to terminate the event.

Ninety-seven (31%) of the 311 children reported at least 1 episode of severe hypoglycemia since their IDDM was diagnosed, 50 (16%) reported at least 1 moderate hypoglycemic episode, and 164 (53%) had no history of either moderate or severe hypoglycemic episodes. Sixty-eight of the 97 children with severe episodes reported 2–20 such episodes, 50 of whom reported such an event in a single year. Of the 285 severe hypoglycemic episodes reported, 39% occurred during sleep and 61% during waking hours. Children with severe hypoglycemic episodes tended to have IDDM of longer duration and to be younger at the time of their first episodes. Of the 285 episodes, 37% occurred in spring, 28% in summer, 22% in fall, and 13% in winter.

Exercise, missed caloric intake, and excess insulin administration were implicated either alone or in combination in most episodes of severe hypoglycemia. Although all families had been taught to use glucagon to reverse severe hypoglycemia, glucagon was available in only 80 of the 97 homes and was used in only 30 of the 80 homes where it was available. The primary modes of therapy for the remainder was oral administration of glucose in 31 patients and intravenous glucose administration at an ED in the remaining 36 patients. No children had significant morbidity associated with a severe episode. Severe hypoglycemia is common among children with IDDM who are treated conventionally.

▶ The emergency physician is likely to see children with IDDM and significant hypoglycemic episodes since these are quite common even in children who are treated conventionally. Knowledge of the predisposing factors associated with these episodes is important to determine a management plan before discharge in the ED. This is also a good opportunity to provide teaching to the patients regarding use of glucagon in future episodes.— K.N. Shaw, M.D.

---

**Hypoglycemic Hemiplegia in an Adolescent With Insulin-Dependent Diabetes Mellitus: A Case Report and a Review of the Literature**
Lala VR, Vedanarayana VV, Ganesh S, Fray C, Iosub S, Noto R (Lincoln Med and Mental Health Ctr, New York; New York Med College, Bronx)
*J Emerg Med* 7:233–236, 1989                                              4–69

---

Hypoglycemic hemiplegia (HH) is the most frequent focal neurologic abnormality in adults with hypoglycemia of various etiology, but it has rarely been reported in children. An adolescent with insulin-dependent diabetes mellitus (IDDM) was seen during an episode of HH.

Girl, 15 years, with IDDM had left facial paresis and muscular weakness of the left upper and lower extremities with a documented blood glucose level of 31 mg/ dL. Rapid infusion of glucose led to a rapid and complete recovery of hemiplegia. The patient remained neurologically intact 6 months later.

Hypoglycemia should be considered in the differential etiology of acute hemiplegia in diabetic patients. The mechanism of this focal neurologic abnormality of hypoglycemia is not clear, but selective neuronal susceptibility is a likely explanation in most patients. Although rare in children and adolescents, clinicians should be aware of HH in pediatric patients because rapid infusion of glucose may prevent irreversible neurologic sequelae and possibly death.

▶ This is an interesting case report. Based on the patient's findings on entrance to the ED and her past medical history, it is unlikely that the diagnosis of hypoglycemia would have been missed. However, without this report, I think most patients like this would be subjected to much more intensive study, including a CT scan and lumbar puncture. It appears that treating the hypoglycemia and waiting 12–24 hours is all that is needed.— S. Ludwig, M.D.

### Calcium Blocking Agents in Pediatric Emergency Care

Shahar E, Sagy M, Koren G, Barzilay Z (The Chaim Sheba Med Ctr, Tel Hashomer, Israel; Hosp for Sick Children, Toronto)
*Pediatric Emerg Care* 6:52–57, 1990                                    4–70

Much evidence indicates that preventing calcium ion from entering tissue cells has therapeutic benefits in various diseases and symptoms. In many EDs, calcium-blocking agents (CBAs) already have become the first line of drug therapy for converting paroxysmal supraventricular tachycardia (PSVT) into normal sinus rhythm and in ameliorating malignant hypertension. Because pediatricians often encounter life-threatening clinical episodes in the pediatric ED, familiarity with the current indications for CBAs in adults is important.

Calcium-blocking agents now used clinically are verapamil, nifedipine, nimodipine, flunarizine, cinnarizine, and diltiazem. Verapamil is highly effective in the treatment of tachyarrhythmias. Diltiazem has been used successfully to treat PSVT in adults, but clinical experience with this drug in children is not yet available. The use of CBAs to protect the heart against myocardial ischemia is still in the experimental stage. Some evidence suggests that both nifedipine and verapamil are somewhat beneficial to patients undergoing cardiopulmonary resuscitation. The use of CBAs to treat and prevent acute asthma is relatively new. Although the results of animal experiments have been promising, studies of human beings have been inconsistent. Increasing evidence suggests that nimodipine effectively decreases cerebral damage after severe head trauma and intracranial hemorrhage. Nimodipine appears promising for a variety of neurologic emergencies, but data for the pediatric age group are still insufficient. Flunarizine has been used as add-on therapy for patients with seizures. However, results are still preliminary. Flunarizine also appears to be effective as prophylactic therapy in common, classic, and complicated childhood migraine.

As investigation of the CBAs for use in EDs continues, additional therapeutic applications for CBAs undoubtedly will find their way into pediatric emergency care.

▶ For the emergency practitioner, CBAs are very commonly used in the care of adult patients. Thus, they are very familiar with the indications and contraindications of CBAs in the adult population.

The majority of pediatric uses has been limited for most of us to the treatment of PSVT in children more than 1 year of age and for children with severe hypertension or complicated childhood migraines. Several articles in the literature have discussed the potential benefits of CBAs in cardiopulmonary and cardiopulmonary-cerebral resuscitation, but the studies have been inconclusive and inconsistent. This article nicely outlines the different effects of the various CBAs. It is important that the clinician understands the actions of verapamil, nifedipine, diltiazem, and flunarizine and continue to watch the literature for additional usages of CBAs in the pediatric practice.

I was disappointed that the article did not cover the other important issue of CBAs, namely, the accidental ingestion of these agents in the toddler. Accidental ingestion of these agents can cause profound cardiovascular collapse or seizures in the pediatric patient, and it is important to keep that in your differential as you resuscitate these patients, because calcium chloride or calcium gluconate is the agent of choice in resuscitating these patients. For the child who has not arrested, it is important to decontaminate the gastrointestinal tract and to have calcium available for infusion.—R.W. Schafermeyer, M.D.

---

**Common Clinical Features as Predictors of Bacterial Diarrhea in Infants**
Finkelstein JA, Schwartz JS, Torrey S, Fleisher GR (Univ of Pennsylvania; Temple Univ, Philadelphia)
*Am J Emerg Med* 7:469–473, 1989                                           4–71

---

Bacterial diarrhea in young infants usually is self-limited, but it can have serious complications. Optimal treatment requires identification of those infants who harbor bacterial pathogens. Clinical features were analyzed in a series of 1,035 infants less than 1 year of age who were seen in a 1-year period with diarrhea. Bacterial pathogens were present in 10.4% of the infants. *Salmonella* species were isolated in 84% of cases and *Campylobacter* in 10%. The infants with and those without bacterial pathogens differed in temperature, a history of blood in the stool, and frequency of stools. A history of fecal blood was the best single predictor. There were significant seasonal variations in prevalence of bacterial pathogens (Fig 4–6). Low-, intermediate-, and high-risk groups were defined by analyzing combinations of clinical factors by season. The findings in infants less than 3 months of age were similar to those in the study group as a whole.

The 3 clinical factors evaluated are not very sensitive or specific predictors of bacterial diarrhea in young infants. A prospective study should focus on discrimination of infants at intermediate risk of bacterial disease.

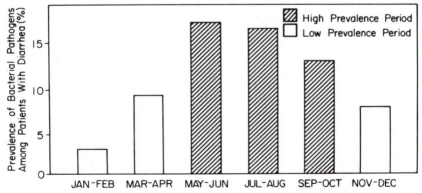

Fig 4–6.—Seasonal prevalence of bacterial pathogens among infants with diarrhea. (Courtesy of Finkelstein JA, Schwartz JS, Torrey S, et al: *Am J Emerg Med* 7:469–473, 1989.)

The usefulness of stool leukocyte estimates in young infants requires further study.

▶ Two other smaller but similar studies are cited by the authors (1, 2). All 3 studies concentrated on developing clinical strategies for predicting bacterial diarrhea. Each study enrolled consecutive patients seen at an ED with acute diarrhea, though there were different age characteristics. The rate of bacterial isolates varied from 10% to 23%. *Salmonella, Campylobacter,* and *Shigella* were the 3 most common bacterial isolates; each study had marked variation in the relative incidence of these 3 etiologies.

The results of testing for fecal leukocytes will tend to mirror the distribution of etiologies of the diarrhea. *Shigella* and *Campylobacter* more commonly are associated with colitis and therefore will have fecal leukocytes, but only about 30% of patients with *Salmonella* will have fecal leukocytes.

A high level of suspicion should be maintained in all children with diarrhea, especially those most at risk for bacteremia (<12 months of age). An infant with fever and bloody diarrhea should have a stool culture performed; depending on the age of the child, a blood culture and even admission may be indicated. A child with vomiting, no fever, and no mucus or blood in the stool would be the least likely to have bacterial gastroenteritis (<5%). The presence of fecal leukocytes increases the possibility of a bacterial isolate, but a negative finding does not rule out bacterial disease, especially in *Salmonella* gastroenteritis. Remember that public health concerns dictate an increased level of screening for children with diarrhea who are enrolled in day care or who have family members employed in food service or health care occupations.

The issue of predicting bacterial disease in children with diarrhea is important partly because of the risk of bacteremia associated with *Salmonella* gastroenteritis. Overall, 35% of all reported *Salmonella* infections occur in children less than 4 years old, with one half of that amount in children less than 12 months of age. Approximately 5%–10% of infants with *Salmonella* gastroenteritis are bacteremic at the time they are seen. Controversy still remains regarding the optimal management of infants with suspected *Salmonella* gastroenteritis, bacteremia, or both. For a good summary of the issues, see the consensus article by St. Geme et al. (3).—R.M. Rutstein, M.D.

*References*

1. Fontana M, et al: *Pediatr Infect Dis J* 6:1088, 1987.
2. DeWitt TG, et al: *Pediatrics* 76:551, 1985.
3. St. Geme JW III, et al: *Pediatric Infect Dis J* 7:615, 1988.

---

**Food-Based Oral Rehydration Salt Solution for Acute Childhood Diarrhoea**
Molla AM, Molla A, Nath SK, Khatun M (Internatl Ctr for Diarrhoeal Disease Research, Dhaka, Bangladesh)
*Lancet* 2:429–431, 1989                                                    4–72

Early oral rehydration with salt solution can prevent progressive dehydration from acute diarrhea in children, but treatment based on sugar or glucose does not reduce the stool output. In this study, 266 children aged 1–5 years with acute diarrhea and moderate to severe dehydration were given either standard glucose oral rehydration solution (ORS) or oral rehydration therapy (ORT) based on maize, millet, wheat, sorghum, rice flour, or potato. Cereal-based ORS has the same salt composition as standard ORS.

Cholera was the most common cause of diarrhea in this study. Most of the children were severely dehydrated when treatment began. Stool output was greatest among the children given standard ORS. It was 30%–50% less in those given food-based ORT. Electrolyte abnormalities present at admission were corrected with both types of treatment. Stool glucose content did not differ significantly between groups at admission or after 24 hours of treatment.

Food-based ORT should prove more acceptable in developing countries because it is similar to the foods traditionally used in weaning. In addition, it reduces stool output substantially, whereas standard ORT does not.

---

**Cereal Based Oral Rehydration Solutions**
Kenya PR, Odongo HW, Oundo G, Waswa K, Muttunga J, Molla AM, Nath SK, Molla A, Greenough WB III, Juma R, Were BN (Kenya Med Research Inst, Nairobi; Ministry of Health, Kakamega, Kenya; Internatl Ctr for Diarrhoeal Disease Research, Dhaka, Bangladesh; Aga Khan Univ Hosp, Karachi, Pakistan)
*Arch Dis Child* 64:1032–1035, 1989                                    4–73

---

Oral rehydration solutions made from various low-cost cereals that are readily available in most parts of Africa were compared to evaluate effectiveness. Solutions made of maize, millet, sorghum, or rice were compared with WHO-UNICEF-recommended oral rehydration solution in 257 boys aged 4–55 months with acute diarrhea and moderate to severe hydration. Those with bloody diarrhea or systemic illness other than malaria were excluded. No antibiotics were prescribed.

All but 3% of the children were successfully rehydrated, and no complications or adverse reactions were noted. Failures were caused chiefly by a persistent refusal to take oral rehydration solution, with consequent negative fluid balance and progressive dehydration. Stool output and weight gain were similar in all treatment groups.

Cereal-based solutions were as effective as standard glucose-based solution in rehydrating children with diarrhea in this study. With the goal of making rehydration possible at homes where diarrhea is a major risk, the next step is to evaluate solutions made with locally available ingredients.

► For those of us in more fortunate countries, the 2 articles reviewed in Abstracts 4–72 and 4–73 serve as a reminder that oral rehydration is effective in all but the most severe cases of dehydration. In 1982, Santosham et al. (1) studied children in Panama and the United States admitted with greater than 5% dehydration. Of the 98 children, 97 were successfully treated with oral rehydration with salt solution (ORS). Patients with signs of shock or more than 10% dehydration were given intravenous fluids until the blood pressure values and heart rate normalized. For the 10% of patients with severe dehydration, the mean length of time for intravenous hydration was 4 hours. Thereafter, the ORS group fared as well as the group maintained on the usual intravenous therapy. The study found comparable results with either ORS tested, 50 or 90 mol of sodium/L.

Oral rehydration is a reasonable and proved method of treatment for all but the most severely dehydrated children. Arguments against the routine use of ORS instead of intravenous hydration have centered on its use in vomiting children and the question of supervision of the child during the rehydration. In these studies, children with vomiting responded just as well to the ORS. All of the studies noted were reviewed hospitalized patients.—R.M. Rutstein, M.D.

*Reference*

1. Santosham M, et al: *N Engl J Med* 306:1070, 1982.

---

**Hypokalemia Complicating Emergency Fluid Resuscitation in Children**
Malone DR, McNamara RM, Malone RS, Fleisher GR, Spivey WH (Bethesda Naval Hosp, Bethesda, Md; Med College of Pennsylvania, Philadelphia; Georgetown Univ, Washington, DC; Boston Children's Hosp)
*Pediatr Emerg Care* 6:13–16, 1990                                    4–74

It has been observed that vigorous fluid therapy in the resuscitation of critically ill or traumatized children often results in hypokalemia. However, hypokalemia secondary to acute volume resuscitation has not been well described in the literature. Because previous studies have shown greater mortality among traumatized and cardiac arrest patients with hypokalemia, a retrospective chart review compared serum potassium concentrations before and after vigorous fluid therapy in critically ill children given treatment in an ED.

During a 4-year period, 29 patients with a median age of 14 months received at least 20 mL of intravenous fluid/kg during their first hour of care in an ED. Indications for vigorous fluid therapy included dehydration, sepsis, and hemorrhage. Serum potassium levels were determined before and up to 6 hours after rehydration.

Pretreatment serum potassium levels ranged from 3.2 to 8.0 mEq/L (mean 4.6 mEq/L). Posthydration serum potassium levels ranged from 1.4 to 4.0 mEq/L (mean 3.3 mEq/L). The difference was statistically significant. Before rehydration, only 2 patients had serum potassium levels less than 3.5 mEq/L, but 16 patients had such levels after hydration therapy. Eleven of these 16 children had serum potassium levels less than 3.0 mEq/L after fluid replacement therapy. A separate analysis of coincidental arterial pH measurements and potassium change revealed that a rise in pH alone could not account for the drop in serum potassium levels.

Aggressive rehydration of critically ill children may result in significant hypokalemia. The actual mechanism responsible for such a phenomenon and its clinical implications have not yet been determined.

▶ The authors document an important finding that must not be forgotten during volume resuscitation in children. Once a patient has been given more than 20 mL/kg, serum potassium levels should be measured and replaced, if necessary. This detail is easily lost in the midst of a vigorous resuscitation effort.— S. Ludwig, M.D.

---

**Iatrogenic Bilateral Tibial Fractures After Intraosseous Infusion Attempts in a 3-Month-Old Infant**
La Fleche FR, Slepin MJ, Vargas J, Milzman DP (Eastern Virginia Graduate School of Medicine, Norfolk, Va)
*Ann Emerg Med* 18:1099–1101, 1989                                    4–75

---

Few serious complications are reported when intraosseous (IO) infusion is used as an alternative to intravenous access in pediatric resuscitation. One female infant had serious complications after IO access was attempted unsuccessfully in both tibias and the right femur.

Girl, 3 months, was seen after 1 week of coughing and nasal congestion when she suddenly became lethargic, with grunting respirations and a brief apneic episode. She was difficult to arouse and irritable. Poor skin turgor and dry mucous membranes were noted, and there were rhonchi in both lung fields. Because intravenous cannulation could not be attained, insertion of an IO needle was attempted on 4 occasions but without success. The right proximal tibia was approached twice, and the left proximal tibia and right distal femur were each approached once. The patient was admitted and treated for *Streptococcus pneumoniae* meningitis. The right leg was tender and swollen 3 days after discharge, and films showed healing fractures of the midshaft of both tibias and a healing nondisplaced fracture of the proximal left tibia. No cause of fracture other than attempted IO infusion could be found.

Use of a large-bore needle and distal insertion sites probably contributed to these injuries. Delayed diagnosis of the fractures would have been prevented by postprocedure radiographs. It may be wise to routinely obtain radiographs after attempting IO needle insertions in infants.

▶ The authors report a known and predictable complication of the IU method of gaining vascular access. Although one would prefer not to produce this complication, it is one worth accepting when weighed against the alternative. The case presented is one that appeared to warrant the risk. The infant was in extremis, and intravenous routes were unattainable. Two retrospective suggestions I would make are (1) use of a more proximal site 1–2 fingerbreadths below the tibial plateau and (2) use of a smaller-gauge IO needle. I applaud the authors' willingness to share their complications with us. (See also Abstract 1–21.)—S. Ludwig, M.D.

---

### Mortality in Children and Adolescents With Sickle Cell Disease

Leikin SL, Gallagher D, Kinney TR, Sloane D, Klug P, Rida W, Cooperative Study of Sickle Cell Disease (Children's Hosp, Natl Med Ctr, Washington, DC)
*Pediatrics* 84:500–508, 1989                                                          4–76

---

Mortality studies of patients with sickle cell disorders have reported that infection with encapsulated microorganisms is a frequent cause of death among infants and young children. However, most of those studies were retrospective reviews of relatively small patient populations with short-term follow-up. In March 1979, the Cooperative Study of Sickle Cell Disease initiated a large prospective study of the natural history of sickle cell disease in children and adolescents.

The study population included patients from 23 U.S. centers representing urban and rural areas with a wide geographic distribution. Enrollment was limited to patients less than 20 years of age with sickle cell anemia (Hb SS), hemoglobin SC disease (Hb SC), or hemoglobin S/β-thalassemia syndrome of either the $\beta^+$ or $\beta^0$ variety.

During the first 8½ years, 2,824 patients less than 20 years of age were enrolled in the study, providing a total of 14,668 person-years of follow-up. By August 1987, 36 boys and 37 girls had died when less than 20 years of age. The highest mortality rates were in children with homozygous sickle disease who were between 1 and 3 years of age. There was no difference in mortality rates between the sexes at any age. No deaths occurred in patients with Hb S/β-thalassemia disease. The overall mortality was 0.5 deaths per 100 person-years, or 2.6%.

Autopsy was performed on 36 of the 73 patients. Bacterial infection accounted for 28 of the 73 deaths and cerebral vascular accidents (CVAs) for 9 deaths. Death from CVAs and traumatic events exceeded infections

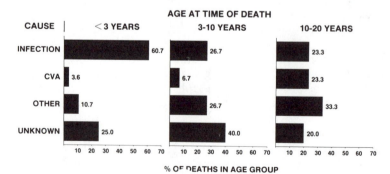

Fig 4–7.—Cause of death by age at time of death in patients with sickle hemoglobinopathies entered at less than 20 years of age in Cooperative Study of Sickle Cell Disease. (Courtesy of Leikin SL, Gallagher D, Kinney TR, et al: *Pediatrics* 84:500–508, 1989.)

as a cause of death in patients more than 10 years of age (Fig 4–7). *Streptococcus pneumoniae* was identified as the causative agent in blood cultures of 23 patients, *Hemophilus influenzae* in 3 patients, and *Salmonella* in 1 patient. Seven patients with *S. pneumoniae* sepsis had concomitant meningitis, and 2 also had splenic sequestration. Ten patients had disseminated intravascular coagulation.

No risk factors for death were identified, although low hemoglobin F levels at entry may have prognostic significance as a survival factor. The 2.6% overall mortality rate because of sickle hemoglobinopathy in this study of patients less than 20 years of age suggests that survival is gradually improving. The highest mortality still occurs among children between 1 and 3 years of age who have the homozygous form of sickle disease.

▶ The report of the Cooperative Study of Sickle Cell Disease Group provides some reinforcement of existing concepts as well as some new information. In addition to the specific data provided, it gives an example of what we need more of in emergency medicine, large cooperative studies. Pediatric hematology and oncology have used the cooperative study technique with great skill and to positive benefit for their patients. This study is a shining example.

The results of the study support the existing notion that the child with sickle cell disease who is younger than 3 or 4 years and who has fever is at high risk for bacterial sepsis. These children are immunocompromised in several different ways and must be identified in the ED, fully cultured, and admitted for intravenous antibiotic treatment, pending culture results. Although sepsis was the singular cause of death in the younger children, it also accounted for 25% of the deaths in older children. The study further supports the notion that for older children, the other mechanism for death is through a CNS event, thrombosis, or bleed. The emergency physician must be alert to patients seen with even minor neurologic findings or with even vague complaints referrable to the CNS.

The surprising findings were the low incidence of splenic sequestration as a cause of death and the fact that there were so many children (>20%) with cause of death unknown. The development of sickle cell centers and their education of parents has been an important advance. Reports from the cooperative study need to continue to educate the physicians on the front lines. (See also Abstract 3–50.)—S. Ludwig, M.D.

## AIDS, Infections

### Human Immunodeficiency Virus and the Emergency Department: Risks and Risk Protection for Health Care Providers

Kelen GD (Johns Hopkins Univ)
*Ann Emerg Med* 19:242–248, 1990                                    4–77

Significant numbers of patients in inner-city EDs have unrecognized HIV infection. Thus, health care providers in the ED are at increased risk of occupational HIV transmission. Reported cases of HIV transmission in

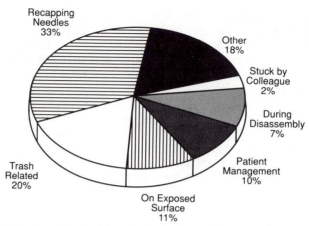

**Fig 4-8.**—Mechanisms of needlestick injuries. (Courtesy of Jagger J, Hunt EH, Brand-Elnaggar J, et al: *N Engl J Med* 319:284-288, 1988. From Kelen GD: *Ann Emerg Med* 19:242-248, 1990.)

the health care setting have occurred mainly from exposure to blood of infected patients caused primarily by injuries from sharp instruments.

Of 169 known health care workers diagnosed with AIDS, investigation of risk factors for HIV infection is still ongoing in 97, is considered incomplete in 28, and failed to identify risk factors in 44. Eighteen of the latter 44 health care workers reported exposures to blood or other body fluids from patients during the past 10 years. However, all of these exposures involved patients whose HIV status was not known. Furthermore, 4 of the health care workers had no patient contact.

At the present time, there are only 18 documented cases worldwide of nosocomial HIV transmission after occupational exposure, 13 of which were reported in the United States. Only 4 of the 18 patients were infected from nonparenteral exposures. Thus, the occupational risk of acquiring HIV infection appears to be minimal. Based on surveillance studies, the best estimate of seroconversion occurring after HIV exposure is about 0.5%.

At the present time, the best protection against HIV infection in the ED remains the use of the universal recommendations for precaution as issued in 1985 by the Centers for Disease Control. Much of these precaution recommendations deal with the appropriate use of barrier technology. Yet 80%-90% of all documented nosocomial HIV transmissions have been from needlesticks or injuries with sharp instruments rather than from actual patient management (Fig 4-8). New workers appear to be at the greatest risk of sticking themselves. Although azidothymidine has been advocated as a prophylactic after HIV exposure in the health care setting, its effectiveness as a postexposure prophylactic against HIV infection has not been shown.

▶ The risk of acquiring AIDS from patients can now be calculated well enough for medical students to factor into their choice of specialty. It is important, if not surprising, to learn that universal precautions are not followed among novice personnel and where incidence of HIV is low. We are still trying to make universal precautions universal; the latest idea is putting a sharps bin between the legs of patients we resuscitate so that needles are less likely to be lost in the bedclothes.—T. Stair, M.D.

---

**Duration of Human Immunodeficiency Virus Infection Before Detection of Antibody**
Horsburgh CR Jr, Ou CY, Jason J, Holmberg SD, Longini IM Jr, Schable C, Mayer KH, Lifson AR, Schochetman G, Ward JW, Rutherford GW, Evatt BL, Seage GR III, Jaffe HW (Centers for Disease Control, Atlanta; Emory Univ; Boston Dept of Health and Hosps; San Francisco Dept of Public Health)
*Lancet* 2:637–639, 1989                                                         4–78

---

To determine how long HIV infection can be present before antibody is detectable the polymerase chain reaction (PCR), with *gag* and *env* region primers, was used to analyze peripheral blood mononuclear cells from 39 men before and after seroconversion to HIV. Twenty-seven homosexual and 12 hemophiliac men were studied. In addition, sera were tested for p24 antigen by antigen-capture enzyme immunoassay.

The HIV DNA was detected in 4 men before seroconversion but only in the sample obtained closest to the time of seroconversion. Three men—all with HIV DNA—had antigen detected before conversion. The median time from infection, as reflected by the finding of HIV DNA, and initial detection of HIV antibody was 2.4 months. In a review of 45 cases, the estimated median time from HIV exposure to detection of antibody was 2.1 months.

Attempts to detect HIV DNA in blood mononuclear cells can be a useful adjunct to diagnosing HIV infection when clinical suspicion is high and an early diagnosis is important. Antibody detection is, however, the standard diagnostic method. Infection for longer than 6 months without detectable antibody would appear to be infrequent.

▶ Exposure of health care workers in the ED has been studied. The added uncertainty addressed in this paper, that HIV-positive patients may remain antibody negative raises some concern that our exposure in the ED may be more frequent than suspected. It also suggests that follow-up screening tests for health care workers exposed to blood from high-risk patients may not be adequate. In this study, 10% of patients (4) with polymerase chain reaction (i.e., positive for the virus) were identified 5–21 months before HIV antibodies were detected. With only 4 patients who were PCR positive and HIV antibody negative, it might be premature to suggest that this test will be a useful adjunct to HIV diagnosis. More statistical power will be required. Furthermore, 18% of patients who were HIV antibody positive tested PCR negative. Should this assay be the gold standard? The most reassuring statistic noted in this study is that 95% of patients who will seroconvert following HIV exposure will do so within 6 months.—H. Unger, M.D.

## Frequency of Puncture Injuries in Surgeons and Estimated Risk of HIV Infection

Lowenfels AB, Wormser GP, Jain R (New York Med College, Valhalla)
*Arch Surg* 124:1284–1286, 1989                    4–79

Surgeons, who work with sharp instruments and are exposed to HIV-positive patients, may well be at increased risk of seroconversion. A total of 202 surgeons working in the New York City metropolitan area, where patients with AIDS and HIV infection are treated frequently, were surveyed regarding their exposure.

Eighty-six percent of the surgeons reported puncture injuries in the past year; the median number of yearly injuries per surgeon was 2. Only 12% of injuries were reported to the hospital health service. Three fourths of the injuries occurred during surgery, a majority of which were self-inflicted. The nondominant hand was the most frequent site of injury, about one half of these injuries involved the index finger. In addition to puncture wounds, the majority of surgeons reported exposure to large amounts of blood or ocular or oral exposure to patient fluids.

Seroconversion after parenteral exposure to HIV-infected blood is infrequent, but the high rate of injury at surgery is disturbing. Any avoidable technical factors associated with these high injury rates should be corrected quickly.

▶ This article underscores what we already know: (1) you can't be careful enough, and (2) make sure the procedure for handling this occupational risk is as effective as possible.— E.H. Taliaferro, M.D.

## Pharyngitis in Adults: The Presence and Coexistence of Viruses and Bacterial Organisms

Huovinen P, Lahtonen R, Ziegler T, Meurman O, Hakkarainen K, Miettinen A, Arstila P, Eskola J, Saikku P (Univ of Turku, Health Ctr Pulssi, Turku, Finland; Univ of Tampere, Tampere, Finland; Univ of Helsinki)
*Ann Intern Med* 110:612–616, 1989                    4–80

Usually only the streptococcal culture or rapid detection technique for group A streptococcal antigen is used to determine the cause of pharyngitis in adults. In an open study, 106 consecutive patients aged 15–62 years with sore throats were evaluated to determine the presence and coexistence of different microbial pathogens in pharyngitis. Various diagnostic techniques, including rapid antigen detection procedures, were used to determine the presence of viruses of the respiratory tract, as well as *Mycoplasma pneumoniae, Chlamydia trachomatis, Chlamydia* species strain TWAR, and β-hemolytic streptococci.

β-Hemolytic streptococci were detected in 24 patients, *M. pneumoniae* was found in 10, the *Chlamydia* species strain TWAR was found in 9, and viruses were found in 27. No microbial pathogens were found in 33 patients. Two microbial agents were identified simultaneously in 10 patients. Diagnosis was made by serologic findings in 7 patients and group C *Streptococcus* was identified in 6.

It appears that diagnostic procedures and treatment for adult patients with pharyngitis may need to be reconsidered. The benefits of treating *Chlamydia* species strain TWAR and *M. pneumoniae* should be carefully examined in further clinical studies of adult pharyngitis.

▶ The diversity of bacterial and viral agents causing pharyngitis demonstrated by this study explains the diverse management regimens that have been advocated for this problem. The authors do not recommend a change in our practice at this time, but the future looks good for a more specific approach to treatment than is currently possible, given the tools we have to work with.— E. Ruiz, M.D.

---

**Human Rabies: Clinical Features, Diagnosis, Complications, and Management**
Udwadia ZF, Udwadia FE, Katrak SM, Dastur DK, Sekhar M, Lall A, Kumta A, Sane B (Bombay Hosp, Bombay, India)
*Crit Care Med* 17:834–836, 1989                                                              4–81

---

India probably has the highest incidence of rabies in the world, with 15,000 deaths reported annually. Nearly all patients die within 3–10 days after the onset of symptoms, but intensive medical care has extended the survival time. The longest survival on record is 133 days. Only 3 cures have been well documented. One man died 25 days after onset of symptoms in spite of intensive medical support.

Man, 45, was scratched on the lip by a rabid dog and 3 days later began a course of vaccination with human diploid cell vaccine. However, he had an allergic reaction to a test dose of equine antirabies serum and was advised against passive prophylaxis. The patient became febrile after 15 days and had bulbar symptoms shortly afterward. Hydrophobia did not occur, and there were no signs of meningeal irritation. Ascending motor paralysis, diabetes insipidus, and adult respiratory distress syndrome (ARDS) ensued despite intensive medical care in a rabies ward. By day 22 the patient was comatose. A second electroencephalogram on day 24 showed flattened background activity with episodic slow-wave complexes at irregular intervals suggestive of burst suppression. At autopsy a large number of Negri bodies were found in the brain, with diffuse inflammation and necrosis throughout the cerebrum, brain stem, and upper part of the spinal cord. Mice inoculated intracerebrally with a brain suspension had typical signs of rabies, and their brain tissue, in turn, had extensive Negri bodies.

This case emphasizes the need for passive serum prophylaxis as well as antirabies vaccine for postexposure management, especially after a facial bite. Concerted effort can lead to prolonged survival.

▶ This report from India serves to remind American and European physicians, who may never have seen a case of rabies, of the clinical features of this gruesome and uniformly fatal disease. I question the wisdom of the authors in lavishing intensive care on a patient in a country with 15,000 cases yearly of a disease from which there have been only 3 confirmed survivors in the world's literature. The "rare" complications they report—neurogenic ARDS, diabetes insipidus, hypothermia, and rabies myocarditis—have been well described previously.

American physicians must expect this disease to present atypically. Between 1980 and 1989, 6 of 10 rabies patients who reported to the Centers for Disease Control had no known exposure to the virus (1, 2). One half of the cases are not diagnosed before death (3). Because of these diagnostic difficulties, rabies must be considered in the differential diagnosis of any encephalitis of unclear etiology.

Our understanding of postexposure prophylaxis continues to evolve (4, 5). Failures have been reported, and strict adherence to published guidelines is mandatory. The risk of rabies from wild and domestic animal exposure varies greatly from area to area (6), and the emergency physician should stay in close touch with the local public health department to keep abreast of current recommendations.—J. Schoffstall, M.D.

*References*

1. Centers for Disease Control: *MMWR* 38:335, 1989.
2. Dempsey D: *Pediatr Infect Dis J* 9:49, 1990.
3. Fishbein DB, et al: *Ann Intern Med* 109:935, 1988.
4. Anonymous: *Lancet* 1:917, 1988.
5. Fishbein DB: *N Engl J Med* 318:124, 1988.
6. Centers for Disease Control: *MMWR* 36:35, 1987.

---

**Toxic Shock Syndrome: Associated With Nasal Packing**
Mansfield CJ, Peterson MB (New England Med Ctr Hosps, Boston)
*Clin Pediatr* 28:443–445, 1989                                4–82

---

Toxic shock syndrome usually is thought of in connection with menstruating women, but by 1984 more than one fourth of reported patients were children or adults without menstruation-related risk factors.

Boy, 10 years, previously in good health, was seen with vomiting, diarrhea, and dehydration 2 weeks after his nose had been injured in a bike accident. Nasal reconstruction and septoplasty had been done 2 days before admission; fever and vomiting began later on the day of surgery. The temperature at admission was 40°C and the pulse was 150 beats/minute, with a blood pressure value of 66/45 mm Hg. Peripheral perfusion was poor. A nasal pack was present without associated drainage. An erythematous macular rash was noted on the abdomen. Mild cervical adenopathy and pharyngeal erythema also were noted. The white blood cell count was 4,900/mm$^3$. The serum sodium level was 146 mEq/L, and the potassium was 2.7 mEq/L. Intravenous saline and antibiotics were administered, and the remaining nasal packing was removed. Renal function deteriorated, and liver and coagulation abnormalities developed. Systolic pressure remained less than 70 mm Hg. Dopamine and calcium gluconate were administered. Rapid volume expansion was carried out with normal saline, packed red blood cells, and plasma. The patient was stable by the fifth day, at which time skin desquamation was noted on the fingertips. A nasal culture taken on hospital day 4 yielded *Staphylococcus aureus.*

This case demonstrates the multisystem nature of toxic shock syndrome and the need for aggressive treatment. Most important is eliminating the source of staphylococcal infection and toxin production.

▶ Toxic shock syndrome has been reported in many conditions that may confront the emergency physician ranging from peritonsilar abscess to osteomyelitis to infected surgical wounds. Add nasal packing to the list.— E. Ruiz, M.D.

## Psychiatric Emergencies

**Risk Factors for Attempted Suicide During Adolescence**
Slap GB, Vorters DF, Chaudhuri S, Centor RM (Univ of Pennsylvania)
*Pediatrics* 84:762–772, 1989                                                                     4–83

Identifying adolescents at risk for suicidal behavior is a growing problem. Most studies on this problem have used data collected from parents or other contacts, and it is not known whether adolescents themselves can provide the information necessary to identify their risk for attempted suicide. Data collected from patients aged 13–19 years hospitalized for medical complications of serious suicide attempts (n = 56) or for acute illnesses unrelated to injuries or ingestions (n = 248) were evaluated to determine whether a model for distinguishing suicidal from nonsuicidal adolescents can be developed. The patients completed self-administered questionnaires on psychosocial function, recent stress, alcohol and drug use, and use of health care.

Compared with ill adolescents, suicidal adolescents had significantly poorer mental health, impulse control, family relationships, and school performance; higher scores for 3-month stress and alcohol use; and more use of 7 of 12 drugs. Suicidal adolescents were more likely to report previous suicide attempts and previous mental health care but less likely to identify a primary care site than ill adolescents. Using a logistic regression model based on previous suicide attempts, previous mental health care, poor school performance, marijuana use, and dependence on an emergency room for primary care, 84% of the suicidal and 55% of ill adolescents were correctly identified.

This model, based on 5 self-reported variables, may help identify adolescents at risk for attempted suicide. The model is simple, plausible, and appropriate in ambulatory settings but must be validated in a prospective study.

▶ I strongly recommend that this article be read by all emergency physicians. The most impressive point in this paper is the fact that even after correction for socioeconomic status, adolescents who depend on the ED for their routine care had a 2.5 times higher risk for attempting suicide. As emergency physicians, particularly in inner-city hospitals, we should carefully approach our adolescent patients and probe for the other 4 major variables identified in this paper: (1) drug use, (2) poor school performance, (3) prior history of mental health problems, and (4) previous suicide attempt. Given the enormous time constraints on emergency physicians in busy inner-city EDs, it is all the more difficult to convince ourselves of the importance of taking that extra few minutes to spend with an adolescent who appears otherwise healthy except for a minor problem such as a upper respiratory tract infection or an ankle sprain. But a few simple questions about their everyday life voiced in a truly concerned tone could give us a lot of information. As we get older, we forget how fragile our egos were when we were adolescents. To have a physician express concern can mean a great deal to these young people, even though they may not express it at the time. With more than 5,000 American youths committing suicide each year, this paper makes me realize that we can have an important impact on this tragic problem.—E.J. Lucid, M.D.

---

**Suicidal Ideation and Suicide Attempts in Panic Disorder and Attacks**
Weissman MM, Klerman GL, Markowitz JS, Ouellette R (Columbia Univ; New York State Psychiatric Inst; Cornell Med School, New York)
*N Engl J Med* 321:1209–1214, 1989                                      4–84

Panic disorder can be found in about 1.5% of the population at some time in their lives. Panic attacks are 2–3 times more prevalent. The risk of suicidal ideation and suicide attempts in persons with panic attacks or panic disorder was determined in a random sample of 18,011 adults from 5 U.S. communities.

Individuals who had panic disorder compared with those with other psychiatric disorders had more suicidal ideation and suicide attempts. The adjusted odds ratio for suicide attempts in this group was 2.62. When persons with panic disorder were compared with those without psychiatric disorder, the odds ratio rose to 17.99. Twenty percent of the subjects with panic disorder had made suicide attempts compared with 12% of those who suffered from panic attacks. The findings could not be explained by coexisting disorders such as major depression or alcohol or drug abuse.

Panic disorder and panic attacks are associated with an increased risk of suicidal ideation and attempts. This increased risk is independent of the presence of coexisting depression, alcohol or drug abuse, or agoraphobia.

► Much attention has recently been given to the recognition of panic attacks, which may affect as much as 3%–5% of the population at some time during their lives. The authors now present data to include this condition with increased suicidal ideation and attempts. Emergency physicians are well advised to be knowledgeable about panic disorders because they permeate our environment. An in-depth evaluation regarding self-destructive tendencies may well be indicated. (See also Abstract 4–88.)—D.K. Wagner, M.D.

---

**Detecting Physical Disorders in Emotionally Disturbed Patients**
Herring ME, Ross J (Ambulatory Health Care Ctr, Stratford, NJ)
*Postgrad Med* 86:135–142, 1989                                              4–85

---

Underdiagnosis of physical causes of mental disorders is common even though physical illness is frequent in mentally ill patients. Such illness may not be detected because of the sharing of symptoms by both neuropsychiatric and physical disorders and omission of a comprehensive physical examination. Other reasons include an absence of cooperation, misleading history, and lack of complaints on the part of the patient.

Four clinical clues should raise suspicion of the presence of organic disorder. The first is atypical clinical presentation. Knowledge of diagnostic criteria for psychiatric disorders is recommended. Behavior that is out of character is another clue. Lack of apparent secondary gain should raise suspicion that an organic disorder may exist.

The presence of multiple target-organ symptoms provides a further clue. An example is a case in which symptoms of diarrhea occurred in a patient who already had adrenalin-response symptoms. Prostosigmoidoscopy demonstrated hyperemic mucosa of the colon, which led to a diagnosis of ulcerative colitis.

The complaints of a patient should not be considered diagnoses until completion of a comprehensive evaluation. Viewing the patient in a biopsychosocial framework may be helpful when a psychologic illness and physical disease coexist.

▶ The authors provide 4 clinical clues to physical disorders in patients with an emotional problem. Of equal importance is the typical clinical appearance of a psychiatric condition. Clues to the diagnosis of the emotionally disturbed patient demand knowledge of typical psychiatric manifestations.—D.K. Wagner, M.D.

---

**The Dangerous Patient**
Lande RG (Walter Reed Army Med Ctr, Washington, DC)
*J Fam Pract* 29:74–78, 1989                                                4–86

---

The clinician has some difficult decisions to make when confronted with the dangerous patient if he or she is to prevent injury and optimize management. Understanding the standards of care that are emerging will enable avoidance of legal injury. The standard of duty to protect the victims of violence has become a legal duty in certain states.

The first step in management is assessment of the dangerous patient. This requires understanding of human aggression and the personality traits of internal inhibition, habit strength, and motivation that, when joined with situational factors, contribute to violence. A history of prior violence, substance abuse, and mental illness all increase the risk. Behavioral clues (e.g., posture, the startle response, speech, and motor activity) can fortell impending loss of control.

Managing the dangerous patient is a process of progression of steps determined by the level of dangerousness. The interview is the first step toward stabilization of the patient. While the clinician is evaluating the threat of violence, the physician's attitude and lack of a confrontational approach will help avoid escalating it. Progression to medication or to restraints is made as the situation demands. Psychiatric consultation may be sought if the indications of violence escalate. The clinician's alertness and flexibility will ultimately help the dangerous patient and protect others.

▶ Security in the emergency center has become a major issue for many urban centers. The authors point out several key guidelines: (1) health professionals must be nonconfrontational in their approach to the aggressive patient, (2) safety considerations must take priority in managing the aggressive situation, and (3) understanding behavioral clues is important. Specifically, early evidence of loss of control as manifest by speech volume, agitated movement, and an easily evoked startle reaction should be addressed before overt, violent behavior ensues. (See also Abstract 6–33.)—D.K. Wagner, M.D.

---

**Rapid Tranquilization of the Violent Patient**
Dubin WR, Feld JA (Philadelphia Psychiatric Ctr; Temple Univ)
*Am J Emerg Med* 7:313–320, 1989                                    4–87

---

Chemical restraint has replaced mechanical restraint in the ED for calming psychotic potentially violent patients. Rapid tranquilization (RT) of violent patients involves administering antipsychotic medication usually for 30–60 minutes.

Most studies of RT have compared various regimens of intramuscular medication, which is the preferred route of administration. However, several studies show that oral concentrate may be an effective alternative to intramuscular medication. Although some studies advocate the use of intravenous antipsychotic medication, its advantage has not been proved.

Psychotic, agitated patients usually respond after 1–3 doses administered in a period of 30–90 minutes; symptoms start to attenuate within 20–30 minutes after the first dose. No ceiling dosage has been established, but patients should not be given more than 6 doses per 24 hours. Although side effects of RT are generally few, mild, and reversible, some patients become akathisic. Patients with dystonia and akathisia may be treated with benztropine or diphenhydramine, intravenously or intramuscularly; this usually provides relief within 1–3 minutes after injection. Although antipsychotic medications are the mainstay of RT, some physicians advocate the use of benzodiazepines rather than antipsychotic agents either alone or in combination with an antipsychotic agent as needed.

The judicious use of RT can significantly reduce morbidity in potentially assaultive psychotic patients. However, RT is not a treatment in itself, and it should be used only after verbal reasoning has failed to calm the patient.

▶ In a violently agitated patient, use of intramuscular haloperidol is a technically simple approach. If it is possible to achieve intravenous access, however, there is abundant evidence of the safety of intravenous haloperidol. The onset of action is 10–30 minutes, with maximum affect at about 45 minutes. The half-life of intravenous haloperidol is surprisingly long, ranging from 10 to 19 hours. Depending on the level of agitation, start with 2–5 mg, with additional doses given at 30-minute intervals, if needed.—W.P. Burdick, M.D.

---

**Panic Disorder in the Medically Ill**
Katon W, Roy-Byrne PP (Univ of Washington, Seattle)
*J Clin Psychiatry* 50:299–302, 1989                                        4–88

---

Panic disorder in the medically ill patient is not infrequent at a busy university consultation service. It usually is inaccurately diagnosed and often amplifies the symptoms of medical illness.

In some cases the development of panic disorder is associated with deteriorating physical illness. Sympathetic arousal may be responsible. An example is precipitation of angina in a patient with coronary artery disease when sympathetic arousal raises the heart rate, blood pressure levels, and cardiac output. A similar mechanism can explain ulceration that follows repeated untreated panic attacks. In other patients, panic disorder can lead to continued symptoms after medical illness has resolved; the symptoms of panic disorder mimic those of the medical illness. Delayed diagnosis and prolonged suffering may result. Organic factors may be causal in these patients but do not maintain the disorder.

Whether medically ill patients are at an increased risk of having panic disorder remains uncertain. Whether primary and secondary panic disorders are identical or disparate, although overlapping, disorders also is not clear.

▶ One should remember that panic disorders mimic medical illness and vice versa. (See also Abstract 4–84.)—S. Repasky, D.O.

## Geriatric Emergencies

---

**Elderly Patients in the Emergency Department**
Eliastam M (Stanford Univ)
*Ann Emerg Med* 18:1222–1229, 1989                                        4–89

---

By the year 2000, the number of persons aged 65 years or older is expected to exceed 35 million, or 13.1% of the total population of the United States. The greatest increase will be in the 85-year-old or older age group, more than doubling in size between 1980 and 2000 (Fig 4–9). These projections have serious implications for the field of health care. Emergency departments will be caring for a greater number of elderly patients and should be prepared to recognize the atypical manifestations of disease in old age.

Several recent findings are important to ED physicians. Although aging is associated with physiologic change, most of its symptoms and disabilities result from disease and many are treatable. Illness in the elderly can be underreported (e.g., anemia) and overreported (e.g., irreversible dementia). Drug-induced disease is more common in this population than was previously thought. Although some laboratory parameters are not altered in the elderly, others show age-related changes.

Elderly persons may be at greater risk for certain diseases because of age-related reductions in lung function and renal function, diminished immunocompetence, and a propensity for falling and osteoporosis. Some diseases, however, are less likely or less severe in later years, including multiple sclerosis and certain types of cancer. Medications present many problems in geriatric patients, including multiple drug use with its potential for adverse side effects. Although patients aged older than 65 years consume more than one third of all prescription medications, these drugs may not have been tested on older persons. The likelihood of multiple disorders in the elderly may make diagnosis and treatment of the presenting problem more difficult.

On admission to the ED, elderly patients are frequently sicker than the general population and are twice as likely to require hospitalization. Their examination may be difficult because of physical or mental disabilities. The ED staff should try to be attentive and patient and must exer-

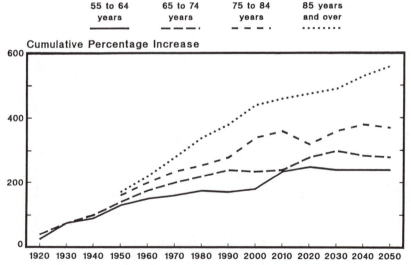

Fig 4–9.—Percentage increase of the older population from 1920 to 2050. (Courtesy of Eliastam M: *Ann Emerg Med* 18:1222–1229, 1989.)

cise special care when administering medication because of the risk of overdosage or interactions.

▶ Although this review article, by necessity, touches only the surface of this subject (considering that the special problems faced by the elderly are protean enough to have generated an entire new subspecialty), it provides a useful introduction and points out the necessity for emergency physicians to consider the impact of an aging general population and the importance of physiologic age in individual patients on our clinical practice.—J.R. Hoffman, M.D.

---

**A Case Control Study for Major Trauma in Geriatric Patients**
Finelli FC, Jonsson J, Champion HR, Morelli S, Fouty WJ (Washington Hosp Ctr, Washington, DC)
*J Trauma* 29:541–548, 1989                                                          4–90

---

Elderly patients are at greater risk of dying of traumatic injury than are younger patients with injuries of similar severity. However, the importance of age as a prognostic factor of mortality after traumatic injury has not been determined. Age was analyzed as a univariate factor in survival after trauma.

During a 4-year period, 46,613 patients with major trauma were admitted to 120 trauma centers. The probability of surviving the injury was estimated based on Trauma Scores, Injury Severity Scores, and autopsy results. A more detailed analysis was performed on the data from 3,918 patients aged younger than 65 years and 180 patients aged 65 years and older admitted to a trauma service in Washington, DC.

Analysis of the national data revealed that mortality increased with age up to 85 years, after which mortality rates tapered off slightly. Mortality rates increased from 10% at age 45 years, to 15% at age 55 years, to 20% at age 75 years. This age-dependent survival decrement occurred at all Injury Severity Score values for all mechanisms of injury and for all body regions. Analysis of the Washington data yielded a mortality rate of 14% for persons younger than 65 years compared with a 27% mortality rate for those older than 65 years. The median length of hospital stay was 7 days for persons younger than 65 years compared with 14 days for those older than 65 years. Analysis of cost data revealed that the Diagnostic Related Groups prospective payment system grossly underestimates the cost of hospital care for trauma patients aged older than 65 years.

To minimize mortality and morbidity among elderly trauma victims, it is suggested that patients aged older than 65 years be triaged to trauma centers at a much lower threshold than similarly injured younger patients.

▶ This study is probably no great surprise to those in emergency medicine, but the higher mortality in those 65 years or older (89%) would indicate that the criteria for admission of these patients to trauma centers should be more liberal.—G.V. Anderson, M.D.

---

## Acute Mesenteric Infarction in Elderly Patients

Finucane PM, Arunachalam T, O'Dowd J, Pathy MSJ (Univ of Wales, Cardiff)

*J Am Geriatr Soc* 37:355–358, 1989                                                4–91

---

The clinical features, the treatment given, the factors governing treatment selection, and the result of such treatment were analyzed in all patients aged 65 years and older in whom a tissue diagnosis of acute mesenteric infarction was made at 1 hospital.

During the 8-year study period, 32 patients with a mean age of 78.5 years met the criteria for ischemia secondary to primary vascular disease. Eighteen patients were women. Mesenteric thrombosis caused bowel infarction in 14 patients (44%), 4 had a mesenteric embolus, 8 had a diagnosis of mesenteric atherosclerosis, and in 6 mesenteric insufficiency was the presumed cause of infarction.

Eighteen patients were admitted to a surgical unit, 13 were admitted to a medical unit, and 1 died in transit to the hospital. Those in the surgical group were more likely to have symptoms typical of bowel infarction, such as abdominal tenderness and pain.

Fifteen from the surgical group and 5 from the medical group underwent bowel resection. All 11 patients who did not undergo surgery died at an average of 4 days after the onset of symptoms. Eight of the surgical group (44%) but only 2 of the medical group (15%) survived to leave the hospital.

Mesenteric vascular disease is an uncommon condition and may go unrecognized, especially in elderly patients admitted to medical wards. Acute confusion was present in 29% of the patients. This sign should be a warning, and the absence of abdominal pain or tenderness should not rule out the possibility of bowel infarction.

▶ The elderly patient who has abdominal pain with or without shock, acidosis, and confusion is a difficult clinical problem. The patient is already compromised by the factors of age and chronic organ dysfunction. The further insult of a surgical procedure presents a therapeutic dilemma in these patients.

In the study period of 8 years at an 836-bed hospital, the authors were able to review only 32 cases of bowel ischemia in the elderly secondary to primary vascular disease. The study population is small, but there are some disturbing factors demonstrated. Only 74% had abdominal pain—was the symptom lacking because of confusion? Leukocytosis was common (83%), but only 35% had diarrhea and 16% gastrointestinal bleeding. In fact, confusion was more common than gastrointestinal bleeding and fever. We are reminded that in older, especially confused patients, the manifestation may be atypical, and a high index with early surgical intervention is warranted.—J.M. Mitchell, M.D.

# Ocular Emergencies

### Welder Eye Injuries

Reesal MR, Dufresne RM, Suggett D, Alleyne BC (Workers' Compensation Board, Alberta; Alberta Occupational Health and Safety)
*J Occup Med* 31:1003–1006, 1989                                    4–92

The 1985 annual survey of claims filed with the Workers' Compensation Board (WCB) of Alberta revealed that 584 (21%) of the 2,821 claims for eye injuries came from welders. To examine why welders still represent the largest proportion of workers who sustain eye injuries in a modern industrial community, the WCB data were examined to identify probable causes, sources, characteristics, and consequences of welder eye injuries in Alberta.

Of the 584 requests for compensation, 478 (82%) fulfilled the criteria for compensability defined as an injury judged to have arisen out of and in the course of employment. The median age of welders who submitted claims was 28 years. All claims were filed by men. Seventy-two welders sustained bilateral eye injuries. For 45% of the compensable claims, workers were off work for only 1 day. Most welders (91%) returned to work within 4 days of injury. After 10 days, all except 7 welders had returned to work. Two of the 7 workers who did not return to work after 10 days had sustained serious permanent disability.

First-aid care was available to less than 25% of the workers who sustained eye injury at work. At least 77% of the injured welders were not wearing appropriate eye protection when the injury occurred. However, most were conscientious about wearing tinted lenses for protection from ultraviolet radiation while using the welding torch. Cold metal particles were responsible for most of the eye injuries (Fig 4–10). Particulate foreign bodies entering the unprotected eye were the cause of 72% of the welder eye injury claims reported to the WCB.

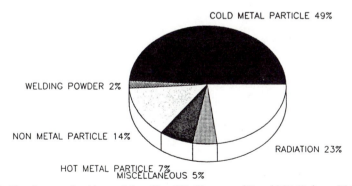

Fig 4–10.—Sources of welder eye injury. N = 395. (Courtesy of Reesal MR, Dufresne RM, Suggett D, et al: *J Occup Med* 31:1003–1006, 1989.)

The importance of wearing eye protection constantly while working with metal pieces and in metal industries should be given greater emphasis.

▶ Welders, at last, know not to gaze at any acetylene arc without protection from the intensive ultraviolet radiation, but perhaps they should also wear goggles under their helmets to protect against flying metal fragments when they are hammering rather than welding.—T. Stair, M.D.

---

**Topical Anesthesia of the Eye as a Diagnostic Test**
Sklar DP, Lauth JE, Johnson DR (Univ of New Mexico, Albuquerque)
*Ann Emerg Med* 18:1209–1211, 1989                                    4–93

---

The corneal surface of the eye has extremely rich innervation, particularly of pain-sensitive fibers. Because topical anesthestics can reach these fibers readily, particularly when there is disruption of the epithelium, the ocular response to topical anesthesia can assist the physician in differentiating between simple corneal injury and other diseases that cause acute eye pain (e.g. conjunctivitis and iritis). To evaluate further, 71 adult patients with complaints of eye pain filled out visual analogue pain scale (range 0–10) before and after use of the topical anesthetic proparacaine 0.5%.

Mean initial scores were higher, final pain scores were lower, and changes in scores were greater among the 50 patients with simple corneal injuries (abrasions and foreign bodies) compared with the 21 patients with other causes of acute eye pain, (e.g., conjunctivitis, iritis, glaucoma, and subconjunctival hemorrhage). When response to topical anesthesia was defined as either a decrease in pain score of more than 5 or a final pain score of less than 1, the sensitivity of this test for simple corneal injury was 80% and the specificity was 86%. The differential pain relief that results from the use of topical anesthesia may assist the physician in diagnosing patients with simple corneal injuries, with or without the benefit of a slit lamp.

▶ This study confirms what I have suspected for some time. If the pain is not dramatically lessened by the initiation of topical anesthetics, one must be extremely careful to look for causes other than simple corneal abrasion. I do have a concern about the converse of this statement, however. Even if the pain is dramatically improved, one cannot totally rule out other causes such as iritis. A careful slit-lamp examination is warranted in every adult patient with eye pain seen in the ED.—E.J. Lucid, M.D.

---

**Eye Injuries in Childhood: Demography, Etiology, and Prevention**
Nelson LB, Wilson TW, Jeffers JB (Wills Eye Hosp, Philadelphia)
*Pediatrics* 84:438–441, 1989                                    4–94

---

The cases of 2,154 children aged 15 and younger treated at the emergency room of Wills Eye Hospital in a 1-year period were reviewed. Children constituted 9% of all emergency patients. Ocular injuries accounted for 38% of all child visits and were twice as frequent in boys as in girls. Ocular trauma was most prevalent in April–June.

Injuries to the anterior globe accounted for more than two thirds of all cases, but only 7% of them were perforating injuries. Only 6% of patients had posterior globe injuries. Twenty-eight percent of the group had extraocular injuries. Another child's hand or foot caused eye injury in 12%. Sports-related injuries and a fall were the next most common causes of injury, followed by a stick or a branch and a foreign body. The sports most often responsible for eye injuries were baseball, basketball, tennis, and hockey. Chemicals caused 4% of the injuries. Two percent of children were burned by an adult's cigarette.

The varied causes of pediatric ocular injuries indicate that parents, teachers, and coaches must be educated regarding the potential for such injuries. Both pediatricians and ophthalmologists should take an active role in making sure that all are aware of the problem and know appropriate preventive measures.

▶ One must suspect that this study from a tertiary care center suffers from a certain degree of referral bias. The author's hospital sees referred patients from throughout the Delaware Valley, a huge catchment area. Most children with minor eye injuries are probably treated by their pediatrician or emergency physician, perhaps in consultation with a local ophthalmologist, and only children with the most serious injuries are sent to such centers. Thus, this series is probably overweighted with serious injuries. Nonetheless, it is useful documentation of the kinds and causes of eye trauma children suffer.

Their recommendations are unexceptionable: Baseball batters and hockey players should wear helmets with eyeshields, dangerous chemicals should be kept out of reach of children, BB guns should not be sold in toy stores, children's play should be supervised by adults, and so forth. This is nothing new or radical but is all sound advice. This is a good article to have around if you are called on, as many of us are, to serve as a medical advisor or team physician for school or extramural sports.—J. Schoffstall, M.D.

---

**Localisation of Intraocular and Intraorbital Foreign Bodies Using Computed Tomography**
Etherington RJ, Hourihan MD (Univ Hosp of Wales, Heath Park, Cardiff)
*Clin Radiol* 40:610–614, 1989                                     4–95

---

Accurate localization of intraorbital foreign bodies is necessary for correct management. The role of CT in localizing foreign bodies in the orbit was studied in 15 patients with suspected intraorbital foreign bodies. Surgical follow-up was obtained in 11 patients.

The presence of foreign bodies was confirmed by CT in all 15 patients and was accurately localized in all but 1. Computed tomography was accurate in differentiating between extraocular and intraocular sites of the foreign bodies and in localization within the globe.

A foreign body that was visible on frontal plain radiographs was demonstrated on contiguous axial 6-mm thick CT sections. If the radiographs were equivocal, the foreign body was visible on 3-mm CT sections. Coronal scans were of limited usefulness.

In patients with suspected ocular injury by a metallic foreign body, CT should be the radiologic procedure of choice after a plain radiograph. Foreign bodies that are visible on plain radiographs can be localized accurately using axial 6-mm CT sections, whereas those that appear equivocal or normal on plain radiographs can be shown by 3-mm thick CT sections.

▶ This study is consistent with previous literature on the subject of intraorbital foreign bodies. Computed tomography is the method of choice, providing a 3-dimensional assessment of the orbit. Magnetic resonance imaging is not recommended, because the foreign objects are often ferrous. Ultrasonography is usually more difficult to perform and interpret. The method described in this paper is simple and can be performed in any hospital with a CT scanner.—G. Ordog, M.D.

---

**Corneal Abrasion in Infancy as a Cause of Inconsolable Crying**
Harkness MJ (Holy Redeemer Hosp and Med Ctr, Meadowbrook, Pa)
*Pediatr Emerg Care* 5:242–244, 1989                                                4–96

An inconsolable infant who emits a high-pitched or shrill cry can be a source of alarm, especially if the crying interferes with feeding or sleep.

Male infant, 6 weeks, began screaming inconsolably after waking from an afternoon nap. He continued screaming for 7 hours; the screaming interfered with a full feeding schedule. Orally administered acetaminophen was ineffective. The eyes appeared normal, but fluorescein staining demonstrated a small central corneal abrasion about 2 mm in diameter on the right cornea. Gentamicin ointment was instilled, and the eye was patched in the closed position. Within 30 minutes the infant slept, and after waking, he returned to normal behavior and feeding. The abrasion had resolved after 12 hours.

A corneal abrasion can lead to inconsolable crying in the preverbal child. If a very irritable but otherwise normal-appearing infant is seen, fluorescein staining can confirm or rule out this lesion. Corneal abrasions can result from fingernails, blankets, or clothing; sponging for fever; various chemical exposures; or the use of a pediculicide to treat head lice.

▶ Harkness alerts the emergency staff to 1 of a long list of causes of inconsolable crying in infants. Corneal abrasions are among the most frequent causes, especially when the onset is sudden and the infant has previously been symptom free. The list of other causes is long but must include incarcerated hernia, torsion testis, otitis media, urinary tract infection, hair tourniquet, acute glaucoma, occult fracture, and colic. The last diagnosis must be considered only after all of the other possibilities have been excluded.—S. Ludwig, M.D.

## Pregnancy-Related Emergencies

**Complications in the Emergency Transport of Pregnant Women**
Katz VL, Hansen AR (Univ of North Carolina)
*South Med J* 83:7–10, 1990                                                4–97

Recent reviews have examined aspects of emergency care for pregnant women. During transport, pregnant women must be placed at a lateral tilt instead of in the supine position to avoid aortocaval compression by the uterus, have adequate volume replacement to ensure uterine perfusion, and have supplemental oxygen.

Woman, 18, was transferred at 31 weeks' gestation from a local emergency room because of premature labor and hypertension. The uterus was not tender. The fetal heart rate was 120/minute. The patient's contractions were mild and irregular. She was taken by ambulance in the supine position to another hospital about 1 hour away. By the time she arrived, the fetal heart rate had dropped to 80/minute. The women had cramping and vaginal bleeding. Results on ultrasonography were consistent with placental abruption. An emergency cesarean section was done. The infant was delivered, weighing 1,500 g, with signs of severe distress. His umbilical arterial pH was 6.6. There was a 70% placental abruption. At the age of 12 months, the child was still hospitalized with severe neurologic deficits and a poor prognosis for recovery. The woman had an unremarkable postpartum course.

Gravid women and their fetuses are particularly vulnerable during transport. As the uterus enlarges, it compresses the vena cava and the aorta of the pregnant woman when she is placed in the supine position. Such compression can result in uteroplacental insufficiency, supine hypotension, and possibly cardiopulmonary arrest. It is also associated with placental abruption.

▶ This case report assumes a cause and effect but does make a point about positioning patients. Pregnant women can sleep supine without ill effect if they are able to change position at will. If patients are comatose, anesthetized, or restrained, a pillow under the right hip should achieve the optimum left-side-down position.—T. Stair, M.D.

**Traumatic Fetal Deaths**
Lane PL (Victoria Hosp, London, Ont)
*J Emerg Med* 7:433–435, 1989                                              4–98

Traumatic fetal death is a tragic consequence of motor vehicle collisions. All traumatic fetal deaths reported to the Chief Coroner's Office in Ontario during a 5-year period were reviewed to determine the incidence of traumatic fetal death and to characterize maternal and fetal injuries, accident factors, and clinical course.

Thirteen traumatic fetal deaths were reported, for an incidence of 2 traumatic fetal deaths per 100,000 live births. All occurred in the third trimester, 5 at the 36th week or more of gestation. Maternal injuries were either very minor or limited solely to the uterus and placenta in 8 mothers, including 4 who were examined in the hospital and discharged home because of no or very minor injuries. The remaining 5 mothers sustained serious injuries. Causes of fetal death were placental abruption in 6, infarction in 1, laceration in 2, and uterine rupture in 4. Five fetuses also sustained other major injuries, usually to the head. Seat belts were used by only 4 mothers.

Traumatic fetal death is a rare and important consequence of motor vehicle collisions. Fetal death may occur despite relatively trivial maternal injuries and primarily in unrestrained mothers. The use of ultrasound to define potential placental injury in mothers even after minor vehicle accidents should be explored.

▶ The authors present rather surprising information on the possibility of fetal death subsequent to relatively minor uterine trauma during pregnancy. Although it is an admittedly uncommon event, 4 of the injuries were considered trivial enough to evaluate and discharge the mother from the emergency center. The authors do not describe the length or the degree to which fetal monitoring occurred at the initial evaluation. Close scrutiny of those cases would be helpful to attempt to identify whether subtle changes might have indicated the use of more sophisticated sonographic evaluation.—D.K. Wagner, M.D.

---

**Evaluation of Blunt Abdominal Trauma Occurring During Pregnancy**
Esposito TJ, Gens DR, Gerber Smith L, Scorpio R (Univ of Maryland)
*J Trauma* 29:1628–1632, 1989                                          4–99

Evaluation of pregnant women who sustain blunt abdominal trauma is problematic. The existing controversy about the safety and accuracy of laparotomy, observation, diagnostic peritoneal lavage, and CT is further magnified when pregnant women are involved, often leading to a delay in diagnosis and in prompt initiation of treatment.

During a 7.5-year period, 40 pregnant women sustained possible blunt abdominal trauma. Thirty women were occupants of motor vehicles involved in collisions, 5 were pedestrians, 4 were injured during falls, and 1 was riding a motorcycle. Ten patients were in the first trimester, 14 were in the second, and 16 were in their last trimester. Pregnancy was confirmed by positive serum human chorionic gonadotropin determination, physical examination, or ultrasonography. Injury Severity Scores (ISSs) were calculated for all patients. Results of diagnostic peritoneal lavage

(DPL) were considered abnormal if 10 mL of blood was aspirated initially or if the effluent contained more than 100,000 red blood cells/mm³, more than 500 white blood cells/mm³, or if bile, bacteria, or fecal material were noted.

Immediate laparotomy for emergency cesarean section or other indications was performed in 3 patients, DPL was performed in 13 patients, and CT was performed in 3 patients. The remaining 22 patients were observed with serial physical examinations and hematocrits. The overall mean ISS was 5.9. None of the patients required exploratory laparotomy for abdominal injury during their hospitalization. The mean ISS for the 13 patients who underwent DPL was 34.6. The results of DPL were abnormal in 5 women and normal in 8. All 5 abnormal results were confirmed by laparotomy. Six maternal deaths occurred. Excluding 4 women having elective abortions and 6 who were lost to follow-up, 14 (47%) of 30 known pregnancy outcomes were unsuccessful.

Pregnant women with suspected intra-abdominal injury should be managed no differently than those who are not pregnant. Women with minor injuries and blunt abdominal trauma may be observed safely, whereas those with major injuries, shock, altered mental status, or neurologic deficits require further testing to rule out intra-abdominal injury. Diagnostic peritoneal lavage is safe and accurate for use in pregnant women. The use of CT and ultrasonography merits additional analysis.

▶ The authors recommend continuous fetal monitoring for 24–48 hours in those patients with a viable fetus. Although it is not clearly presented in the paper, it appears that at least 1 of the 22 patients observed required an emergency cesarean section for fetal distress. A more recent study with 84 patients documented 2 cases of absorption and a 28% rate of preterm labor in third-trimester patients with blunt abdominal trauma (1). This study concluded that all such patients should receive an ultrasound and fetal monitoring to rule out preterm labor, and if normal, the patient may be discharged within "hours" of admittance. The emergency physician should refer all patients in the late stages of pregnancy with abdominal trauma for obstetric evaluation.—R.M. McNamara, M.D.

*Reference*

1. Williams JK, et al: *Obstet Gynecol* 75:33, 1990.

---

**Diagnosis of Acute Appendicitis in Pregnancy**
Richards C, Daya S (McMaster Univ, Hamilton, Ont)
*Can J Surg* 32:358–360, 1989                                    4–100

---

The diagnosis of acute appendicitis in pregnancy may be difficult because of the associated physiologic changes in pregnancy. The records of 28 pregnant patients who underwent appendectomy for a presumptive diagnosis of acute appendicitis were studied to determine whether there is a specific feature of acute appendicitis in pregnancy that would aid in establishing the diagnosis.

The most consistent symptom was abdominal pain, and two thirds of patients had nausea, vomiting, abdominal guarding, rebound tenderness, and positive Rovsing's sign. Mean leukocyte count in women with histologically confirmed appendicitis was $15.3 \times 10^9/L$, and 80% of women in the study had a count greater than $12.5 \times 10^9/L$. However, compared with age-matched nonpregnant women with appendicitis, pregnant patients did not differ significantly in symptoms, physical signs, and laboratory parameters. Overall false positive rate was similar in both groups (18%), but there were significantly more false positive cases in the third trimester.

The diagnosis of acute appendicitis in pregnancy is no more difficult than in the nonpregnant state. Acute appendicitis should be suspected in pregnant patients with abdominal pain with a leukocyte count greater than $12.5 \times 10^9/L$, particularly in the presence of nausea and abdominal guarding.

▶ This interesting article covers an important, albeit relatively uncommon, condition. When false positive cases are eliminated, the survey's results are based on 23 histologically proved cases of appendicitis over a 5-year period. When these cases were compared with nonpregnant controls, no differences in signs, symptoms, or laboratory results could be detected. Significantly, the time from admittance to surgery, the false positive rate, and the frequency of perforation was the same in both groups, though the numbers are small.

On the face of it, this study suggests that the diagnosis of appendicitis is no more difficult in the pregnant than in the nonpregnant state. However, the real problem is making the diagnosis in the third trimester. The authors report that there were more false positive cases in the third trimester, and yet 50% (2 of 4) of the cases diagnosed in the third trimester had already perforated at the time of surgery.

What this study really demonstrates is that the diagnosis of appendicitis is relatively straightforward early in pregnancy and becomes more difficult as pregnancy advances.

Clearly, better diagnostic aids, especially in the third trimester, would be helpful. Ultrasonography is a modality that appears to be relatively safe and offers some promise (1,2). Unfortunately, this retrospective study was not designed to address this issue. A final answer to this question must await a large-scale prospective study. In the meantime, pregnant women with persistent abdominal pain, leukocytosis, or abdominal guarding have to be taken very seriously, especially in the third trimester.—H.H. Osborn, M.D.

*References*

1. Ruylaert JS, et al: *N Engl J Med* 317:666, 1987.
2. Kniskern JH, et al: *Ann Surg* 53:222, 1986.

## Ectopic Pregnancy: Duplex Doppler Evaluation

Taylor KJW, Ramos IM, Feyock AL, Snower DP, Carter D, Shapiro BS, Meyer WR, De Cherney AH (Yale Univ)

*Radiology* 173:93–97, 1989                                     4–101

The incidence of ectopic pregnancy, a major cause of maternal mortality, has increased dramatically in the last 2 decades. Early diagnosis has been accomplished by means of sonography and determination of the serum human chorionic gonadotropin (hCG) level. To improve the accuracy and timeliness of diagnosis, the clinical value of the flow patterns around a developing pregnancy as measured by duplex Doppler imaging was assessed.

Six women who were undergoing elective abortion in the first trimester agreed to take part in a determination of baseline criteria. Doppler waveforms were recorded in the main uterine artery, the ovarian arteries, and the uterine contents of the volunteers. In a study group of 398 patients with suspected ectopic pregnancy, 96 (24%) had the condition. Seventy of those women underwent Doppler imaging as well as ultrasound.

High-velocity flow suggestive of ectopic pregnancy was detected in 38 patients, yielding a preoperative sensitivity for the combined 2 methods of 73%. Positive predictive values were 47% for ultrasound alone and 85% for Doppler imaging; negative predictive values were 60% and 81%, respectively. The value of Doppler flow imaging was particularly evident in 1 patient, in whom a confirmed ectopic pregnancy was initially missed during laparoscopy.

Although sonography can be a valuable diagnostic tool, it is limited by the nonspecific appearance of many adnexal masses. Duplex doppler imaging can display luteal and placental flow as well as structure. The addition of color and pulsed Doppler imaging to the transvaginal probe should improve the accuracy of the test and limit the number of false positive studies.

▶ Ectopic pregnancy is one of the boogeymen of emergency medicine, both difficult to diagnose and potentially lethal, and it is on the increase. The rapid β-hCG assay on serum or urine has made diagnosis much easier, but a test that is more specific would be welcome. The authors of this paper believe that duplex Doppler is such a test.

This paper is difficult to evaluate. The selection and exclusion criteria are not well described. Ultrasound, a notoriously operator-dependent technique, had a sensitivity of only 53% in the authors' hands, whereas other studies using transvaginal ultrasound have reported sensitivities up to 95% and specificities up to 99.7% (1), which is better than the authors' results using both ultrasound and duplex Doppler together. It is difficult to rule out an ectopic pregnancy when one is relying on a test with a sensitivity of only 85%.

This is a technique in its infancy. We need to see more reports on the use of duplex Doppler in this situation before we will know whether it is truly useful in ruling out ectopic pregnancy. (See also Abstract 3–66.)—J. Schoffstall, M.D.

*Reference*

1. Rempen A: *J Ultrasound Med* 7:381, 1988.

---

### Lack of a Tachycardic Response to Hypotension With Ruptured Ectopic Pregnancy

Snyder HS (Albany Med Ctr Hosp, NY)
*Am J Emerg Med* 8:23–26, 1990                                        4–102

---

The role of tachycardia as a reliable indicator of hypovolemic shock in patients with hemoperitoneum is controversial. The records of 154 patients with documented ectopic pregnancy were retrospectively reviewed to establish the chronotropic response to hypotension and to correlate the hemodynamic response with the estimated blood loss resulting from the hemoperitoneum.

Hypotension, defined as systolic blood pressure 90 mm Hg, was present in 20 patients (13%). Of the 9 patients (45%) with tachycardia, defined as a pulse rate greater than or equal to 100 beats/minute, 5 had only minimal tachycardia with pulse rates of 100–110 beats/minute, and 3 had pulse rates of 100 beats/minute. The other 11 patients had no tachycardia. All but 1 patient had consistent tachycardia or lack of tachycardia with hypotension during the entire preoperative course. The quantity of hemoperitoneum varied widely in each group and did not correlate with hypotension and chronotropic response.

The absence of tachycardia in response to hypotension should not obscure the diagnosis of hypovolemic shock in patients with ruptured ectopic pregnancy. It appears that hemoperitoneum may trigger a parasympathetic reflex, resulting in a pulse rate inappropriate for the degree of hypotension. A vasovagal reflex, along with mechanoreceptor stimulation, may play a role in some patients without significant hemoperitoneum.

▶ This is an important study, pointing out the frequent absence of tachycardia in cases of ruptured ectopic pregnancy. Emergency physicians should not rely on the presence of tachycardia and postural changes to diagnose hemoperitoneum; conversely, in a patient who looks like she is in shock but is normocardiac or even bradycardic, one should strongly consider hemoperitoneum to be present.—G. Ordog, M.D.

---

### Transvaginal Ultrasonography in Patients at Risk for Ectopic Pregnancy

Stiller RJ, Haynes de Regt R, Blair E (Bridgeport Hosp, Bridgeport, Conn)
*Am J Obstet Gynecol* 161:930–933, 1989                                        4–103

---

Ectopic pregnancy is diagnosed by the β–human chorionic gonadotropin (β-hCG) plasma levels above a discriminatory value when there is no ultrasonographic evidence of an intrauterine pregnancy. However, 40%

of patients at risk for an ectopic pregnancy do not have elevated initial β-hCG values. Furthermore, pelvic ultrasound is not reliable for determining an ectopic pregnancy. Preliminary studies report that transvaginal ultrasound provides enhanced imaging of the intrauterine and adnexal anatomy.

During a 9-month period 139 pregnant women at risk for ectopic pregnancy underwent transvaginal ultrasound. Quantitative β-hCG levels were measured at the time of ultrasonography. A β-hCG plasma concentration of 1,300 mIU/mL was used as the discriminatory value for which an intrauterine pregnancy was expected to be visualized.

Overall, 117 women had confirmed intrauterine pregnancies and 22 had confirmed ectopic pregnancies. Transvaginal ultrasound identified 18 of the 22 ectopic pregnancies at initial evaluation by either direct visualization of an ectopically placed gestational sac (14 patients) or failure to visualize an intrauterine gestational sac combined with a β-hCG reading of more than 1,300 IU/mL (4 patients). Transvaginal ultrasound identified 103 of the 117 intrauterine pregnancies at initial evaluation. In the remaining 18 patients the diagnosis could not be made by transvaginal ultrasound at initial evaluation because a gestational sac was not visualized and the initial β-hCG value was less than 1,300 mIU/mL. Repeat ultrasonography, β-hCG measurement, or both, confirmed ectopic gestations in 4 patients and early intrauterine pregnancies in another 4. Ten patients had complete abortions.

Transvaginal ultrasound is more useful than conventional transabdominal ultrasound in detecting intrauterine and ectopic pregnancies in patients at risk for ectopic pregnancy.

▶ The new technique of transvaginal ultrasonography locates more than 82% of the gestational sacs associated with β-hCG levels greater than 1,300 mIU/ mL, whereas transabdominal ultrasound locates the majority of sacs only at β-hCG levels greater than 6,500 mIU/mL. This added sensitivity for gestational sac localization has made the transvaginal probe a valuable tool, particularly in the patient seen very early in pregnancy. (See also Abstract 4–101.)—W.P. Burdick, M.D.

---

**Advances in Pelvic Ultrasound: Endovaginal Scanning for Ectopic Gestation and Graded Compression Sonography for Appendicitis**
Marn CS, Bree RL (Univ of Michigan)
*Ann Emerg Med* 18:1304–1309, 1989                                         4–104

---

Ectopic gestation and acute appendicitis are common diagnoses in the ED. The precise diagnosis of these disorders is sometimes difficult, particularly in atypical manifestations. Until recently, imaging was of limited use in these diagnoses, but the recent introduction of endovaginal sonography and graded compression sonography now offers significant diagnostic information in the imaging evaluation of the pelvis.

Woman, 30, with crampy abdominal pain, nausea, and bilious vomiting for 20 hours, was seen in the ED. She had experienced a similar episode 4 weeks earlier, but the symptoms had resolved spontaneously. Her last menstrual period was 4 weeks earlier. She had been using the rhythm method for birth control. There was mild right lower quadrant tenderness on both abdominal and pelvic examination. Laboratory evaluation revealed a white blood cell count of 15,500/mm³ and a positive serum pregnancy test result. The β-human chorionic gonadotropin (β-hCG) quantitative analysis was 1,994 IU/L. Routine pelvic ultrasound scanning showed a tiny fluid collection within the uterus. Scanning of the right lower quadrant demonstrated a tubular 6-cm structure at the point of maximal tenderness. Endovaginal ultrasound scanning was then performed, which revealed a fluid-filled structure within the uterus with an echogenic margin representing a trophoblastic reaction. No fetal pole was observed within this sac, and no adnexal mass was evident. Based on these findings, appendicitis and probable coexistent intrauterine gestation were diagnosed. The patient was taken to the operating room where appendectomy was performed under epidural anesthesia. An inflamed nonruptured appendix was removed. Recovery was uneventful. The patient carried the fetus to term and had an uncomplicated vaginal delivery.

The use of endovaginal ultrasound enables detection of morphologic changes related to intrauterine gestation at least 1 week in advance of transabdominal scanning. In this patient, endovaginal ultrasound conclusively confirmed an intrauterine pregnancy and excluded a diagnosis of ectopic pregnancy.

▶ Transvaginal sonography in skilled hands holds promise in the evaluation of ectopic pregnancy. If a fetal sac is detected earlier, it may obviate the current need for further evaluation or close follow-up of the patient with the "potential" unruptured ectopic pregnancy. Refinement of this correlation between serum hCG levels and presence of an intrauterine gestational sac by transvaginal ultrasound likewise could lead to early diagnosis of ectopic gestation.

It is hard to believe that less than 1 decade ago emergency physicians basically approached the "potential ectopic" armed with a poorly sensitive urine test and a long needle on the end of a 20-mL syringe. (See also Abstract 4–47.)—R.M. McNamara, M.D.

---

## Outcomes of Pregnancy in Adolescents With Severe Asthma
Apter AJ, Greenberger PA, Patterson R (Northwestern Univ)
*Arch Intern Med* 149:2571–2575, 1989                                      4–105

---

Asthma in adolescent pregnancies is not rare and can complicate patient management, especially because mortality from asthma is of particular concern in adolescents. The outcomes of 28 pregnancies in 21 adolescents with severe asthma were studied to identify factors associated with the worsening of asthma and to document the major issues that confront managing physicians. There were 56 exacerbations of asthma, including 22 hospitalizations and 20 emergency room visits. For 18 of the

28 pregnancies (64%), corticosteroids were administered systemically on an outpatient basis, and inhaled corticosteroids were prescribed for 8 patients (29%). Respiratory tract infection and noncompliance with medical regimens were associated with exacerbations. There were no maternal or fetal deaths, nor was there evidence of intrauterine growth retardation. Two infants were born prematurely, 1 of whom had acute respiratory distress syndrome.

Pregnant adolescents with severe asthma may have a variety of problems. Aggressive management of asthma and infection and careful follow-up to improve patient compliance may result in better outcomes.

▶ It is really hard to conclude much from this paper, which merely demonstrates that a small group of young women with previous history of asthma of unknown severity seemed to tolerate their pregnancies well, despite both acute and chronic medication regimens, excluding inhaled β-adrenergic agents. The word "severe" in the title is misleading, because no definition of severity is given, nor is any prior or current clinical characteristic required for inclusion into the "study."—J.R. Hoffman, M.D.

---

### The Intrauterine Hematoma: Diagnostic and Clinical Aspects
Mandruzzato GP, D'Ottavio G, Rustico MA, Fontana A, Bogatti P (Istituto per l'Infanzia "Burlo Garofolo," Trieste, Italy)
*J Clin Ultrasound* 17:503–510, 1989                                          4–106

---

Because intrauterine hematoma may have serious consequences for the outcome of pregnancy, 62 patients in whom the fetus was viable were followed up until conclusion.

The condition occurred in 12% of patients with threatened abortion. Diagnosis was based on ultrasound examination. The frequency of spontaneous abortion was similar in patients with threatened abortion with and without hematoma. Delivery occurred before week 37 was completed in 13% of patients with nonaborted pregnancies. Both the abortion rate and the frequency of delivery at a menstrual age of 35 weeks or less were significantly related to volume of the hematoma greater than 15 mL.

In 22% of the infants, the birth weight was low; there was a perinatal mortality rate of 2%. The rate of cesarean section was 26%. The placenta had to be removed manually in 7% of patients.

In patients with bleeding in early pregnancy, intrauterine hematoma is common. Diagnosis requires ultrasound examination. Spontaneous abortion may occur if the volume of the hematoma is greater than 15 mL. Careful monitoring of fetal growth is necessary, and premature delivery is more likely. The perinatal outcome is favorable, although complications should be anticipated.

▶ Now that ultrasound is used so frequently in cases of threatened abortion (usually to rule out ectopic pregnancy), it has been learned that intrauterine hematoma commonly accompanies the vaginal bleeding. Neither this nor the associated discovery that small hematomas of this kind tend not to have any significance in those patients who successfully carry the pregnancy past the first trimester is likely to have much impact on emergency medical (or even obstetric) practice.—J.R. Hoffman, M.D.

## Foreign Bodies

### How Accurate Is Chest Radiography in the Diagnosis of Tracheobronchial Foreign Bodies in Children?

Svedström E, Puhakka H, Kero P (Turku Univ Central Hosp, Finland)
*Pediatr Radiol* 19:520–522, 1989                                                      4–107

Respiratory problems in pediatric patients are frequently caused by inhalation of a foreign body. When a tracheobronchial foreign body is suspected, chest radiography is almost always performed. The accuracy of this procedure was analyzed retrospectively in 108 children with suspected inhalation of a foreign body.

The most common radiologic findings were air trapping, infection, and atelectasis. In 23 examinations (28%) no abnormality was detected. Compared with bronchoscopy, radiography was 67% accurate. The sensitivity of radiography in demonstrating a foreign body was 68% and the specificity was 67%. A foreign body was identified by radiography in 34 of 83 bronchoscopied patients (41%); however, 16 of these patients, all showing signs of atelectasis or air trapping, had no foreign body. A false negative result was obtained by radiography in 11 patients (32%).

Plain film radiology is not sufficiently sensitive or a specific method for the diagnosis of foreign body aspiration.

▶ One of my cardinal rules is always suspect a foreign body in the child with signs of respiratory distress or dysphagia. This can be a very tough diagnosis if the ingested item is not radiopaque. A significant percentage of these children do not have a history of foreign body ingestion or coughing spell. The child may be in another room away from the parent or caretaker when the event occurs. We all know how fast toddlers move and that they explore the environment with all of their senses, including taste. The physical examination is helpful if there is asymetric chest wall movement or unilateral wheezing or decreased breath sounds, but the majority of patients do not exhibit these findings. Inspiratory and expiratory films are suggested as 1 way to identify a child with a foreign body that causes air trapping. However, a recent article by Losek et al. illustrated the difficulty of identifying a foreign body in the toddler's airway. In their retrospective review of 42 children with foreign body aspiration, 20% were unwitnessed, and 57% were asymptomatic at the time they were seen. Twenty percent had a totally normal physical examination, and 24 percent had normal inspiratory and expiratory chest x-ray films. The most common objects that children aspirate include peanuts, peas, small plastic objects, pearls, and other small miscellaneous food products.

Identifying which child has a foreign body is difficult for the clinician. One should always consider the possibility of a foreign body and document a thorough history and physical examination. One should obtain inspiratory and expiratory chest x-ray films and, most important, assure appropriate consultation for admission or close follow-up. Sometimes it takes several weeks to months to identify which children need to have bronchoscopy for retained respiratory foreign bodies.

One last caveat to remember is that esophageal foreign bodies trapped at the thoracic inlet or carina can manifest as respiratory distress in the pediatric patient.—R.W. Schafermeyer, M.D.

---

**Tracheobronchial Foreign Bodies: A Persistent Problem in Pediatric Patients**
Puhakka H, Svedström E, Kero P, Valli P, Iisalo E (Univ Central Hosp, Turku, Finland)
*Am J Dis Child* 143:543–545, 1989                                    4–108

---

Although foreign body inhalation by a child is usually accompanied by severe coughing, stridor, wheezing, or dyspnea, it is frequently followed by an asymptomatic period. Because the acute episode may escape notice by parents or caretakers, the incident may not be discovered for several weeks. Data on 83 children with confirmed foreign body inhalation treated during an 18-year period were studied.

The patient population consisted of 27 girls (mean age 1 year 9 months) and 56 boys (mean age 3 years 1 month). Forty-six children were younger than age 2 years when aspiration occurred. Sixty-four children had a transient or persistent cough, 31 had signs of infection, and 12 were cyanotic when seen. Symptoms had started suddenly in 77 children, and the parents were aware of aspiration. The time lag between inhalation and extraction of the foreign body was less than 12 hours in 27 children. Radiologic examination before endoscopy showed 16 radiopaque foreign bodies and evidence of bronchial obstruction by 19 foreign bodies. A peanut was the most commonly inhaled foreign body (30%).

Endoscopic extraction was successful in 81 of the 83 children. Only 2 patients required thoracotomy—1 for removal of a pin and the other for removal of a piece of a spike that had perforated the bronchial wall. Three children required 2 attempts on 2 subsequent days to remove the foreign body. There were only 3 patients who had residual foreign bodies, 2 of whom had first been treated in another hospital. There were no deaths, cardiac arrests, or pneumothoraces associated with foreign body extraction procedures, and none of the patients required tracheostomy.

Except for emergency conditions, only an experienced endoscopist with the support of skilled anesthesiologists should attempt foreign body extraction in children. All healthy children who suddenly have abnormal stridor or cough should undergo open tube bronchoscopy to rule out foreign body aspiration, because foreign body inhalation may be hazardous or even fatal to the child.

▶ The differential diagnosis of a child with the acute onset of cough and stridor includes foreign body aspiration, spasmodic croup, and severe allergic reaction. The history will frequently suggest the correct diagnosis. (Aspirations occur during waking hours, whereas many patients with spasmodic croup present late at night.) More than 90% of the parents in this study were aware of the aspiration episode. In this series, the initial x-ray film failed to identify a foreign object in 54%.

In the presence of a history strongly suggestive of aspiration, bronchoscopy would be the diagnostic and therapeutic intervention of choice, even with normal radiographs. The authors review their experience with foreign object aspiration in children treated with bronchoscopy. They were successful in 81 of 84 patients, without significant morbidity.

Much more difficult for the clinician is the child with stridor and no observed aspiration or the patient with the 3 weeks of intermittent cough after an apparent aspiration. In these cases, clinicians must weigh the history, physical examination, and results of chest x-ray films in reaching a decision on bronchoscopy. The authors suggest an empiric trial of antibiotics and that a lack of response indicates the need for bronchoscopy. Unfortunately, this is only a retrospective review of "positive" cases, and we have no data on the number of procedures performed that failed to identify foreign objects. The authors' conclusion that a "bronchoscopy should be performed whenever abnormal stridor or cough is observed in a healthy child and when appropriate antibiotic therapy is unsuccessful" appears unjustified at this time. Foreign object aspiration must be entertained in such patients, but the extent of the evaluation requires careful assessment of each patient.

And, once again, remind parents of the dangers of peanuts and other small foods around young children. Seventy-four percent of these patients were less than 4 years old. Peanuts and apples were the offending objects in 42%.— R.M. Rutstein, M.D.

---

**Pediatric Coin Ingestion: A Prospective Study on the Utility of Routine Roentgenograms**
Caravati EM, Bennett DL, McElwee NE (Intermountain Regional Poison Control Ctr, Salt Lake City; Univ of Utah)
*Am J Dis Child* 143:549–551, 1989                                              4–109

---

Routine roentgenograms have been recommended in all pediatric patients with a history of coin ingestion, regardless of symptoms. A prospective study of 162 children aged 9 months–12 years was undertaken to determine the risk of a coin being lodged in the esophagus of asymptomatic vs. symptomatic children at the time of ingestion and to assess the need for routine roentgenography. All cases were reported to the Intermountain Regional Poison Control Center, and patients were referred for immediate roentgenography and followed up daily by telephone for 5 days. Of these, 66 complied and 96 did not comply with the recommendation.

A coin was seen in the esophagus in 13 patients; 11 were symptomatic and 2 were asymptomatic. The risk of a coin later being located in the esophagus by roentgenography was 42% in symptomatic patients vs. 5% in asymptomatic patients. Ten patients passed the coin uneventfully following administration of oral fluids, whereas 3 symptomatic patients had the coin removed by esophagoscopy. Of the patients who did not comply with the recommendation, 18 were symptomatic at the time of ingestion, and all became asymptomatic within 24 hours. The incidence of morbidity did not differ between the 2 groups, demonstrating that children who are asymptomatic at the time of coin ingestion may not need immediate roentgenography if they can tolerate oral fluids and close follow-up by telephone is available.

▶ This report seeks to challenge the existing x-ray localization of the coin despite the absence of symptoms. It fails to change that standard of practice for me. I have serious concern with any research in which more than half of the study population is lost. Even the initial selection of the study population are those who call a regional poison control center. Is this reflective of the population at large? The report further documents a significant number of asymptomatic children with esophageal coins. The incidence of serious complication from an entrapped foreign body is low. However, the possible complications are life threatening. Thus, the authors need much larger numbers to report no impact from their proposed change in management. It would be comforting to be able to tell the parents of these coin eaters not to worry and not to bother getting an x-ray film. Unfortunately, this report does not allow us to feel that comfort.—S. Ludwig, M.D.

---

**Button Batteries in the Ear, Nose and Cervical Esophagus: A Destructive Foreign Body**

McRae D, Premachandra DJ, Gatland DJ (St Bartholomew's Hosp, London; Kent and Sussex Hosp, Tunbridge Wells, England)
*J Otolaryngol* 18:317–319, 1989                                    4–110

---

Because of their small size and shiny surface, button batteries are attractive to children and are consequently potentially dangerous as foreign bodies.

Button batteries generally contain a zinc anode and a mercury or a silver oxide cathode immersed in a potent alkaline solution, usually 45% potassium hydroxide. A burn may occur from low-voltage direct current passing between the anode and the cathode, which is potentiated in the external auditory meatus by the high conductivity of cerumen. The tissue fluid that results from an electric burn creates moisture in the ear while moisture is present physiologically in the nose and esophagus. The moisture not only potentiates the generation of an electric current but also causes leakage of the battery's alkaline electrolyte solution, which can penetrate deeply into tissue, causing liquefaction necrosis. Dissolution of protein and collagen, saponification of lipids, dehydration of tissue cells, and extensive tissue damage result.

Two boys, aged 30 months and 10 years, with a button battery in the external auditory meatus that resulted in skin, bone, and tympanic membrane necrosis were treated. Nasal and otic drops must be avoided before removal of button battery foreign bodies. After removal, irrigation of the impaction site with sterile water will remove precipitate and dilute the residual alkali. The site should be kept dry. Close follow-up is necessary in the event that further débridement of necrotic tissue is needed. The authors recommend that antibiotic and corticosteroid therapy be used in alkaline esophageal burns.

▶ Previous articles have documented the danger of button batteries when they become lodged in the esophagus (1). This article points out the potentially serious consequences of button battery lodgement in the ears or nose. Significantly, in 2 cases of nasal septal perforation reviewed by the authors, the button batteries had been in the nostrils for less than 24 hours. Their admonition should be heeded by all emergency physicians: A button battery lodged in the esophagus, nose, or ear should be removed immediately by the appropriate specialist.

The article points out that nasal and otic scopes should be avoided before removal because they can potentiate battery electrolysis and leakage. The recommendation to treat all alkaline esophageal burns with antibiotics and corticosteroids is somewhat more controversial. The efficacy of this approach has not yet been scientifically established (2).

Parents should be able to keep those button batteries (and wristwatches, cameras, hearing aids, etc.) out of the reach of young children.—H.H. Osborn, M.D.

*References*

1. Kuhns DW, Dire DJ: *Ann Emerg Med* 1989; 18:293–300.
2. Tintinalli JE, et al (eds): *Emergency Medicine: A Comprehensive Study Guide*, ed 2. New York, McGraw-Hill Book Co, 1988, pp 733–737.

## Fish Bones in the Throat
Knight LC, Lesser THJ (Royal Gwent Hosp, Newport, Wales)
*Arch Emerg Med* 6:13–16, 1989                                    4–111

Seventy-one patients with sharp pain in their throat after eating fish were studied to determine the site and frequency of impacted fish bones. All patients underwent direct examination of the oral cavity and oropharynx and mirror examination of the pharynx and larynx.

Fish bones were found in 15 patients (21%), and in 14 (93%) they were in the oropharynx or hypopharynx. The base of the tongue was the most common site of an impacted fish bone (53%), followed by the tonsil

(20%), posterior pharyngeal wall, aryepiglottic fold, and upper esophagus. Symptoms resolved within 48 hours in 73% of patients in whom no fish bone was found.

If no fish bone is evident after initial examination of the pharynx, a lateral neck x-ray film is required and should include the region of the cricopharyngeus, which is the most common site of impaction of esophageal foreign bodies. If findings at initial examination and on x-ray films are normal, the patient should be observed to see if symptoms resolve. Immediate referral for endoscopy is not mandatory.

▶ This paper gives an excellent approach for retrieving fish bones in the throat. The authors contend that only 1 of 5 patients who complain of a fish bone in the throat will actually have 1. Of those that have a fish bone in the throat, more than 90% are seen by an adequate physical examination, which includes direct laryngoscopy. Indirect laryngoscopy appears to be becoming a lost art with the advent of fiberoptic nasopharyngoscopy. Nevertheless, for evaluation of foreign bodies in the throat, indirect visualization with a mirror is easy to perform. To provide anesthesia for indirect laryngoscopy, the patient must inhale an aerosol of 4 cc of 4% xylocaine solution through a nebulizer. This also diminishes gag response and may relieve any sensation of discomfort. If a foreign body cannot be seen on initial examination, soft-tissue cervical radiographs have a low yield. If there are suspicious findings on soft-tissue cervical x-ray film, or the patient still complains of symptoms 48 hours later, otolaryngologic referral is warranted. If there is gas in the soft tissues of the prevertebral space of the neck, otolaryngologic involvement is more urgent.—E.J. Reisdorff, M.D.

---

**A Prospective Study on Fish Bone Ingestion: Experience of 358 Patients**
Ngan JHK, Fok PJ, Lai ECS, Branicki FJ, Wong J (Univ of Hong Kong)
*Ann Surg* 211:459–462, 1990                                              4–112

---

Fish bone remains 1 of the most common foreign bodies to be ingested and carries the hazard of bowel perforation. The bones usually are radiolucent and therefore difficult to detect. Of 358 patients reporting ingestion of fish bones, their mean age was 41.5 years. Fish bones were found in 117 persons; 83% of the bones were above the cricopharyngeal sphincter.

Twenty-one fish bones were located and removed without further procedures being needed. Flexible endoscopy was tolerated by all except 2 patients. Of 94 bones seen with endoscopy, 82 were retrieved endoscopically with the immediate cessation of symptoms. No abdominal complications occurred in 12 patients whose bones were dislodged and not retrieved. Two bones were missed with endoscopy. One patient had a cervical esophageal tear when a triangular bone was trailed from the hypopharynx through the cricopharyngeal sphincter. In 1 of 35 patients who refused endoscopy, a retropharyngeal abscess developed. Neck radiographs were specific but not sensitive in detecting fish bones. The only relatively predictive symptom was a sharp pricking sensation on swallowing.

Flexible endoscopy with a patient under local pharyngeal anesthesia is indicated if fish bone ingestion is reported and a bone is not found on oral examination. If a bone is lodged in the hypopharynx, rigid laryngoesophagoscopy with general anesthesia should be considered.

▶ The authors present an extensive experience with fish bone ingestion. Their experience is enhanced by the large amount of fish ingested in that part of the world as well as by custom; often the fish head is eaten. This provides particularly onorous problems when the bone becomes impacted. The authors suggest that in the presence of symptoms suggesting the presence of a foreign body, both direct oral examination as well as fiberoptic endoscopic evaluation be carried out. Of 117 identified foreign bodies, 115 were located at or above the hypopharynx. Such foreign bodies should be visualized by use of the fiberoptic nasopharyngoscope, an instrument rapidly becoming routinely available to the emergency physician. When identified, the majority of fish bones located in this area can be removed by the direct forceps approach. The authors caution against removal of triangular-shaped bones wedged in the hypopharynx. Such are best removed in an operating room environment. Of interest is their data on the natural history of retained foreign bodies in patients refusing extraction. Only 1 developed a complicating abscess. All others subsequently became asymptomatic because of spontaneous dislodgement. Not unexpectedly, radiographic evaluation provided little help in most cases.—D.K. Wagner, M.D.

# 5 Emergency Procedures, Techniques, and Instrumentation

## Airway Control

**Acute Airway Management: Role of Cricothyroidotomy**
DeLaurier GA, Hawkins ML, Treat RC, Mansberger AR Jr (Med College of Georgia, Augusta)
*Am Surg* 56:12–15, 1990                                                        5–1

Cricothyroidotomy as a surgical procedure in the management of upper airway obstruction was condemned for several decades until its safe use as an emergency procedure was reconfirmed in 1976. The records of all patients who underwent cricothyroidotomy during a 4-year period were studied.

Emergency cricothyroidotomy was performed on 31 acute trauma patients in whom intubation was considered unsafe because of associated head and neck injury or in whom attempts at intubation had failed. Another 3 patients who had not sustained acute trauma underwent the procedure when oral or nasal intubation could not be accomplished. Ten patients underwent laryngoscopy and 2 patients underwent bronchoscopy after cricothyroidotomy or subsequent tracheostomy.

Fourteen of the 31 acute trauma patients died of their injuries, 13 of whom died within the first several hours after injury. The 20 surviving patients were evaluated in 2 groups. The first group comprised 11 patients whose cricothyroidotomy tube remained in place until decannulation; the second group included 9 patients who underwent formal tracheostomy subsequent to emergency cricothyroidotomy.

One patient in the first group has remained in a vegetative state because of severe head injury, and the cricothyroidotomy has remained in place for 4 months. In the remaining 10 patients, decannulation was performed after an average of 6.3 days. Six patients underwent laryngoscopy within 10 days of decannulation. After an average follow-up of 67 days, 3 patients had minor complications consisting of stomal granulation and minimal tracheal erosion. In the second group, tracheostomy was performed 30 minutes–9 days after cricothyroidotomy and left in place for 8–270 days. After an average follow-up of 83 days, 6 patients had complications, including 2 patients who required reoperation because of a partial airway obstruction. Decannulation was never performed on one patient before his death from oral cancer 9 months after tracheostomy. The other 3 complications were considered minor and included bleeding, supraglottic inflammation, and stomal granulation. In all, only 2 of the 20 survivors experienced significant morbidity as a result of surgical airway management. Tracheostomy subsequent to emergency cricothyroidotomy does not necessarily reduce airway-related morbidity in these patients.

▶ In this small group of patients (20) who underwent emergency cricothyroidotomy, only 2 had significant complications as a direct result of the surgical airway management. It is interesting that a no. 6 or 8 Shiley tracheostomy tube was used in their patients (Tintinalli et al. [1] recommend a no. 4 tracheostomy tube to avoid laryngeal injury). Either way, when the other options—no airway at all or emergency tracheostomy under less than optimal conditions—are considered, the benefits of cricothyroidotomy outweight the risks.—J.M. Mitchell, M.D.

*Reference*

1. Tintinalli JE, et al (eds): *Emergency Medicine: A Comprehensive Study Guide*, ed 2. New York, McGraw-Hill Book Co, 1988, p 16.

---

**Surgical Cricothyrotomy in the Field: Experience of a Helicopter Transport Team**
Miklus RM, Elliot C, Snow N (Case Western Reserve Univ; Cleveland Metropolitan Gen Hosp)
*J Trauma* 29:506–508, 1989                    5–2

---

Cricothyrotomy has been advocated by the American College of Surgeons as an appropriate alternative to endotracheal intubation for emergency airway access. Its role in emergency airway access in the field was studied in a retrospective analysis of 3,500 helicopter missions of the Metro Life Flight.

Cricothyrotomy was performed in 20 patients in the field for emergency airway access. The standard cricothyrotomy technique was used by the medical crew consisting of a flight nurse and physician. Despite adequate airway control, 5 patients in cardiopulmonary arrest died. Autopsies revealed no laryngotracheal pathology of airway compromise. Cricothyrotomy was required in 12 patients because of severe oral, maxillofacial, or cervical trauma; of these, 7 survived and none had bleeding episodes, subglottic stenosis, airway obstruction, or dysphonia after decannulation.

Surgical cricothyrotomy can be successfully performed in the field by a well-trained helicopter transport team. Cricothyrotomy is recommended for emergency airway access in the field when conventional airway maneuvers are unsuccessful.

▶ An experienced helicopter team brings rapid medical support to a victim and rapid transport back to the ED. On arrival, the team is capable of advanced airway support. The findings of this study are, therefore, not a surprise. A similar study should be performed when the team does not include a physician (assuming the nurse or nurse-paramedic team is appropriately trained in the technique of cricothyrotomy). Indeed, studies that have shown the importance of the physician as a member of the team have frequently indicated the need for advanced airway support as a reason. This does not mean that this same service could not be performed by another trained individual.—J.T. Amsterdam, M.D.

---

**Fiberoptic Intubation in the Emergency Department**
Mlinek EJ Jr, Clinton JE, Plummer D, Ruiz E (Hennepin County Med Ctr, Minneapolis)
*Ann Emerg Med* 19:359–362, 1990                                    5–3

---

Fiberoptic-aided endotracheal intubation has been shown to be effective in difficult intubations involving various anatomical and traumatic conditions. However, because the technique has not been widely adopted for use in EDs, an experience with fiberoptic-aided scope intubation in an ED was reviewed.

During a 30-month period, 35 patients underwent fiberoptic-aided endotracheal intubation in an ED; 31 had treatment for medical conditions, and 4 were trauma patients. Indications included failed nasotracheal intubation, anatomical abnormalities, and the initial airway attempted. Identified anatomical conditions that influenced the decision to use the fiberoptic scope in 6 medical patients included kyphosis, clenched teeth, and trismus. Ten medical patients had fiberoptic-aided nasal intubation attempted after blind nasotracheal intubation had failed.

All 4 trauma patients had successful nasal intubation. The fiberoptic technique failed in 6 patients with medical conditions. Causes of failure included secretions, blood, or vomitus and persistent scope swallowing. The overall success rate was 83%: 81% for medical patients and 100% for trauma patients.

Fiberoptic equipment is expensive and fragile, and fiscal restraints may limit its use in EDs. During an 8-year period, $17,000 was spent on maintenance and replacement of worn equipment. Because of the expenses associated with the use of fiberoptic scopes, specific indications should be developed for which the use of fiberoptic equipment in the ED is justified. The development of a more durable scope would contribute further to keeping costs at an acceptable level.

▶ In emergency medicine, sheer fright is the difficult and elusive airway that defies intubation while the patient slips away. Any helpful technique quickly finds a trial.

Unfortunately, crash intubations are usually messy with the difficult, recalcitrant airway disappearing in the blood, vomitus, or copious secretions that cake the tip of the fiberoptic laryngoscope. Landmarks blur into dim red light. Given these obstacles, it is likely that the fiberoptic laryngoscope provides little help in the true crash intubation.—E.H. Taliaferro, M.D.

## Correct Positioning of an Endotracheal Tube Using a Flexible Lighted Stylet

Stewart RD, LaRosee A, Kaplan RM, Ilkhanipour K (Univ of Pittsburgh)
*Crit Care Med* 18:97–99, 1990                    5–4

The traditional methods for insertion of an endotracheal (ET) tube in critically ill or injured patients have recently been expanded to include placement with the aid of a lighted stylet, or light wand, in which transillumination of the soft tissues of the neck helps guide the ET tube to a position within the trachea. A more recent development is the design of a flexible stylet to facilitate nasotracheal intubation using the transillumination method to distinguish correct intratracheal from inadvertent esophageal tube placement. Correct positioning of an ET tube is usually defined as the placement of the tube within the trachea approximately 5 cm above the carina. Chest radiography is most commonly used to demonstrate correct positioning of the ET tube. This study was done to determine whether transillumination could position an ET tube consistently within 5 cm of the carina.

Ten fresh, unembalmed human cadavers of varied body weight and habitus were used. Each cadaver was measured for height and neck circumference; weight was estimated. Intubation under direct vision was performed on all cadavers, and a radiopaque dye was injected down the tube as a marker for the carina. A premeasured flexible lighted stylet was then inserted into the in-place tube and advanced distally so that the bulb was positioned at the tube's distal opening. The tube and stylet combination was then adjusted to the point at which the bright circumscribed glow of the stylet began to disappear beneath the sternum at the sternal notch. The distance of the bulb of the stylet from the carina was calculated from a control chest radiograph.

By observing the maximal transilluminated glow at the sternal notch, the tube tip could be placed accurately and consistently at a level 5 cm from the carina. Use of this method in critically ill and injured patients could reduce the need for routine radiographic confirmation of ET tube position.

▶ A light at the sternal notch can obviate a chest x-ray film taken purely to verify tube placement. This trick could also be performed with a bronchoscope.—T. Stair, M.D.

## Cricoarytenoid Subluxation: Complication of Blind Intubation With a Lighted Stylet

Debo RF, Colonna D, Dewerd G, Gonzalez C (Uniformed Services Univ of the Health Sciences, Washington, DC)
*Ear Nose Throat J* 68:517–520, 1989                    5–5

A lighted stylet is used to transilluminate the soft tissues of the neck during blind intubation. Complications from use of the light wand are rare.

Man, 29, with a chronic left tympanic membrane perforation and conductive hearing loss, was admitted for elective tympanoplasty. He was otherwise healthy and had no evident upper airway abnormality. Blind orotracheal intubation was carried out with a lighted stylet, but 3 attempts were necessary. The patient later underwent extubation uneventfully but had a very hoarse voice and reported moderate odynophagia. Laryngoscopy showed an edematous right arytenoid cartilage that was displaced anteromedially. The true vocal cord was bowed and fixed in the paramedian position. Direct laryngoscopy subsequently was done with general anesthesia to reduce the cricoarytenoid cartilage. Marked vocal improvement ensued.

Only 11 cases of postintubation arytenoid subluxation have appeared in the English language literature. Anterior dislocation of the arytenoid tends to cause marked hoarseness in adults but respiratory compromise in children. Posterior dislocation produces severe sore throat, odynophagia, and hoarseness.

▶ The light wand is an available adjunct to the emergency physician for airway control of the upper airway. Although cricoarytenoid subluxation is relatively uncommon, it can certainly occur following any attempted intubation of the larynx. Emergency physicians will be well to consider this possibility in the postintubated patient with unusual hoarseness and odynophagia. Careful evaluation with the nasopharyngoscope should allow diagnosis of this unusual condition. Reduction should be carried out by an appropriately trained specialist in the operating room setting.—D.K. Wagner, M.D.

---

**Pharyngeal Tracheal Lumen Airway Training: Failure to Discriminate Between Esophageal and Endotracheal Modes and Failure to Confirm Ventilation**
Hunt RC, Sheets CA, Whitley TW (East Carolina Univ, Greenville, NC; Wright State Univ, Dayton)
*Ann Emerg Med* 18:947–952, 1989                                             5–6

---

A new airway control device, the pharyngeal tracheal lumen (PTL) airway, which can function as an esophageal obturator airway or an endotracheal tube, was developed (Fig 5–1). Because training for this device had not been standardized, a 10-step training protocol was developed and tested.

The 70 insertion attempts by 32 emergency medical technicians and paramedics all resulted in placement in the esophageal obturator mode, so discrimination between endotracheal and esophageal placement could not be practiced. With the model in the esophageal mode, 4 trainees could not select the esophageal port to ventilate 6 weeks later. When the

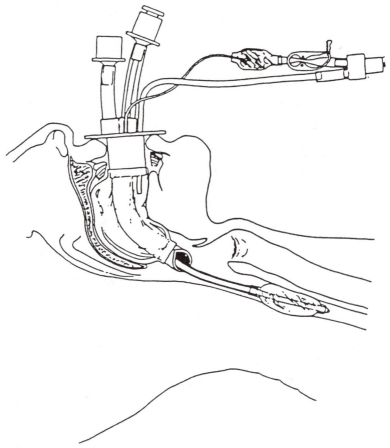

**Fig 5–1.**—The PTL airway positioned in the esophagus. (Courtesy of Niemann JT, Rosborough JP, Myers R, et al: *Ann Emerg Med* 13:591–596, 1984. From Hunt RC, Sheets CA, Whitley TW: *Ann Emerg Med* 18:947–952, 1989.)

model was in the endotracheal mode, 1 paramedic could not discriminate between the 2 modes, and 2 emergency medical technicians tried ventilation with the esophageal port when the tracheal balloon occluded the airway. Ventilation could be confirmed by chest auscultation in only one half of the attempts.

The protocol outlined is insufficient to teach discrimination between endotracheal and esophageal modes. Because practice in insertion of the airway in both modes is essential, training intubation models or the device should be modified accordingly. Ability to confirm ventilation needs more emphasis in training.

▶ The PTL airway device has two theoretical advantages over the esophageal obturator airway and esophageal gastric tube airway. The first is that with esophageal placement, the pharyngeal balloon allows for automatic maintenance of a seal eliminating the inherent difficulty with the face mask seal during use of the esophageal obturator airway and esophageal gastric tube airway. Second, if it is placed in the trachea, ventilation can be accomplished by removing a stylet and using a second port.

This device is designed for prehospital providers who either are insufficiently trained or who have infrequent opportunity to use standard endotracheal intubation. This important study highlights the prehospital danger of this device in just such hands. This is not a simple, foolproof method, and serious errors may occur. The device does seem to be an improvement over the esophageal obturator airway and esophageal gastric tube airway, but careful training and frequent review of proper use must be ensured if chosen by a prehospital care system. Standard endotracheal intubation, of course, is the standard to which all systems should aspire.—R.M. McNamara, M.D.

## Vascular Access/Volume Replacement

### A Prospective Study of Femoral Versus Subclavian Vein Catheterization During Cardiac Arrest

Emerman CL, Bellon EM, Lukens TW, May TE, Effron D (Case Western Reserve Univ)
*Ann Emerg Med* 19:26–30, 1990                                     5–7

Femoral venous catheterization interferes minimally with ongoing cardiopulmonary resuscitation, and the risks are less than those of subclavian catheterization. A prospective comparative study was carried out in 94 patients having cardiopulmonary resuscitation. Each route was utilized in 47 patients. Catheter placement was confirmed by injection of opaque contrast material.

Femoral catheterization was successful in 77% of attempts and subclavian vein catheterization in 94%. No pneumothoraces occurred when the subclavian vein was catheterized. No learning curve was apparent.

Subclavian venous catheterization was successful more often than femoral vein catheterization in this prospective study of patients undergoing cardiopulmonary resuscitation. The subclavian route is preferable for use in cardiac arrest. Femoral catheterization is used when neither peripheral nor subclavian vein catheterization is possible.

▶ The femoral approach to percutaneous venous and arterial cannulation is often difficult, as this study demonstrates. But the advantages of the femoral route, especially for arterial cannulation, should stimulate innovative approaches to overcoming these difficulties. A rapid, easily accomplished method of establishing a percutaneous femoral arterial line would be very helpful in the management of cardiac arrest.—E. Ruiz, M.D.

### A Modified Wire-Guided Technique for Venous Cutdown Access

Shockley LW, Butzier DJ (Fairview Southdale Hosp, Minneapolis)
*Ann Emerg Med* 19:393–395, 1990                                     5–8

Vascular access is important in resuscitating severely ill or injured patients, but intravenous access via the percutaneous route often is not possible in such patients. Venous cutdown is therefore an essential skill for an emergency physician, but because the classic cutdown technique is often difficult to carry out, particularly in children, a new wire-dilator-catheter assembly was designed to facilitate the placement of an intravenous cannula through venous cutdown. This new assembly was compared with the classic technique for placement of intravenous cutdown catheters.

Twenty-four inexperienced medical students and first-year residents were taught both the classic and modified cutdown techniques for placement of catheters into femoral veins in dogs. The techniques were taught in 7 sessions to small groups consisting of 3 or 4 novice operators. The mean times required to successfully complete cannulation were measured. No hands-on assistance by the instructor was allowed.

The students and residents successfully cannulated the femoral veins of the dogs using the classic technique 7 times, with 1 failure, for which the modified technique then was used to correct the problem. The times required to complete all tasks ranged from 5 minutes 50 seconds to 15 minutes 43 seconds (mean 10 minutes 11 seconds). The same students and residents successfully carried out the modified technique in all 7 attempts. The times required for completing all tasks ranged from 3 minutes 55 seconds to 11 minutes 26 seconds (mean 7 minutes 58 seconds). The modified guide wire–aided technique was performed 22% faster, on average, than the classic technique.

▶ When equipment is preassembled, this procedure is faster and more successful than the classic techniques.

The small vein in the deep hole presents a challenge that this new technique addresses.—E.H. Taliaferro, M.D.

---

**Rapid Venous Access Using Saphenous Vein Cutdown at the Ankle**
Rhee KJ, Derlet RW, Beal SL (Univ of California, Davis)
*Am J Emerg Med* 7:263–266, 1989                                    5–9

---

Peripheral access usually is available in injured adults, but alternate methods such as vein cutdown may be necessary for those who are hypotensive. Seventy-three cutdowns were attempted in 56 adults in a 1-year period at a major trauma center. The general policy was to initiate a saphenous vein cutdown at the ankle of any hypotensive patient with suspected major injury. An attempt at large-bore access in an upper extremity usually is made at the same time.

Sixty-two of 73 attempts led to venous cannulation with free flow. The average time required was 5 minutes. Surgical residents in years 2–5 and ED staff were successful significantly more often than first-year residents. Local cellulitis developed in 1 patient, but none had deep venous thrombosis or septic thrombophlebitis.

Saphenous vein cutdown at the ankle usually provides venous access in adult trauma patients who are hypotensive. Some degree of experience is needed to perform cutdowns reliably and expeditiously. If a catheter is removed within 24 hours, the risk of complications is low.

▶ With the advent of sophisticated, over-the-needle and wire-guided catheters and an interest in cervically placed vascular access, the cutdown catheter placement has been often abandoned. The authors point out some distinct advantages of a saphenous vein cutdown. First, it does not disrupt other resuscitative maneuvers, nor does it inhibit attempts at upper extremity peripheral access. If coincident with the upper extremity approach, saphenous vein catheterization is attempted, an immediately available route is provided should the peripheral attempt fail, and in the event of upper extremity access, with the additional saphenous vein entry, access both above and below the diaphragm has been obtained. To be strongly supported is the authors' technique that provides vein exposure with direct cannulation with large-bore tubing and direct insertion of a cutoff intravenous connecting tubing. The vein is not sacrificed, and catheter withdrawal occurs within 48 hours of the resuscitative event—a technique in many training programs in sore need of resuscitation.—D.K. Wagner, M.D.

---

### Feasibility of Intracardiac Injection of Drugs During Cardiac Arrest

Jespersen HF, Granborg J, Hansen U, Torp-Pedersen C, Pedersen A (Copenhagen County Univ Hosp, Glostrup, Denmark)
*Eur Heart J* 11:269–274, 1990                                    5–10

---

The purpose of intracardiac injection (ICI) during cardiopulmonary resuscitation (CPR) is to rapidly introduce potentially life-saving drugs into the coronary circulation. However, wider application of ICI has been hampered by repeated warnings of its dangers. On the other hand, practical experience with the systematic use of ICI in small series of patients has found the risk quite acceptable for the circumstances. A 7-year experience with ICI in a larger series of patients in a coronary care unit (CCU) is reported.

Since 1967, ICI has been done routinely for administering inotropic drugs for cardiac arrest with ECG asystole or electromechanical dissociation occurring in the CCU. Trained nurses usually give ICI with the parasternal approach into the right ventricle, followed by continued external cardiac massage. In 7 years, 543 ICIs were administered to 247 patients in cardiac arrest. Thirty percent of the patients had only 1 injection each, 41% had 2 injections, 18% had 3 injections, and 12% had between 4 and 8 injections. Isoproterenol and epinephrine were the drugs used most commonly.

Of the 247 patients having ICI, 122 could not be resuscitated, 45 died within 1 hour after CPR, and 80 survived for more than 1 hour, 19 (7.7%) of whom were discharged alive. Autopsies were performed in 182 of the 228 fatal cases. Left-sided pneumothoraces were discovered in 9 of the 80 patients who survived CPR for more than 1 hour, and right-sided pneumothoraces were found in 2 patients. Eight of these 11 patients had pleural drainage. Hemothorax never was shown. Minor hemopericardiums with no visible rupture of the myocardium or the aorta were found in another 3 patients who survived for more than 1 hour after ICI. Lesions of the coronary artery or myocardium attributable to the ICI never were seen.

During cardiac arrest, drug treatment by ICI carried out by experienced staff with good technique carries with it a low risk that is quite acceptable for the circumstances.

▶ Confusion regarding what to do when is often eliminated in the clinical setting by considering proposed actions in light of benefit vs. risk.

It is difficult, if not impossible, to determine the true beneficial advantages of this delivery route. However, the risk can be studied, and these authors conclude that the risk of this delivery route is quite acceptable when good technique is used in the patient with asystole or electromechanical dissociation. We may never know if benefits outweigh costs, but this article concludes that the cost of this procedure is acceptable in this setting.— E.H. Taliaferro, M.D.

---

**The Safety of Intraosseous Infusions: Risks of Fat and Bone Marrow Emboli to the Lungs**
Orlowski JP, Julius CJ, Petras RE, Porembka DT, Gallagher JM (Cleveland Clinic Found)
*Ann Emerg Med* 18:1062–1067, 1989                                         5–11

Intraosseous infusion is a practical and effective alternative route when intravenous access is impossible or will be critically delayed, particularly in children. Because concerns about its safety remain, especially on the risk of bone marrow and fat emboli to the lungs, representative sections of lungs from normotensive dogs who received intraosseous infusions of common emergency drugs and solutions into the distal femur were examined for the presence of fat and bone marrow emboli. In addition, lung sections from 2 children who received intraosseous infusions during resuscitation attempts were also studied. The animals were killed 4 hours after intraosseous infusion of epinephrine, sodium bicarbonate, calcium chloride, atropine, lidocaine, 6% hydroxyethyl starch in normal saline, or 50% dextrose in water. Control dogs received intraosseous infusions of normal saline.

Fat and bone marrow emboli to the lungs were found in all animals and both pediatric patients. The number of emboli varied from 0.11 to 4.48 emboli/mm$^2$ of lung (mean 0.91) for the emergency drugs and solutions compared with 0.06–0.53 emboli/mm$^2$ of lung (mean 0.29) for the controls; the difference was not significant. The 95% confidence limits for estimating the proportion of the population to develop bone marrow and fat emboli after intraosseous infusions was 0.89–1.00. Pressurized maintenance infusion into the intraosseous needle did not increase the incidence of emboli. Despite the universal finding of fat and bone marrow pulmonary emboli in the animals, there were no significant alterations in arterial oxygen pressure (tension) or intrapulmonary shunt during the 4-hour study.

Fat and bone marrow emboli occur frequently after intraosseous infusions, and their occurrence is not related to the drug or solution infused. Their occurrence is not of acute clinical importance and should not interfere with the success of resuscitation. However, pulmonary fat embolism may complicate postresuscitation care, and bone marrow and fat emboli may be of clinical importance in patients with intracardiac right-to-left shunts.

▶ Intraosseous infusion into the femur of any kind causes some fat and marrow embolization to the lung. No new intrapulmonary shunting occurred, however, so the clinical sequelae will probably not be significant. It does reinforce the need to replace an intraosseous line as soon as possible with an intravenous catheter, because it seems possible that ongoing microembolization could eventually be detrimental. (See also Abstracts 4–75 and 4–11.)—W.P. Burdick, M.D.

---

**Intraosseous Infusions in Adults**
Iserson KV (Univ of Arizona, Tucson)
*J Emerg Med* 7:587–591, 1989                                              5–12

---

Intravascular access is a vital component of emergency care and resuscitation. The use of lower extremity intraosseous (IO) infusions for emergent intravascular access has recently been reintroduced for pediatric resuscitation. All studies of IO infusions have been conducted in pediatric patients or animal models. Intraosseous access in adults through the distal tibia has never been a widely accepted technique, but there have been some occasional reports of its successful use in adults. To determine the value of IO infusions through distal tibial access in adult patients, including those in cardiac arrest, 17 men and 5 women aged 36–84 years who arrived in the ED in cardiac arrest from a nonhypovolemic cause and in whom an intravenous line could not be established were studied over a 4-year period.

After arrival in the ED, a 13-gauge IO needle was placed just above the midline of the medial malleolus at a 90-degree angle to the bone. The IO needle was connected to standard intravenous tubing, with an external pressure bag or pressure device delivering 300 mm Hg to the solution bag. The resultant flow rate through the intravenous line ranged from 5 to 12 mL/minute. Medications were administered through either the needle hub or through the attached intravenous line.

The IO needle was placed and flow was established in less than 1 minute in all patients. Six needles were placed by individuals who had never used the technique before. Of the 22 patients, 20 died in the ED; the other 2 patients died in the hospital within 24 hours. No complications from IO access were noted in the 2 short-term survivors. There was an apparent effect of the sodium bicarbonate administered through the

IO route in the 4 patients in whom a subsequent arterial blood gas value was obtained. Other temporally related pharmacologic effects were observed within 1 minute after IO administration of lidocaine, atropine, and vasopressors. However, blood levels of the IO administered medications were not obtained.

In adults, IO vascular access for instilling medications when intravenous access is not available can be quickly and easily obtained through the medial supramalleolar position. The technique is not suitable for rapid fluid replacement.

▶ This is an important paper in that it allows the emergency physician another vascular access in tough situations. Although IO access is now routinely used in advanced pulmonary life support, it has not been recommended in the adult. The authors provide convincing data for its utilization in the non-volume-depleted patient in need of vascular access.—D.K. Wagner, M.D.

---

**Comparison of Intraosseous, Intramuscular, and Intravenous Administration of Succinylcholine**
Moore GP, Pace SA, Busby W (Madigan Army Med Ctr, Tacoma, Wash; Maricopa Hosp, Phoenix)
*Pediatr Emerg Care* 5:209–210, 1989                                            5–13

---

Intraosseous drug administration is being used more often to resuscitate pediatric patients. This route was compared with the intramuscular and intravenous routes for administering the depolarizing paralyzing agent succinylcholine in sheep that were anesthetized with halothane and subsequently intubated. The dose of succinylcholine was 1 mg/kg.

Intraosseous access was achieved in less than 30 seconds in all attempts. The average time from succinylcholine administration to respiratory arrest was 31 seconds with intravenous administration, 57.5 seconds with intraosseous administration, and 230 seconds with intramuscular injection. The average times to 100% loss of forefoot twitch were 93, 101, and 291 seconds, respectively. All of the group differences were significant.

The intraosseous route appears to be an acceptable alternative to intravenous administration of succinylcholine. The needle traditionally is directed away from the epiphysis, but trials in pigs have revealed no adverse effects from either epiphyseal injection or the infusion of alkaline solution.

▶ This is another article showing that intraosseous access is a good alternative to intravenous access. (See also Abstract 1–21.)—T. Stair, M.D.

---

**Comparison Study of Intraosseous, Central Intravenous, and Peripheral Intravenous Infusions of Emergency Drugs**
Orlowski JP, Porembka DT, Gallagher JM, Lockrem JD, Van Lente F (Cleveland Clinic Found)
*Am J Dis Child* 144:112–117, 1990                                            5–14

Intraosseous infusion of emergency drugs is a lifesaving alternative to intravenous administration when intravenous access cannot be established or will be critically delayed. The pharmacokinetics of emergency drugs and solutions administered by the intraosseous, central intravenous, and peripheral routes were compared in normotensive anesthetized dogs. Each animal was treated with each of the following drugs and solutions using all 3 routes of administration: epinephrine hydrochloride, 0.01 mg/kg; sodium bicarbonate, 1 mEq/kg; calcium chloride, 10 mg/kg; lidocaine hydrochloride, 1 mg/kg; 6% hydroxyethyl starch in normal saline, 10 mL/kg; and 50% dextrose in water, 0.25 g/kg.

The intraosseous route demonstrated equivalent magnitudes of peak effect or drug level and equal or longer duration of action as the central and peripheral intravenous routes for all emergency drugs and solutions. Time to placement of the needle varied from 2 to 10 minutes among individuals without experience in bone marrow needle insertions to less than 60 seconds among those who had had at least 5 insertion attempts.

The intraosseous route is a very effective alternative to intravenous administration of emergency drugs.

▶ There is no more haunting a task for the emergency physician than obtaining venous access in a small child in cardiac arrest. Sadly, in many of these resuscitations, venous access takes far too long to achieve and is never obtained (1). Using an animal model, the authors demonstrate the efficacy of the intraosseous route for drug administration and plasma expansion in normotensive dogs.

One might take issue with the design of the study: The authors used a 2-in. intravenous catheter in the femoral vein as a "central intravenous" line, the dogs were not in cardiac arrest, and even the animals that bled to 50% of blood volume were allowed to stabilize hemodynamically before the study began. All of these exceptions notwithstanding, the intraosseous route remains an excellent method for venous access until a proper intravenous line can be obtained. With practice, an intraosseous line can be secured quite rapidly (all ED staff, nurses, and physicians should be trained).

Although this technique has been available since the 1940s, it is still underutilized. Thankfully, it is enjoying a resurgence. Emergency physicians can help train others in this lifesaving procedure.—H.H. Osborn, M.D.

*Reference*

1. Rosetti V, et al: *Ann Emerg Med* 13:405, 1984.

**Effects of Pneumatic Antishock Garment Inflation in Normovolemic Subjects**

Rubal BJ, Geer MR, Bickell WH (Brooke Army Med Ctr, Fort Sam Houston, Tex)

*J Appl Physiol* 67:339–345, 1989
5–15

The pneumatic antishock garment (PASG), an inflatable pair of vinyl trousers, is commonly used in the prehospital management of posttraumatic hypotension. The uses of the PASG have been expanding, and controversy over its benefit has arisen. The hemodynamic consequences of PASG inflation in normovolemic persons during graded PASG inflation and the mechanisms whereby PASG augments systemic arterial pressures were investigated.

Ten normovolemic men (mean age 44 years) undergoing diagnostic catheterization were studied. Seven had normal heart function and no evidence of coronary artery disease (CAD), and 3 had CAD. Right- and left-sided heart pressures before and after PASG inflation to 40, 70, and 100 mm Hg were simultaneously recorded. Pulmonary capillary wedge pressure and cardiac output were measured. Counterpressure rises of 40 mm Hg or more were associated with significant changes in left- and right-sided heart pressures. At maximum inflation in normal persons, right and left ventricular end-diastolic pressures rose 100%. Mean pulmonary arterial pressure increased 77%, and mean aortic pressure increased 25%. Systemic vascular resistance rose by 22%. Pulmonary vascular resistance was unchanged. Neither group had a change in heart rate, cardiac output, and aortic and pulmonary arterial pulse pressure during inflation. Right and left ventricular end-diastolic pressures and pulmonary capillary wedge pressure were greater in the patients with CAD than in normal persons during inflation.

Pneumatic antishock garment inflation appears to induce changes in central hemodynamics in normovolemic persons primarily through an acute increase in left ventricular afterload. Pneumatic antishock garment changes in afterload and pulmonary capillary wedge pressure suggest that the PASG should be used with caution in patients whose cardiac function is compromised.

▶ The PASG, also known as military antishock trousers (MAST), was first described by Dr. George Crile more than 80 years ago and has been in wide use in this country for almost 20 years, abetted by legislative fiat. Despite its age and ubiquity, physiologic effects of the PASG remain poorly understood, and the sphere of its proper use, if any, in trauma and medical emergencies, is an area of growing controversy.

This study is limited by the small number of subjects (10), the fact that they are inhomogeneous, (3 have heart disease and 7 do not), and by its use of subjects who are normovolemic. Any conclusion based on a subgroup of 3 subjects should be regarded cautiously. Nonetheless, this study agrees with what has been known for some time (1, 2): the PASG "autotransfuses" blood from the lower extremities and abdomen.

In a sense, then, using the PASG is similar to giving a vasopressor. The use of vasopressors to treat hemorrhagic shock has been thoroughly discredited, and thus the use of PASG in trauma has come under increasing scrutiny. Recent clinical trials have not supported its use (3), and the outspoken Dr. Kenneth Mattox has branded it "a tool of the devil." The future of its routine use in trauma management is unclear.—J. Schoffstall, M.D.

*References*

1. Bivens HG, et al: *Ann Emerg Med* 11:409, 1982.
2. Goldsmith SR: *Ann Emerg Med* 12:348, 1983.
3. Mattox KL, et al: *J Trauma* 29:1104, 1989.

**MAST-Associated Compartment Syndrome (MACS): A Review**
Aprahamian C, Gessert G, Bandyk DF, Sell L, Stiehl J, Olson DW (Med College of Wisconsin, Milwaukee)
*J Trauma* 29:549–555, 1989                                                5–16

The use of pneumatic military antishock trousers (MAST) has been implicated in the development of MAST-associated compartment syndrome (MACS), which has contributed to amputation and mortality in patients both with and without lower extremity trauma. Whether compartment syndromes develop as a consequence of the trauma that leads to the use of MAST or whether the syndrome results from the extrinsic compression and ischemia produced by the inflated MAST was investigated in 15 patients who were treated for vascular injuries at the authors' institution during an 8-year study period and 12 previously reported cases identified from a literature review.

Duration of MAST use varied between the 2 groups; it was used for 60 minutes or less in 5 of the 15 (33.3%) hospital cases, whereas it was used for a mean of 16 hours in 10 of the 12 literature cases. In the other 10 hospital cases and 2 literature cases, the MAST had been removed during or at the completion of surgery.

Five of the 15 hospital patients and 5 of the 12 literature patients died of multiple organ failure. Three hospital patients and 4 literature patients required amputation. Two of the 5 hospital patients who died may have had ischemic and infected limbs that contributed to their death. The other 3 patients had viable limbs at the time of their deaths.

It appears that lower extremity trauma and systemic hypotension are cofactors responsible for the development of compartment syndromes. However, MAST use contributes to this process by prolonging muscle ischemia. It is suggested that complications of lower limb compartment hypertension may be avoided by early diagnosis and fasciotomy.

▶ The authors present the literature's most complete review of MACSs. Although the use of the MAST has recently declined, there are persistent, selected situations where its use may prove a valuable adjunct to volume stabilization. Consequently, an awareness that compartmental injury may ensue in the presence of prolonged usage or may occur early on in the patient with traumatic or acquired vascular insufficiency to the lower extremity is worth remembering.—D.K. Wagner, M.D.

### Prospective MAST Study in 911 Patients

Mattox KL, Bickell W, Pepe PE, Burch J, Feliciano D (Baylor College of Medicine, Ben Taub Gen Hosp, Houston)

*J Trauma* 29:1104–1112, 1989                                              5–17

During the 1970s, the use of military antishock trousers (MAST) in the prehospital care of hypotensive trauma patients received unqualified support from emergency medical service providers, emergency physicians, and surgeons. In a 1985 prospectively randomized study of MAST, no benefit was demonstrated. A review was made of the findings of a continuation study in 911 injured patients with systolic blood pressures (BP) of 90 mm Hg or less.

Of 784 evaluable patients, 345 were randomly assigned to MAST and 439 were assigned to no-MAST protocol on an alternate-day protocol. Patients randomized to receive MAST were treated the same as no-MAST patients except that the MAST garment was applied before intravenous catheter placement. All patients were taken to the same level I trauma center. The population cohorts were statistically identical. The principal sites of injury were the thorax (41%), abdomen (32%), extremity (16%), head (7%), and neck (4%).

Among 185 patients with initial systolic BP between 51 and 70 mm Hg, survival in the no-MAST group was 11.4% higher than in the MAST group. Mortality rates among 320 patients with thoracic injuries were 31.7% in the no-MAST group and 41.8% in the MAST group. Prehospital mortality rates among patients with thoracic injuries were 5.2% in the no-MAST group and 16.4% in the MAST group. Among 484 patients who had total prehospital times of 30 minutes or longer, MAST application did not increase survival rates. Of the 784 patients, 222 died. The overall mortality rates were 31% in the MAST group and 25% in the no-MAST group. Because the survival rate of no-MAST patients was significantly better, the garment is no longer used on ambulances of the Houston Fire Department, and all inventory has been removed from the emergency center at the Ben Taub General Hospital.

▶ Numerous debates have transpired concerning the use of the MAST. This article helps confirm what these authors have been saying for some time: Use of the MAST should be discontinued. Although its application does increase blood pressure, in many cases such an increase in blood pressure, before bleeding has been adequately controlled, can increase the morbidity and mortality. Patients with thoracic trauma have a greater chance of dying if it is applied, and those with abdominal injuries have no proved increase in survival. When I was an intern 1 decade ago, the MAST was the end-all; you were made to feel inadequate if you did not consider using it in the emergency center. Subsequently, many realized that it made examination of the patient more difficult, it precluded venous and arterial access in the groin, and premature or uncontrolled removal could be devastating. Research should be put to use. It's time to let this device join the esophageal obturator airway in extinction or develop distinct criteria for its use (e.g., pelvic fractures). In any case, this article would certainly support its routine use in the prehospital setting.—J.T. Amsterdam, M.D.

## Diagnostic Procedures/Instrumentation

### Oligoanalgesia in the Emergency Department
Wilson JE, Pendleton JM (Akron City Hosp; Northeastern Ohio Univs, Akron)
*Am J Emerg Med* 7:620–623, 1989                                              5–18

To determine the analgesic prescribing practices of physicians in the emergency room for patients with acutely painful medical and surgical conditions who required hospital admission through the ED, the charts of 198 patients were reviewed.

No analgesic medication was prescribed in the ED for 56% of patients; of 131 patients with moderately severe or severe pain, 50% were given analgesic medication. Patients least likely to be given pain medication were those with pain from intrathoracic structures. In the 44% of patients who received pain medication, 69% waited longer than 1 hour and 42% waited longer than 2 hours before narcotic analgesia was administered. The initial dose of narcotic was given intramuscularly in 60% of patients, although intravenous administration might have been more appropriate. In addition, 32% of patients initially received less than an optimal equianalgesic dose of narcotic compared with morphine.

Suboptimal management of pain is prevalent. The probable reasons for this prevalence of oligoanalgesia are hospital dogma, physicians' misconceptions, and tradition. New information on pain management should be emphasized to help all physicians overcome their reluctance to treat acute, severe pain appropriately.

▶ This important paper highlights a critical problem still prevalent in many (most) EDs: the inappropriate withholding of timely and adequate analgesics for patients with significant pain. This appears to be even more true when those patients are children but is certainly not limited to that group or to patients with abdominal pain. This last group typically has treatment withheld because of the very mistaken assumptions that accurate diagnosis cannot be made, nor legal consent for surgery obtained, once analgesia has been provided. On the contrary, appropriate medication helps to elucidate diagnosis by allowing a reasonable physical examination, which is typically obscured by severe pain. At the same time, a consent form can hardly be considered uncoerced when delivery of pain medication is contingent on its being signed.

Patients' agendas are not always the same as those of their physicians: We want to know "what they have," whereas they are often much more concerned with feeling better. Fortunately, these 2 objectives are not mutually exclusive, and papers like this do a great service in reminding us how important it is to pay attention to the analgesic needs of our frequently hurting patients.—J.R. Hoffman, M.D.

### The Safety of Fentanyl Use in the Emergency Department
Chudnofsky CR, Wright SW, Dronen SC, Borron SW, Wright MB (Univ of Cincinnati Med Ctr)
*Ann Emerg Med* 18:635–639, 1989                                                        5–19

Fentanyl appears to be safe in various outpatient settings, including the repair of facial trauma in children; however, its safety for emergency care of adult patients remains uncertain. Experience with fentanyl in 841 adult patients seen at an ED in 1985–1988 was reviewed. The average age of the patients was 33 years. The average dose of fentanyl given was 180 μg and the maximum was 1,400 μg. Nearly one half of the patients received medications in addition to fentanyl.

Indications for fentanyl were fracture or joint reduction and incision and drainage of an abscess in 69% of cases. Six patients (0.7%) had mild side effects, such as nausea and urticaria. Nine (1.1%) had more serious complications. Six patients had some degree of respiratory compromise, and 3 had hypotension. One patient had both respiratory depression and hypotension.

Fentanyl is a safe agent for use in producing sedation and analgesia in adult patients in the ED. The initial dose limit is 1 μg/kg, and further treatment should be titrated to the desired clinical effect. Naloxone and resuscitation equipment should be available. Fentanyl should be used cautiously in intoxicated patients and those given other drugs that have CNS or respiratory depressant activity. Slow intravenous administration of fentanyl may prevent muscular rigidity.

▶ Fentanyl is an excellent drug for use in the manner described by the authors. The popularity of the drug in anesthesia is well deserved. It is effective, short-acting, and easily reversed. The precautions described by the authors must be assiduously observed to avoid complications.

We have used fentanyl in our pediatric ED with excellent results. It is apparent that the drug should be used in adults under appropriate circumstances as well.

Turf issues are raised in a letter to the editor about this article (1). The letter has a very interesting and well-written response from the authors. The authors clearly win the debate in this reviewer's mind.—J.E. Clinton, M.D.

*Reference*

1. Eckhardt WF: *Ann Emerg Med* 19:839, 1990.

### Safety of Invasive Procedures in Patients With the Coagulopathy of Liver Disease
Friedman EW, Sussman II (Albert Einstein College of Medicine, Bronx)
*Clin Lab Haematol* 11:199–204, 1989                                                    5–20

A prolonged prothrombin time (PT) is the most frequent coagulation abnormality in patients with chronic liver disease. The need for prophylactic treatment with fresh frozen plasma was assessed in 39 consecutive patients with PT values of 15–29 seconds who underwent 71 invasive procedures. A large majority of patients had cirrhosis of the liver caused by alcoholism.

Thirty patients underwent 57 procedures without prophylactic plasma, cryoprecipitate, platelets, or blood. The PT exceeded 20 seconds in 13% of this group. Although 43% of the patients had platelet counts less than 100,000/mm$^3$, the mean count was only minimally depressed. The most common procedures were paracentesis, lumbar puncture, and thoracentesis. In patients given blood product support preoperatively, treatment was chiefly for unrelated gastrointestinal bleeding. Repeat PT estimates did not show improvement despite plasma use. One patient in this group had 2 bleeding complications that required no further treatment.

Treatment with fresh frozen plasma is not recommended for preventing an elevated PT before patients with chronic liver disease undergo invasive procedures. Bleeding is infrequent and is readily controlled when it does occur.

▶ Patients with known or suspected liver disease are seen in EDs with gastrointestinal bleeding, dehydration, altered mental status, and sepsis. As a result, they may occasionally need rapid venous access in the presence of poor peripheral veins.

This study took patients with severe liver disease resulting in significant coagulopathy and looked at bleeding complications following invasive procedures performed without prior correction of the coagulopathy. Unfortunately, paracentesis accounted for two thirds of the procedures. Only 4 patients had central venous lines placed at unspecified sites, and 5 had lumbar puncture performed. Interestingly, despite the control group receiving an average of 5 units of fresh, frozen plasma, there was no improvement in PT. Neither group had any complications beyond persistent oozing.

The message from this paper is that if you must achieve venous access quickly, it has been done safely in patients with uncontrolled coagulopathy. However, I would recommend using the posterior approach to the internal jugular or femoral vein so that the blood vessels are accessible to compression, if necessary.—W.P. Burdick, M.D.

---

**Complications Associated With Thoracentesis: A Prospective, Randomized Study Comparing Three Different Methods**
Grogan DR, Irwin RS, Channick R, Raptopoulos V, Curley FJ, Bartter T, Corwin RW (Univ of Massachusetts, Worcester)
*Arch Intern Med* 150:873–877, 1990                                                    5–21

---

In a previous prospective study of thoracentesis, nearly one half of the procedures had complications, 14% of which were major. The role of technique now has been studied prospectively by assessing 3 sampling methods: needle, needle with catheter, and needle with direct sonographic guidance. Fifty-two patients with free-flowing effusions that obliterated more than one half of the hemidiaphragm on upright postero-anterior chest x-ray films were randomized in the study.

Pneumothorax occurred in 14 of 18 needle-catheter procedures, in 6 of 15 needle procedures, and in none of 19 sonography-guided thoracenteses. Minor complications also were most frequent with needle-catheter thoracentesis and least frequent with the sonographically guided procedure.

Sonography-guided thoracentesis appears to be the safest diagnostic technique. The needle-catheter method should be avoided. If needle thoracentesis is unproductive or yields inadequate fluid, the procedure should be repeated with sonographic guidance. Needle-catheter thoracentesis still is practiced for therapeutic reasons, but risk studies are needed.

▶ A concerning statistic revealed in this paper is the alarmingly high morbidity rate in nonultrasound-guided thoracentesis (10 of 33 major and 17 of 33 minor complications) when performed by house staff who received more intense training for this procedure because of this study than most house staff ever will. Most interns learn how to perform a thoracentesis from the next most senior-level resident. One can only guess at their morbidity rates. Several EDs have begun using ultrasound within the emergency center. In addition to its other emergent applications, this paper would strongly suggest the use of ultrasound for ED thoracentesis.—H. Unger, M.D.

---

**Diagnostic Peritoneal Lavage in Evaluation of Acute Abdominal Disease**
Bailey RL, Laws HL (Carraway Methodist Med Ctr, Birmingham, Ala)
*South Med J* 83:422–424, 1990                                          5–22

Diagnostic peritoneal lavage (DPL) commonly is used in the evaluation of blunt thoracoabdominal trauma. It recently has been used in critically ill patients with altered mental status in whom acute intra-abdominal disease is suspected. The usefulness of DPL in this setting was reviewed retrospectively.

Between 1984 and 1988, 15 women and 11 men with an average age of 64.6 years underwent DPL because acute intra-abdominal disease was suspected and the usual radiographic studies had been nondiagnostic. The use of DPL indicated sepsis in 10 patients, which was confirmed at celiotomy or autopsy in 7 patients. Only 1 patient whose DPL indicated sepsis survived for more than 2 weeks without laparotomy. The results of DPL in this patient were considered false positive. In 16 patients, DPL indicated no sepsis, which was confirmed by operation in 3 patients, autopsy in 4 patients, or survival longer than 2 weeks in 7 patients. The results of DPL in these 14 patients were considered true negative. In 1 patient whose DPL showed sepsis, the small bowel was entered inadvertently at the time of DPL, requiring repair at laparotomy. However, the patient had improvement and could be discharged to a nursing home 6 days later. Overall, 22 patients were evaluated. Because only 1 patient had a false positive result and no patient had a false negative result, the diagnostic accuracy of DPL in this group of patients was 95%.

The use of DPL in critically ill patients with a suspected acute intra-abdominal disease process appears most useful for patients in whom an unnecessary operation would hasten their death. Diagnostic peritoneal lavage is not performed if a patient's family would not allow celiotomy in any case.

▶ The findings presented in this article are of only peripheral concern when surgeons are readily available for consultation. However, in smaller EDs, this procedure might well facilitate the course of treatment in this selected group of patients. Therapeutic intervention can be hastened when the DPL is performed while the surgeon is en route to the hospital.

Unfortunately, 26 patients is a small study group when you consider introducing a procedure to your practice that provides valuable information at the expense of a very costly 5% complication rate. (See also Abstract 2–37.)—E.H. Taliaferro, M.D.

---

**Bedside Cerebrospinal Fluid Glucose Analysis**
Slovis CM, Negus RA, Amerson SM, Kutner MH (Emory Univ)
*Ann Emerg Med* 18:931–933, 1989                                     5–23

---

The glucose concentration in CSF provides the emergency physician with important information, but its determination may take hours. The reliability and accuracy of 2 bedside methods used to estimate CSF glucose levels in an emergency setting, a 2-minute glucose reagent strip (Chemstrip bG) and a hand-held bedside autoanalyzer (Accu-Chek II), were investigated.

For estimating the CSF glucose concentration with the reagent strip, the color of the strip is compared with a color-coded chart corresponding to glucose values of 0–800 mg/dL. The Accu-Chek II reading is obtained by following the manufacturer's instructions. A total of 237 different CSF samples obtained in the emergency room were studied. Chemstrip bG and Accu-Chek II readings were compared with values obtained in the laboratory.

There was a high correlation over a wide range of values between the laboratory CSF glucose determinations and the readings obtained with the Chemstrip bG and the Accu-Chek II. There was no significant difference in accuracy between the 2 methods. The Chemstrip bG and the Accu-Chek II are both highly reliable and accurate for the quick determination of a patient's CSF glucose concentration.

▶ These 2 bedside methods of evaluating CSF glucose levels within minutes after the specimen is available are shown to be sufficiently accurate to be very useful in helping the emergency physician diagnose and initiate treatment for bacterial meningitis in a timely manner. However, as stated, a Gram stain of CSF is quick and should be done also.—G.V. Anderson, M.D.

## Infrared Tympanic Thermography in the Emergency Department

Green MM, Danzl DF, Praszkier H (Univ of Louisville)
*J Emerg Med* 7:437–440, 1989                                                    5–24

The accurate assessment of body temperature is an integral component of patient evaluation in the ED. The failure to diagnose hypothermia and hyperthermia has profound clinical implications. Oral temperatures are most commonly obtained but may not reflect core temperatures. Although rectal measurements are considered more reliable, they may also not reflect core temperatures. To determine the practicality and comparative accuracy of using tympanic thermography to measure core temperatures, oral, rectal, and tympanic temperature measurements were obtained in 411 patients aged 14–91 years. Oral and rectal temperatures were measured with self-calibrating temperature probes using liquid crystal thermography. Tympanic temperatures were measured with an infrared tympanic thermometer.

Temperatures ranged from 35° C to 40.6° C for rectal temperatures (mean 37.637° C), from 35.4° C to 40.7° C for tympanic temperatures (mean, 37.632° C), and from 32.4° C to 39.7° C for oral temperatures (mean 37.019° C). The difference between rectal and tympanic temperatures was not significant. The difference between rectal and oral temperatures was significant, as was the difference between tympanic and oral temperatures. There were no complications associated with the use of the tympanic probe. Infrared tympanic thermography is a rapid, accurate, efficient, and noninvasive alternative means for measuring body temperature in patients in the ED.

▶ The authors describe an interesting device that provides rapid "core" temperature evaluation. Some questions remain unanswered: First, how much cerumen is too much to allow an accurate reading? Second, does 1 size instrument fit all ages? Third, is continuous monitoring possible? Finally, does the instrument hold up to typical rough and tough emergency center activities?—D.K. Wagner, M.D.

## An Evaluation of Clinical Predictors to Determine Need for Rectal Temperature Measurement in the Emergency Department

Kresovich-Wendler K, Levitt MA, Yearly L (Thomas Jefferson Univ Hosp, Philadelphia)
*Am J Emerg Med* 7:391–394, 1989                                                 5–25

It is believed that there are patients whose fevers are detected only by rectal temperature measurements. A cross-sectional study was conducted in an urban ED to determine if there are predictive criteria that can identify patients who are febrile by rectal temperature measurement but afebrile by oral temperature measurement.

Of the 366 patients evaluated, 39 were afebrile orally but febrile by rectal temperature measurement. Univariate analysis showed that mouth breathing, respiratory rate, supplemental oxygen, pulse, and supplemental oxygen through a mask were predictive of fever by rectal temperature measurement but not by oral measurement. Placing these variables in a logistic regression model showed that pulse and mouth breathing significantly explained the variance between patients afebrile by both rectal and oral temperature measurements and those afebrile by oral measurement but febrile by rectal measurement. Contrary to the previous concept that rectal temperature is 0.6° C higher than oral temperature, the data showed poor linear correlation between oral and rectal temperatures.

If a patient is afebrile orally, a rectal temperature should be taken, particularly in patients with unexplained tachycardia, breathing by mouth, or both. In addition to being more selective in the use of rectal temperature measurements, identifying these patients would reduce the number of rectal temperature measurements in the ED and minimize the number of patients whose fever would be missed with oral temperature measurements alone.

▶ Although this study appears to have been performed prospectively, it has the significance of a retrospective study because the protocol for doing a rectal temperature was neither preestablished nor evenly applied to all patients. The study group who received oral and febrile temperatures constituted 39 patients whose need for a rectal temperature was determined by the ED staff on duty. This does not define which clinical indicators will predict the need for a rectal temperature but, rather, describes the differences between patients whose rectal temperature was higher. It does not tell us what respiratory rate will predict a difference between the 2 methods of temperature measurement.—W.P. Burdick, M.D.

---

### Evaluation of a Tympanic Membrane Thermometer in an Outpatient Clinical Setting

Ros SP (Loyola Univ, Maywood, Ill)
*Ann Emerg Med* 18:1004–1006, 1989                                        5–26

---

Temperature measurement, an integral part of patient assessment, is usually time consuming and cumbersome. Recently, a tympanic membrane thermometer was introduced. It records infrared energy emitted from the tympanic membrane and may simplify and shorten the process of taking temperatures. The correlation between the tympanic membrane and glass-mercury thermometers in an outpatient setting was determined.

A total of 102 patients completed the study. The mean difference between the tympanic membrane and glass-mercury thermometers was −0.311° C. According to linear regression analysis, the relationship between the 2 methods was shown by the following equation: tympanic

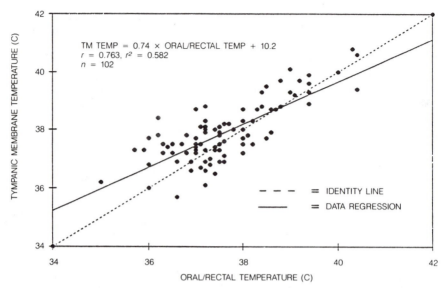

TM TEMP = 0.74 × ORAL/RECTAL TEMP + 10.2
$r = 0.763$, $r^2 = 0.582$
$n = 102$

Fig 5–2.—Correlation between tympanic membrane and oral/rectal temperature measurements. (Courtesy of Ros SP: *Ann Emerg Med* 18:1004–1006, 1989.)

membrane temperature = 0.74 × oral/rectal temperature + 10.2. The correlation between the measurements was poor (Fig 5–2).

Replacing the glass-mercury thermometer with the infrared tympanic-membrane device is not recommended. The correlation between the 2 devices is poor. More studies are needed to develop standards for the tympanic membrane thermometer.

► Every new medical innovation enjoys an initial period of delirious enthusiasm and uncritical acceptance, followed by a phase of increasingly critical reappraisal and reports of complications and side effects, followed by a denouement in which the innovation is either accepted on a more rational basis or discarded. We have seen this cycle happen in the 1970s and early 1980s to coronary artery bypass grafts and external pacemakers, and it is evident that both high-dose epinephrine and military antishock trousers (see Abstract 5–5) have recently entered the reappraisal stage.

Tympanic membrane thermometry is a minor technology compared with the others mentioned earlier, but it too is following this cyclic pattern. The first reports on its use were quite positive (1, 2), but in this paper and others (3) doubts have begun to emerge.

My own experience using this device leads me not to fully trust it; I do occasionally find serious discrepancies between the tympanic and rectal temperatures that can significantly change patient evaluation and care.—J. Schoffstall, M.D.

*References*

1. Green MM, et al: *J Emerg Med* 7:437, 1989.
2. Shinozaki T: *Crit Care Med* 16:148, 1988.
3. Rhoads FA, et al: *Clin Pediatr* 19:112, 1990.

## Bedside Diagnosis of Alcohol Intoxication With a Pocket-Size Breath-Alcohol Device: Sampling From Unconscious Subjects and Specificity for Ethanol

Falkensson M, Jones W, Sörbo B (Linköping Univ Hosp, Linköping, Sweden)
*Clin Chem* 35:918–921, 1989                                          5–27

A new mouth-cup device developed for sampling breath from unconscious persons and used with a hand-held breath-alcohol analyzer, the Alcolmeter SD-2, was assessed in healthy volunteers after ingestion of a moderate dose of alcohol. Three types of breath were analyzed: end-expired air from a conventional mouth tube, breath from the mouth cup, and air from a nasal tube supplied with the breath analyzer.

Six healthy persons aged 28–62 years who weighed 55–78 kg were given ethanol, 800 mg/kg, in a drink made from 930 mL of ethanol/L diluted in orange juice, for a total volume of 300 mL, about 2–3 hours after their last meal. This liquid was consumed within 30 minutes, and at 30- to 60-minute intervals, blood was drawn through an indwelling needle into 5-mL Vacutainer tubes that contained sodium fluoride and heparin. At approximately the same time that blood was sampled, the blood alcohol concentration (BAC) was evaluated with the Alcolmeter SD-2. Breath specimens were taken directly from the nasal cavity with the use of the nasal tube supplied with the instrument.

In the 30- to 180-minute interval after the individuals began to drink, the BAC evaluated from analysis of end-expiratory air was higher than in venous blood; however, the concentrations later became approximately equal. The BAC according to the results with the mouth-cup device and the nasal tube were lower than venous BAC for the complete concentration–time profile. It appears possible that breath samples collected by aspiration from a nasal cavity might easily become diluted with alcohol-free room air, thus producing lower values. This possibility prompted the development of an improved sampling system based on the mouth-cup device for use in unconscious individuals. Breath analysis with the Alcolmeter is not a specific method for determination of ethanol.

The Alcolmeter SD-2 is a useful instrument for bedside analysis of alcohol in hospital emergency units. Results obtained with the mouth-cup device coincided with venous BAC and end-expired breath much better than did samples taken through the nasal tube. Skill and training are required to obtain breath samples from unconscious persons.

▶ The ability to distinguish between alcohol intoxication and other potentially life-threatening causes of an acute change in mental status is crucial to the practice of emergency medicine. Although available for some time, breath analysis for a rapid estimate of blood alcohol levels has not enjoyed widespread use in most EDs.

The authors of this study show that 1 such device to measure BACs in exhaled breath can give reasonably accurate results when compared with blood alcohol levels. Although the number of subjects in the study was small, the dose of ethanol administered was low, and most of the blood alcohol levels were less than the legal level of intoxication. Their results argue for greater use of this technique, even in patients who are comatose or unable to cooperate. The lack of specificity of the breath analyzer may be of benefit in that it could also be used to screen cases of suspected methanol or propanol poisoning.

Clinicians should be aware that the breath/blood ethanol ratio varies between individuals and within the same individual over time (1). Also, the following factors can influence the breath analysis: recent use of alcohol or alcohol-containing products (i.e., within 15-30 minutes), belching or vomiting, inadequate and expiratory specimen, chronic lung diseases, and poor technique (2).—H.H. Osborn, M.D.

*References*

1. Jones AW: *J Stud Alcohol* 39:1931, 1978.
2. Ellenhorn MJ, Barcelon DE: *Med Toxicol* 33:793, 1988.

---

**Evaluation of Colorimetric Dipstick Test To Detect Alcohol in Saliva: A Pilot Study**
Schwartz RH, O'Donnell RM, Thorne MM, Getson PR, Hicks JM (Fairfax Hosp, Falls Church, Va; Children's Hosp Natl Med Ctr, Washington, DC)
*Ann Emerg Med* 18:1001–1003, 1989                    5–28

---

Screening patients for ingestion of ethyl alcohol usually involves breath or blood analysis, which may require expensive equipment. There have been no studies of the sensitivity, specificity, and efficiency of dipstick alcohol tests published in emergency medicine journals. The Alco Screen Saliva Dipstick, an inexpensive, easy to use, colorimetric test that gives a semiquantitative estimation of the blood alcohol value by measuring the relative concentration of salivary alcohol was compared with blood alcohol tests in patients suspected of having ingested too much alcohol.

Fifty-three patients seen in an emergency room for evaluation of possible intoxication were studied. Alco dipstick results were strongly correlated with blood alcohol values. At blood alcohol concentrations of 0.1 g/dL or higher, the Alco dipstick test results were 90.9% sensitive, 71.4% specific, and 92% efficient. However, the semiquantitative concordance was unsatisfactory at Alco dipstick values of 0.02 and 0.05 g/dL. Nevertheless, the test was still useful as a screen of de facto alcohol ingestion even at the 0.05 g/dL value of salivary alcohol.

The Alco dipstick test seems potentially valuable as an objective determinant of either absolute ingestion of alcohol or for detection of excessive alcohol in amounts that meet the legal definition of intoxication. The definitive diagnosis of relative alcohol intoxication needs to be confirmed by breath or blood alcohol concentrations by standard methodologies.

▶ The idea of being able to do a rapid dipstick test of a patient's alcohol level, as we now do a dipstick test for blood glucose, is appealing. A number of semiquantitative salivary alcohol tests currently are marketed or about to be released; which will prove to be best is unknown. The Alco dipstick that this paper evaluates is not especially impressive. It reliably detected the presence of alcohol at a blood level of 0.1 g/dL or more, but most of us can do that just smelling the patient's breath! Lower levels of blood alcohol produced an unacceptable number of false positives and false negatives. It was useless as a semiquantitative measure.

I would wait until there is more experience with this device and its competitors before purchasing 1 of them.—J. Schoffstall, M.D.

---

**Emergency Department Sonography by Emergency Physicians**
Jehle D, Davis E, Evans T, Harchelroad F, Martin M, Zaiser K, Lucid J (Allegheny Gen Hosp, Pittsburgh)
*Am J Emerg Med* 7:605–611, 1989                                    5–29

---

Recent advances have made real-time sonography an excellent screening tool for various cardiac, gynecologic, biliary tract, and abdominal vascular disorders. With a moderate amount of training, emergency physicians can probably reliably perform sonography, which may influence the diagnosis and treatment of selected disorders. A retrospective study was conducted to determine if emergency physicians can perform accurate ultrasonography to aid in the diagnosis and treatment of selected disorders in the ED.

Through a series of practical demonstrations and lectures, emergency physicians acquired a moderate level of expertise in sonography. Patients with symptoms suggesting cardiac, gynecologic, biliary tract, or abdominal vascular disease were studied periodically by sonography. Emergency physicians correctly diagnosed the presence and approximate size of pericardial effusions, the presence or absence of organized cardiac activity in patients with clinical electrical mechanical dissociation, the presence or absence of intrauterine pregnancy in pregnant women with lower abdominal or pelvic complaints, the position of intrauterine devices in women with suspected uterine perforation, the presence of gallstones in patients suspected of having biliary tract disease, and the presence and size of abdominal aortic aneurysms in those with pulsatile masses or unexplained abdominal pain.

Emergency physicians with a moderate amount of training can perform dependable sonography of certain disorders. The positive sonographic studies performed in this series were very reliable. Ultrasound should become a standard diagnostic procedure in all EDs.

▶ Ultrasonography is an extremely important ED tool with regard to such critical and varied problems as ectopic pregnancy, cholelithiasis, abdominal aortic aneurysm, and pericardial tamponade. Furthermore, there is no reason its use needs to be restricted to any 1 group of physicians (e.g., radiologists). On the other hand, it can have value only when used with expertise, which requires both appropriate training and ongoing experience.

This paper reports successful ultrasound identification by a group of emergency physicians following an undefined "moderate" training period of almost 100 normal (intrauterine pregnancy) and abnormal (gallstones, pericardial effusion, abdominal aneurysm) findings. Unfortunately, information regarding how many other times ultrasound done by emergency physicians failed to find these conditions when they were present (false negatives) is "not available." Since the most important characteristic of an emergency test is its sensitivity, we cannot even begin to evaluate how globally successful this group of physicians was in their initial use of ED ultrasonography.

There is no reason why, with the cooperation and assistance of expert ultrasonographers, emergency physicians cannot learn to use this technique to make basic yes and no decisions in a variety of emergent conditions. This should certainly not be undertaken lightly, however, because the accuracy of ultrasound is extremely operator dependent, and casual use by poorly trained or inexperienced physicians (of whatever primary specialty) would be far more detrimental (and even catastrophic) than useful.—J.R. Hoffman, M.D.

---

### The Role of Ultrasound in the Detection of Non-Radiopaque Foreign Bodies

Gilbert FJ, Campbell RSD, Bayliss AP (Aberdeen Royal Infirmary, Aberdeen, Scotland)
*Clin Radiol* 41:109–112, 1990                                      5–30

---

The detection and localization of nonradiopaque foreign bodies in soft tissues remains a problem in the ED. The accuracy of high-resolution ultrasound scanning in detecting nonradiopaque foreign bodies was evaluated in a retrospective study of 50 consecutive ultrasound examinations performed for suspected nonradiopaque foreign bodies in the extremities.

Ultrasound detected a foreign body in 24 patients. A foreign body was found on operation in 21, but none was found in 3. The sensitivity of the test was 95.4%, specificity was 89.2%, positive predictive value was 87.5%, and negative predictive value was 96.2%. The foreign body was seen as a bright hyperechoic focus in all patients and was clearly demonstrated with the scan plane parallel to the long axis of the foreign body or at right angles to its axis.

High-resolution ultrasound is a valuable method for detecting nonradiopaque foreign bodies with a high sensitivity and specificity.

▶ This is a useful technique, especially since ultrasound can guide excision. Who has tried CT and magnetic resonance imaging for foreign bodies? Several have—often effective—always expensive.—T. Stair, M.D.

---

### Clinical Value of Ultrasonography in the Detection and Removal of Radiolucent Foreign Bodies

Crawford R, Matheson AB (Aberdeen Royal Infirmary, Aberdeen, Scotland)
*Injury* 20:341–343, 1989                                      5–31

---

The ED sometimes is confronted with a patient with a suspected foreign body in the hand that cannot be detected by conventional soft-tissue radiography. Thirty-nine patients with a suspected foreign body in the hand were evaluated by real-time, high-resolution ultrasonography.

Scanning revealed a foreign body in 21 patients, 19 of whom had a radiolucent foreign body at operation. Ultrasonography did not detect a foreign body in 18 patients, but at subsequent operation in 7 of these patients, 1 foreign body was found. This false negative result occurred in a patient with swelling of the hand and pus in the web space. The size of the 18 wooden splinters and 2 thorns removed at surgery ranged from 2 to 24 mm (Figs 5–3 and 5–4). The mean difference between the size of the foreign body on ultrasonography and that found at surgery was 5 mm. Ultrasound scanning also showed the foreign body's depth, relationship to hand structures, and 3-dimensional aspect. The ultrasound examination usually took 10 minutes but sometimes took 30.

The sensitivity and reliability of real-time, high-resolution ultrasonography in detecting radiolucent foreign bodies in the hand are affirmed. Examination by this method provides 3-dimensional localization of a foreign object but takes time and patience. Nevertheless, it is the best investigation when a foreign body is suspected but is not visualized by standard radiography.

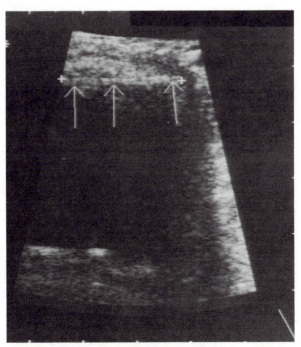

**Fig 5–3.**—Ultrasound scan of the hand showing 2.23-cm foreign body *(arrows)*. (Courtesy of Crawford R, Matheson AB: *Injury* 20:341–343, 1989.)

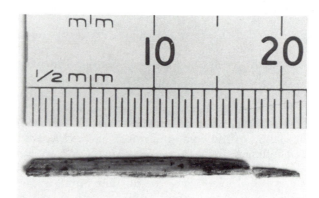

Fig 5–4.—The foreign body shown in Figure 5–3 after removal. (Courtesy of Crawford R, Matheson AB: *Injury* 20:341–343, 1989.)

▶ The suspicion of a retained foreign body, especially in the hand, is a real dilemma and a potential risk management issue for the emergency physician. We often do soft-tissue radiographs knowing before the study is done that small pieces of wood or other material would not be demonstrated. This is a small study of 39 patients, but the findings suggest strongly that real-time, high-resolution ultrasonography is a useful technique in finding foreign bodies not demonstrated by routine radiography. In only 1 of 18 patients with normal ultrasound results was a foreign body found. I have recently used ultrasonography in a patient who was convinced an intravenous catheter had been left in a hand vein. Results of the study were normal, and the patient improved with therapy for aseptic thrombophlebitis. In this risk management case, our other option would have been surgical exploration of the vein, which was not done because of the normal ultrasound results. With further experience and larger numbers of patients, ultrasonography may become the routine second step, or perhaps first step, in evaluation of soft-tissue foreign bodies.—J.M. Mitchell, M.D.

## Treatment Modalities

### Computer-Assisted Optimization of Aminophylline Therapy in the Emergency Department

Gonzalez ER, Vanderheyden BA, Ornato JP, Comstock TG (Medical College of Virginia, Richmond; Univ of Maryland)
*Am J Emerg Med* 7:395–401, 1989                    5–32

The use of bayesian-guided drug dosing is appealing for EDs. To study its value, 67 patients were randomized into group 1, which received aminophylline doses according to population-based guidelines, or group 2, which received doses according to bayesian-guided pharmacokinetic estimates.

Both groups had similar baseline theophylline concentrations and aminophylline loading doses. Aminophylline maintenance infusion and serum theophylline concentrations at 1 and 4 hours after loading doses were significantly higher in group 2 than in group 1. Group 1 had significantly higher peak flow rates than group 2 at baseline but the rates became similar thereafter.

The strongest predictor of treatment outcome was the peak flow rate 1 hour after loading dose: When the rate was 100 L/minute or less, no patients were discharged from the department. The next strongest predictor of outcome, baseline theophylline concentration, was inversely related to outcome. The third strongest predictor was theophylline concentration 4 hours after loading dose. Measured theophylline concentrations were significantly correlated with bayesian-derived estimates but not with those based on population.

▶ The authors attempt to develop a mathematical model to assist in optimized aminophylline therapy in the emergency center. Although the development of a theoretically ideal aminophylline level is desirable in the asthmatic patient, clinical experience indicates that a wide individual variation occurs in correlating level to control of bronchospasm. Since asthma is such an individual disease with connotations unique to the patients themselves, patients' own evaluation of their course remains the single best determinant for decision making and predictor of outcome. The authors provide sophisticated dosage analysis; by their own admission, the clinician must correlate this information with clinical decision making.—D.K. Wagner, M.D.

---

**Lack of Effect of Changing Needles on Contamination of Blood Cultures**
Isaacman DJ, Karasic RB (Univ of Pittsburgh; Children's Hosp of Pittsburgh)
*Pediatr Infect Dis J* 9:274–278, 1990                                         5–33

---

A common practice at many institutions when blood cultures are collected is to replace a needle used for venipuncture with a fresh, sterile needle before the culture media are inoculated. This routine came into use in an effort to reduce culture contamination but has never been validated in formal studies.

To examine the effect of changing needles on the contamination of blood cultures, 303 children were randomly allocated to 3 study groups that differed only in the number of needle changes performed after venipuncture. In the first group, blood samples were instilled directly into the culture bottles through the butterfly needles used for venipuncture. In the second group, clean straight needles were substituted for the butterfly needles before blood was instilled into the aerobic and anaerobic culture bottles. In the third group, needles were changed twice, once before inoculation of an aerobic culture bottle and again before inoculation of an anaerobic culture bottle. Each patient's skin was cleansed with povidone-iodine for 60 seconds according to a standard protocol before venipuncture.

The rates of contamination were 2.2% for the group that had no needle changes, 0% for the group that had 1 needle change, and 1.9% for the group that had 2 needle changes. The difference did not reach statistical significance. Thus, the practice of changing needles after venipuncture before blood culture collection does not influence the contamination rate. The standardized skin-cleansing process used in the study probably eliminated potential contaminants from the venipuncture site and thus prevented their transfer to culture media.

In view of the potential risks associated with the handling of needles, abandoning the practice of changing needles when blood is collected for culture appears justified.

▶ The growing exposure to AIDS adds hazard to the practice of emergency medicine. Any opportunity to diminish the risk must be rapidly and firmly propagated.— E.H. Taliaferro, M.D.

## Evaluation of Skin Stapling for Wound Closure in the Emergency Department

Brickman KR, Lambert RW (St Vincent Med Ctr—The Toledo Hosp, Ohio)
*Ann Emerg Med* 18:1122–1125, 1989                                    5–34

Automatic skin staplers are commonly used for surgical wound closure. They are an attractive alternative to suture repair of certain lacerations seen in the ED. However, emergency physicians have been reluctant to use automatic skin staplers. The efficacy of skin stapling for traumatic lacerations in patients in the ED was investigated.

Eighty-seven lacerations to the scalp, trunk, or extremities, excluding hands and feet, in 76 patients were treated. The patients were seen again at 2 and at 7–10 days for follow-up in the ED. Results were assessed for efficiency, appearance, complications, and cost effectiveness. There was only 1 significant complication—a dehiscence of a scalp laceration caused by hematoma collection. A minor dehiscence of a superficial leg laceration resulted from inadequate primary closure, but it did not produce any cosmetic deformity. There were no infectious complications, delayed wound healing, or cosmetic problems. Skin stapling was found to be easier, quicker, and overall less costly than suture repair.

▶ The craftsman's pleasure we all experienced as medical students when we did a loving, painstaking, time-consuming plastic closure of a laceration has doubtless moderated over the years as we became more concerned about how to keep up with an increasing volume of patients and avoid ED logjam. Skin stapling is 1 way to speed up laceration repairs. We use these devices in our ED, and I cannot count the number of hours they have saved me.

This paper is glowing in its recommendation of skin staplers, as most previous reports have been (1, 2). The infection rate is no worse than that from synthetic, nonabsorbable suture (although the authors' infection rate of zero should be considered a statistical fluke), and the cosmetic results preclude its use on the face. Patient acceptance is good, although it is prudent to carefully sound out the parents before making their little darling look like a Hammer

Films star. At least 1 brand of stapler is even less expensive than suture and disposable instruments.

If you are not using skin staplers yet, you owe it to yourself to try them.—J. Schoffstall, M.D.

*References*

1. Roth JH, et al: *Can J Surg* 31:19, 1988.
2. Ritchie AJ, et al: *Injury* 20:217, 1989.

---

**Skin Stapling of Wounds in the Accident Department**
MacGregor FB, McCombe AW, King PM, Macleod DAD (Bangour Gen Hosp, West Lothian, England)
*Injury* 20:347–348, 1989                                                          5–35

---

Traditionally, skin lacerations treated in the ED are closed by sutures. The use of staples and sutures for skin closure was compared in a randomized prospective study of 100 patients with skin lacerations. Both methods were scored on ease of removal, healing, infection, cosmetic results, method acceptability, and appearance by either medical and nursing staff or the patient.

A total of 253 sutures and 286 staples were inserted. Both techniques were similarly accepted by the staff and patients, and end results were similar. The skin stapling technique was 6 times faster than suturing and was simpler to use, but it was also more expensive than sutures.

The use of staples to close traumatic skin lacerations compares favorably with sutures. Skin stapling is recommended as the standard method of skin closure, particularly in busy accident departments and EDs.

▶ Local anesthetics were not used in the patients receiving staples in this study. This practice would preclude the digital exploration of wounds in alert patients. I prefer to anesthetize wounds before exploration to thoroughly examine them regardless of the method of closure. Staples are easy to use and well tolerated.—E. Ruiz, M.D.

---

**The Use of Chromic Catgut in the Primary Closure of Scalp Wounds in Children**
Start NJ, Armstrong AM, Robson WJ (Royal Liverpool Children's Hosp, England)
*Arch Emerg Med* 6:216–219, 1989                                                   5–36

---

Children with scalp wounds requiring closure are frequently seen in the ED. Suturing is invariably traumatic for the child, and the use of nonabsorbable sutures adds the trauma associated with removal. In addition, a return to hospital is an inconvenience for the parent and child and augments the department's workload. Absorbable sutures were evaluated in comparison with silk in alternate children seen with a scalp wound requiring closure. In both instances 4–0 sutures were employed.

Forty-eight patients who underwent suturing with silk and 42 who had chromic catgut sutures were reviewed after 5 days. More than 75% of the parents would have preferred not to return. No healing complications occurred in either group. Sutures occasionally were retained for a few weeks, but this caused no problems.

Chromic catgut is an acceptable material that can be used to close scalp wounds in children, and it has definite advantages over silk sutures with respect to convenience and expense.

▶ Scalp wounds heal well because of excellent blood supply. Infection and premature lysis of sutures are the only possible complications of absorbable material, and neither was observed in this prospective study. Why bring a child back when absorbable sutures work just as well? A repeat neurologic assessment may be appropriate in cases where there is loss of consciousness, but aside from that situation, I agree with the authors: Use of absorbable suture material is an acceptable alternative for scalp lacerations.—W.P. Burdick, M.D.

---

### Management of Hemorrhage From Severe Scalp Lacerations With Raney Clips

Sykes LN Jr, Cowgill F (Univ of Maryland Med System, Baltimore; Cleveland Metropolitan Gen Hosp)
*Ann Emerg Med* 18:995–996, 1989                                    5–37

---

Severe hemorrhage or even hypovolemic shock can occur after extensive scalp lacerations. Plastic Raney clips are commonly used by neurosurgeons to control bleeding from craniotomy incisions. Raney clips were used to control massive bleeding from scalp lacerations.

Man, 23, was assaulted about the head and face with a wrench, resulting in multiple severe scalp lacerations. The patient remained in hypovolemic shock despite resuscitative efforts. At the ED, Raney clips were applied to the edges of the scalp lacerations. Thereafter, hemodynamic stability was achieved with blood transfusions and crystalloid infusions, whereupon he was admitted to the intensive care unit for definitive management of the scalp lacerations. The patient was discharged on the third hospital day for outpatient treatment.

Application of Raney clips permits quick, atraumatic control of scalp hemorrhage. It can be safely left in place for hours as diagnostic and therapeutic procedures are performed. Because of its simplicity, effectivity, and ease of application, a separate pack of Raney clips and a clip applier should be part of the armamentum in the resuscitation room.

▶ Emergency physicians would be wise to be familiar with Raney clips and to keep them on hand in their trauma carts.—G. Ordog, M.D.

# 6 Emergency Medical Service Systems

## Prehospital Care, ACLS

**Dispatcher-Assisted Cardiopulmonary Resuscitation: Validation of Efficacy**
Kellermann AL, Hackman BB, Somes G (Univ of Tennessee, Memphis)
*Circulation* 80:1231–1239, 1989                                    6–1

Although community training programs in cardiopulmonary resuscitation (CPR) have been promoted for many years, participation in those programs has been limited. Middle-aged and older women are most likely to witness a cardiac event but are the group least likely to have CPR training. Several studies have shown that CPR instruction given by telephone to the person reporting cardiac arrest can be effective. The efficacy of dispatcher-assisted CPR was tested in a group of community volunteers.

Volunteers were recruited to attend a first-aid workshop. When they agreed to take part in a trial of telephone CPR training, they wre subjected to a stressful study environment designed to approximate an emergency situation. Professional ambulance dispatchers delivered the instructions to the volunteers as they performed CPR on a manikin. Instructions were given to volunteers both with (group B) and without (group A) previous CPR training. The performance of both groups was compared with that of previously trained volunteers (group C) who did not receive the telephone message.

The initiation of CPR was significantly delayed in groups A and B, who started ventilation an average of 1.5 minutes later than group C participants. During the 5-minute study period, however, all 3 groups completed an average of 10 or more cycles of ventilations and compressions. Groups B and C were more successful than group A at fully extending the manikin's neck, a maneuver necessary for successful ventilation. The groups receiving telephone instruction were significantly better at performing chest compressions.

Few of the volunteers met the American Heart Association's demanding criteria for adequate resuscitation, but even poor CPR can improve a victim's chances of survival. Thus, telephone instruction is an important adjunct but not a substitute for community-based CPR training. Telephone training can be a valuable, cost-effective means of increasing the rate of bystander CPR and can also improve the performance of those who have had previous training.

▶ The authors have nicely demonstrated the feasibility of dispatchers providing CPR instruction to citizens via telephone. On average, a period of 4 minutes was required until compressions were initiated, and this delay may affect outcome. It is important to reiterate a number of points mentioned by the authors in their discussion: (1) optimal survival is dependent on advanced life support response within 10 minutes; (2) because telephone CPR instruction requires 4–5 minutes, dispatch center staffing must be adjusted to allow uninterrupted time; and (3) this activity should come under the authority of the medical director.—P.T. Pons, M.D.

### Implementation of a Computerized Management Information System in an Urban Fire Department

Valenzuela TD, Keeley KT, Criss EA, Spaite DW, Meislin HW (Univ of Arizona Health Sciences Ctr, Tucson; Tucson Fire Dept)
*Ann Emerg Med* 18:573–578, 1989                                            6–2

To maintain effectiveness, an emergency medical services (EMS) program must be reviewed regularly for performance. Standardized record keeping is a necessary part of any monitoring program. A computerized data collection system resulted from collaboration between the Tucson Fire Department (TFD) and the emergency medicine section of the University of Arizona College of Medicine.

The TFD used a widely adopted computer program, the Uniform Fire Incident Reporting System (UFIRS), for collection of data. Firefighters completed a standarized form with code numbers appropriate to each emergency incident. The information requested in the forms included a description of injuries, illnesses, injury mechanisms, incident location, and the type of property on which the incident took place. In a modification of this form, additional information was provided, such as patient vital signs, the use of seat belts or head protection, initiation of bystander CPR, and prehospital treatment interventions.

All TFD personnel attended training sessions on implementing the new form. The basic system was familiar, however, ensuring a smooth transition and complete and accurate data collection. The new system has improved the quantity and quality of information available to the fire department administration for EMS management. Upgrading the manually coded UFIRS did not require a major form redesign or new computer software or hardware. The forms can be processed and the data base maintained by a half-time employee. Optically scanned forms were considered but proved more limited than the manually coded system.

▶ The need to critically evaluate EMS systems will continue to grow over the next decade, prompted by the necessity to provide medical quality assurance, financial responsibility, and assessment of system response. An important factor in the success of the system described by the authors is the joint effort of the medical director and, in this case, fire department administrator to determine their needs and then to develop and implement the data collection system.—P.T. Pons, M.D.

**A Computer-Assisted Quality Assurance Audit in a Multiprovider EMS Sytem**
Swor RA, Hoelzer M (William Beaumont Hosp, Royal Oak, Mich)
*Ann Emerg Med* 19:286–290, 1990                                           6–3

Evaluating the quality of care in a large emergency medical services (EMS) system is difficult, especially when multiple agencies provide advanced life support (ALS). The prehospital care delivered by multiple agencies and their paramedics in a suburban EMS system were compared in a review of patients seen at 1 member of a 10-hospital system in an 18-month period. Care given by 4 agencies and 100 paramedics in a total of 2,406 ALS runs was assessed.

The mean number of deficiencies declined between the first 6 months of the study and the second 9-month period. The most frequent deficiencies in the later period were failure to totally document run times; failure to reassess vital signs if abnormal or after treatment; and inadequate recording of the incident. Inappropriate treatment was noted in 1.5% of cases.

An EMS quality assurance audit, performed by the receiving hospital, has helped document problems in the performance of member agencies and of individual paramedics. It also has promoted compliance with protocol for patients delivered to the receiving hospital.

▶ Quality assurance and the assessment of EMS system performance involve numerous analyses, including chart review, run tape review, compliance with protocol, technical capability, time evaluations, and patient outcome. These may be accomplished manually or with the aid of computer programs but invariably are time intensive. Unfortunately, this aspect of prehospital care is all too often not performed, or physician involvement is minimal or nonexistent. Some states are now adding language to their EMS laws that mandate quality assurance and EMS audits.— P.T. Pons, M.D.

---

**Effect of Standing Orders on Field Times**
Pointer JE, Osur MA (City and County of San Francisco Emergency Med Services; Alameda County Emergency Med Services District, Oakland, Calif)
*Ann Emerg Med* 18:1119–1121, 1989                                         6–4

One of the 4 base hospitals in an emergency medical services (EMS) district discontinued participation in the system. As a result, the EMS district declared an emergency for that zone. All paramedics serving that base hospital operated on standing orders. When the base hospital resumed medical control function, limited standing orders were in operation. Times at scene and total prehospital care times were compared before standing orders (control period), with standing orders, and with limited standing orders.

Under standing orders, base hospital contact was not required for paramedic practice. Three patient groups were included under limited

Scene Times and Total Prehospital Times by Group

| Group | No. | Scene Time (min) (Mean ± SD) | Prehospital Time (min) (Mean ± SD) |
|---|---|---|---|
| Control | 1,466 | 17.01 ± 7.87 | 25.82 ± 8.94 |
| Standing order | 1,812 | 13.29 ± 6.84 | 21.14 ± 7.83 |
| Limited standing order | 1,628 | 12.45 ± 6.65 | 20.92 ± 8.31 |

(Courtesy of Pointer JE, Osur MA: *Ann Emerg Med* 18:1119–1121, 1989.)

standing orders. Base hospital contact was canceled for cardiac arrest patients using the standard advanced cardiac life support, those needing only an intravenous line, and patients requiring only intravenous administration of naloxone or 50% dextrose.

Compliance with protocols was 95% in the control period, 97% during standing orders, and 98% during limited standing orders. Prehospital care time was assessed during the 3 periods. Total prehospital care and scene times differed significantly between the standing order group and the control group and between the limited standing order group and the control group (table). Outcome criteria for the 3 patient groups were not assessed.

Standing orders can save time in the field and be cost effective, but a potentially negative result is a decrement in on-line medical control. Ideally, standing orders should be used only in cases in which on-line physician direction is not necessary. Although time spent in contact between paramedics and hospital staff may often be better spent, it is important that cost considerations do not override those of medical control.

▶ A great deal of controversy exists regarding the amount of time spent by paramedics on the scene of an emergency situation, particularly as it relates to the trauma victim and the need for delivery of the patient to an appropriate hospital. The authors demonstrated that 1 way to minimize scene time is to use standing orders, and more important, they showed no increase in protocol deviation. Concerns about decrements in on-line medical control may be artificial in that the real issue is overall quality assurance, which many systems lack in any form. It has been shown several times that on-line medical control changes the patient care decision making in only a small percentage of cases. Decisions about routine interventions such as intubation, intravenous line placement and first-round advanced cardiac life support procedures (defibrillation, atropine, epinephrine, lidocaine) can and should be made by prehospital personnel before base station contact.—P.T. Pons, M.D.

**Predicting Demand for Emergency Ambulance Service**
Cadigan RT, Bugarin CE (Massachusetts Dept of Public Health, Office of Emergency Med Services, Boston)
*Ann Emerg Med* 18:618–621, 1989                                    6–5

Adequate planning for emergency medical services (EMS) depends on accurate estimates of demand. Two rule-of-thumb numbers predict emergency transports: 3.5% of the population and 1 transport per 10,000 population per day. Other more scientific models of demand are based on sociodemographic characteristics. Study of community demand for EMS found a number of relevant variables.

In a study of Massachusetts communities with a population of less than 65,000, 5 variables were included in the regression analysis: population, percentage of population age 65 years or older, median income, percentage living below the poverty level, and number of highway miles.

All of these variables except number of highway miles significantly improved accuracy of the prediction for EMS needs. The overall average transport rate corresponded to the rule-of-thumb estimate based on 3.5% of population. Emergency responses per 100 population were 50% higher and more variable. In the communities surveyed, each increase of 1,000 in population resulted in an increase of 39.1 responses and 31.9 emergency transfers. The "Cape Cod" effect, that is, the nonresident demand generated by vacationers, also was predictive.

The single best equation for predicting responses and transports combined population, median income, and Cape Cod effect. Poorer communities with the greatest budget restraints also have the greatest demand for EMS. For example, a community in the 25th percentile of median income may generate 103 more responses than a community of similar size in the 75th percentile of median income, creating a serious problem at a time of limited federal funding.

▶ The authors present a formula to estimate ambulance transports, something most services have determined by experience. Of particular importance is the fact that this formula was derived from an analysis of relatively small residential communities, and its applicability to urban environments was not tested. The next step in any evaluation is to translate that estimate into actual ambulance coverage by using analysis such as utilization per unit hour, peak demands, and geographic considerations to determine the needed hours and distribution of service. This paper did not perform that aspect of system planning and thus is limited in its usefulness.— P.T. Pons, M.D.

---

**Vital Signs as Part of the Prehospital Assessment of the Pediatric Patient: A Survey of Paramedics**
Gausche M, Henderson DP, Seidel JS (Harbor–Univ of California, Los Angeles, Med Ctr, Torrance, Calif)
*Ann Emerg Med* 19:173–178, 1990                                        6–6

---

Paramedics are required in most emergency medical services systems to take vital signs of all patients. There is a lack of research on provider compliance with the use of field assessment parameters in the pediatric age group.

A two-part study was conducted to determine (1) which vital signs, if any, were taken and under what circumstances and (2) the attitudes of paramedics toward assessment of the pediatric patient. In the first study, Los Angeles County prehospital care records on 6,756 pediatric patients were reviewed retrospectively. The sample covered the 3 months of September–November 1984. The pediatric patients ranged in age from 0 to 18 years and were divided into the following age groups for data analysis: 0–6 months, 7 months–2 years, 3–6 years, 7–12 years, and 13–18 years.

Review of the 6,756 prehospital care records revealed that the frequency of vital assessment varied with the age of the pediatric patient, that is, the frequency increased with the age of the patient. Base hospital contact had occurred in 26% of the cases. Vital signs were not often assessed in children less than 2 years of age, even when the patient's chief complaint suggested possible major illness or trauma.

The survey of the prehospital care provider's attitudes demonstrated that paramedics were less confident in their ability to evaluate vital signs in children less than 2 years old. They responded that pulse and respirations were equally important in the assessment of the pediatric trauma or medical patient. Temperature was believed to be useful in pediatric medical patients but not in pediatric trauma patients. More than 80% of the paramedics surveyed were convinced that more continuing education lectures in pediatric emergency medicine, more field experience with pediatric patients, more clinical training, more clinical experience, and more frequent reviews of reports at base station meetings were needed to improve the prehospital care of children.

Paramedics are not as confident in evaluation of vital signs in pediatric patients as in adult patients. Recognition of the difference in field assessment may provide the necessary impetus to improve prehospital provider education in pediatrics to stimulate further research on emergency medical services.

▶ Prior studies by Dr. Seidel indicate an increased need for emphasis on pediatric training for prehospital personnel. The fact demonstrated in this article that paramedics performed vital signs less frequently on children in the younger age groups may not simply be addressed by increased time devoted to training. My suspicion is that because of the short transport times in the Los Angeles system, the paramedics' perceived value of this tool in assessing and managing the patient is small. As the authors suggest, evaluating critically the impact of taking each component vital sign in the field should precede devoting large amounts of training time to teaching prehospital how to perform them accurately and comfortably. Regardless of the outcome of future studies, some conclusions are inescapable: Reliable assessment of the pediatric patient can result only from appropriate training and adequate clinical exposure.—W.J. Koenig, M.D.

---

**Prehospital Advanced Trauma Life Support for Penetrating Cardiac Wounds**

Honigman B, Rohweder K, Moore EE, Lowenstein SR, Pons PT (Univ of Colorado, Denver; Denver Gen Hosp)
*Ann Emerg Med* 19:145–150, 1990                                                6–7

The risks and benefits of prehospital advanced trauma life support are unknown. The records of 70 patients with penetrating cardiac injuries were reviewed retrospectively to ascertain the relationships among prehospital procedures, time in the field, and ultimate patient outcome. The patients were transported by the well-trained paramedical technicians of the Denver Department of Health and Hospitals.

Thirty-one patients sustained gunshot wounds, and 39 had stab wounds, with a mean Revised Trauma Score of 2.8. Paramedical technicians spent an average of 10.7 minutes at the scene, during which 71% of the patients underwent endotracheal intubation, 63% had pneumatic antishock garments (PASGs) applied, 93% had at least 1 intravenous line inserted, and 57% had 2 intravenous lines inserted.

Twenty-one patients (30%) survived, and excluding the patients with no vital signs at the scene, the overall survival was 66.7%. There was no significant correlation between on-scene time and either total number of procedures performed or placement of intravenous lines. On-scene times were similar whether endotracheal intubation or application of a PASG was performed or not. On-scene times did not correlate with the trauma score and did not differ between survivors and nonsurvivors.

Well-trained urban paramedical technicians can perform multiple life support procedures with very short on-scene times and high patient salvage. It appears that prehospital trauma systems require a minimum of "obligatory" time at the scene to find the patient, assess the clinical and environmental situations, and prepare the patient for transport. A prospective randomized trial is necessary to validate the findings.

▶ The importance of rapid delivery of trauma victims to definitive care is widely espoused, and the justification of the performance of prehospital procedures should be on the improvement of care to the patient demonstrated in prospective randomized trials (as espoused by the authors). Although this retrospective study presents some interesting concepts, I believe that it was generated as an answer to those studies that have indicated that the performance of procedures are unnecessarily long in trauma. Rather than demonstrate that what we do does not take more time or does not adversely impact patient care, it is incumbent on all of us to show the decrease in morbidity and mortality that occur with appropriate prehospital intervention. Improvement in intravenous solutions and the use of rapid infusion devices may make the prehospital initiation of intravenous therapy even more compelling in the future. Appropriate evaluation of therapy must take into account the fixed time at the scene and the increment in time added by additional procedures as astutely pointed out in this article.—W.J. Koenig, M.D.

---

**The Effect of Urban Trauma System Hospital Bypass on Prehospital Transport Times and Level 1 Trauma Patient Survival**
Sloan EP, Callahan EP, Duda J, Sheaff CM, Robin AP, Barrett JA (Cook County Hosp, Chicago; Univ of Illinois Affiliated Hosps, Chicago)
*Ann Emerg Med* 18:1146–1150, 1989                6–8

Paramedics in urban trauma systems bypass closer hospitals to take critically ill patients to a more distant trauma center. There has been concern that the additional time required to reach a trauma center could increase mortality either before or after arrival at the center. The total run time needed for bypass and the effect of bypass on patient survival were determined in 258 trauma patients.

Patients meeting level I trauma criteria (life- or limb-threatening injury or a field trauma score of 12 or less) were taken by the Chicago Fire Depart-ment to the closest trauma center. Of the 258 patients who were transported and arrived with vital signs during the 9-month study, 66 (32%) were direct patients and 137 (68%) were bypass patients. Bypass required a mean total run time that was 3 minutes longer than that for direct transport. The overall prehospital time was 60 minutes for direct transport and 63 minutes for bypass. No significant difference in survival was noted between the direct and bypass patients. Survivors were distinguished from nonsurvivors only by age, Injury Severity Score, and hospital Trauma Score.

Although bypass does not adversely affect prehospital times relative to direct transport, in both methods, much of the "golden hour" is consumed with delay time (the time between the injury and paramedic contact) and total run time. Public education stressing the importance of the rapid use of 911 may lower delay time and increase the survival of critically ill patients.

▶ The authors have nicely demonstrated that directing trauma victims to a trauma center and bypassing nontrauma hospitals in an urban environment has no adverse effect on outcome and that the time cost in minutes is small. Great attention has been focused on the prehospital care provided to victims of trauma and the amount of time the patient spends in the field. Numerous authors have advocated abandoning standard resuscitation efforts for trauma victims because of excessive prehospital times. A critical evaluation of prehospital trauma must differentiate those components of total prehospital time over which the paramedic has little or no control (fixed or obligatory times) vs. those that can be controlled by the prehospital provider. Response and transport times are clearly fixed. However, the on-scene time also has intervals that are obligatory and will vary, depending on the environment. These include, first, the time it takes to find and, later, evacuate the patient to the ambulance. These intervals will differ if the patient is found lying in the street vs. a multistory building without elevators, thus affecting on-scene time. Assessing a prehospital system must involve critical evaluation of these logistic variables.— P.T. Pons, M.D.

**Time-Dependent Risk of and Predictors for Cardiac Arrest Recurrence in Survivors of Out-of-Hospital Cardiac Arrest With Chronic Coronary Artery Disease**

Furukawa T, Rozanski JJ, Nogami A, Moroe K, Gosselin AJ, Lister JW (Miami Heart Inst, Miami Beach, Fla)
*Circulation* 80:599–608, 1989                     6–9

Survivors of out-of-hospital cardiac arrest unassociated with acute myocardial infarction have an increased risk of subsequent life-threatening ventricular tachyarrhythmias. To assess the risk of cardiac arrest recurrence with time and the influence of various clinical, angiographic, and electrophysiologic parameters on subsequent cardiac arrest recurrence with time, 101 patients with chronic coronary artery disease who had survived out-of-hospital cardiac arrest were followed prospectively for a mean period of 27 months (range 6 days—63 months).

In the control state, 76 patients (75%) had inducible ventricular tachyarrhythmias that could be suppressed by antiarrhythmic drugs or surgery in 32 (42%). During follow-up, cardiac arrest recurred in 21 patients, including 2 of 25 patients without inducible ventricular tachyarrhythmias in the control state, 3 of 32 patients with inducible ventricular tachyarrhythmias in the control state that were suppressed after treatment, and 16 of 44 patients with inducible ventricular tachyarrhythmias in the control state that could not be suppressed after treatment. Cumulative cardiac arrest recurrence at 4 years was significantly higher among patients with inducible ventricular tachyarrhythmias in the control state that could not be suppressed by treatment.

Actuarial rate of cardiac arrest recurrence was 11.2% during the first 6 months of follow-up (high-risk early-phase) and then decreased to less than 4% for each subsequent 6-month period. Multivariate Cox proportional hazard analysis showed that an ejection fraction less than 35% was the only significant predictor for early-phase ($\leq 6$ months) recurrence, whereas persistent inducibility of ventricular tachyarrhythmia was the strongest predictor for late-phase ($>6$ months) recurrence, with an ejection fraction less than 35% having only marginal predictive value.

In patients with chronic coronary artery disease who survive out-of-hospital cardiac arrest, poor ejection fraction and persistent inducibility of ventricular tachyarrhythmias are significant predictors of early- and late-phase recurrence, respectively. Time-dependent risk factor analysis allows an ongoing assessment of risk on an individual basis.

▶ Every emergency physician caring for a patient with a history of cardiac arrest is acutely aware of the potential of increased risk of recurrence. I would suspect most of us have a low threshold for admitting these patients. Although this article elucidates some features that may be important to note in the past medical history to assist us in further defining those at highest risk, there is still a statistically significant increase in arrest in survivors without the identified risk factors that must be taken into consideration when the disposition of these patients is considered..—W.J. Koenig, M.D.

---

**Outcomes in Unsuccessful Field Resuscitation Attempts**
Bonnin MJ, Swor RA (William Beaumont Hosp, Royal Oak, Mich)
*Ann Emerg Med* 18:507–512, 1989                                    6–10

---

Because some advanced life support (ALS) emergency medical systems declare that adult victims of nontraumatic cardiac arrest who do not respond to prehospital advanced cardiac life support (ACLS) efforts may be declared dead at the scene, the outcomes of 232 adult patients who sustained nontraumatic out-of-hospital cardiac arrest and who did not regain and sustain vital signs after standard prehospital ACLS were reviewed retrospectively.

A total of 181 patients, with an average age of 71 years, had no vital signs on arrival to the ED. Of these, 10 (6%) survived to hospitalization, and 1 (0.6%) was discharged neurologically intact. This 1 survivor who failed prehospital resuscitation was not endotracheally intubated in the field. Survival to hospital admission did not correlate with age, witness, location, cardiopulmonary resuscitation initiator, advanced life support unit response time, initial field rhythm, and initial ECG rhythm. Regaining but not sustaining vital signs in the field was not predictive of survival.

Analysis of the data showed 2 limitations: field rhythm strips were not reviewed for accuracy, and electromechanical dissociation was defined as "any rhythm interpreted as electromechanical dissociation by the paramedic." There may have been differences in outcome if these 2 entities were considered. Any adult nontraumatic cardiac arrest victim who does not respond to prehospital ACLS efforts should be pronounced dead at the scene. Rushing these patients to the ED may endanger the paramedical personnel and the surrounding community and takes away time from potentially salvageable patients. However, whenever endotracheal intubation or intravenous cannulation cannot be successfully accomplished in the field, the arrest victim should be transported to the ED for further resuscitation attempts.

▶ As the economic pinch is felt more and more by emergency medical services, the appropriate utilization of our resources becomes increasingly critical. Efficient system management demands that we evaluate both sides of the coin and clearly define areas of significant impact on patient care and those areas that consume resources without benefiting the patient. Although the medical community has been appropriately hesitant to implement policies discontinuing resuscitation on potentially viable patients, many systems have been more comfortable in defining the obviously dead patient who should not have resuscitation measures started. This paper is an attempt to validate what practicing emergency physicians already intuit. The 1 survivor in this study demonstrates that if therapeutic maneuvers are available in the ED that have not been successful in the field, the patient should be aggressively resuscitated. This also implies that once policies are implemented to withhold further field resuscitation, providers must be kept constantly aware of advances that may become available in the ED and influence decisions to discontinue field resuscitation.—W.J. Koenig, M.D.

---

**Prehospital Intraosseous Infusion by Emergency Medical Services Personnel: A Prospective Study**
Seigler RS, Tecklenburg FW, Shealy R (Greenville, SC)
*Pediatrics* 84:173–177, 1989                                    6–11

Intraosseous infusion was widely used in the 1940s and 1950s in pediatric emergencies before newer intravenous techniques made it outdated. Intraosseous infusion is finding new acceptance, however, particularly when conventional intravenous access is difficult. A 1-year pilot study evaluated the application of intraosseous infusion in children by paramedics who were given a 3-hour training course in the technique.

Intraosseous lines were used by paramedics in 17 children (aged 21 days–3 years) with cardiopulmonary arrest; 16 had no respiration or heart rate. Conventional intravenous access was unsuccessful in 16 attempts in 10 patients. Intravenous access was not attempted in another 7 patients after no apparent venous sites could be found.

Intraosseous access was successful in 16 of 17 patients after 22 bone marrow attempts. In 13 successful first attempts, intraosseous access was established within 1 minute. A second attempt was necessary in the other 3 successful intraosseous infusions. The single failure, attributed to lack of experience with the technique, occurred in a 5-month-old girl with sudden infant death syndrome. Fifteen patients underwent successful intubation by paramedics; 3 patients regained a palpable pulse and survived treatment in the ED but died 2–4 days later in the intensive care unit. None of the other children survived emergency treatment.

The poor outcome of pediatric patients who sustain prehospital cardiac arrest is well documented. The intraosseous access technique for establishing intravascular access could have widespread application in children who have not deteriorated to the point of cardiac arrest.

▶ Intravenous access in children in prehospital care is difficult and may result in prolonged scene times while personnel make multiple, unsuccessful attempts. The estimated time of arrival and the expected impact of the intervention always has to be weighed before any therapy is instituted in the field. The use of interosseous infusion for both volume replacement and the administration of medications is readily learned by paramedical personnel and has minimal complications associated with its use. Once the decision to institute therapy has been appropriately made, the use of the interosseous route can significantly reduce the time to access the vascular compartment. I found it particularly interesting that the greatest fear expressed by emergency medical services personnel was of improper needle placement, yet the most commonly taught method of verification is bone marrow aspirate, and that was seen in only 2 of the 16 successful placements in this study. Other authors have also found that multiple attempts at placement in the same bone may reduce the effectiveness of the procedure. (See also Abstract 4–75.)—W.J. Koenig, M.D.

## Prehospital Blind Nasotracheal Intubation by Paramedics

O'Brien DJ, Danzl DF, Hooker EA, Daniel LM, Dolan MC (Univ of Louisville, Louisville, Ky)
*Ann Emerg Med* 18:612–617, 1989                                    6–12

Blind nasotracheal intubation (BNTI) is ideally suited for emergency management of compromised airways in spontaneously breathing trauma patients, particularly those who are cervically immobilized. Prehospital BNTI when performed by experienced emergency physicians has been found to be a safe procedure. However, the ability of paramedics to successfully perform field BNTI in spontaneously breathing patients has not been evaluated.

During a 19-month study period, BNTI was attempted by trained paramedics in 324 patients and successful in 231 patients (71.3%). Medical patients accounted for 270 BNTI attempts, of which 195 (72%) were successful. Trauma patients accounted for 54 BNTI attempts, of which 36 (67%) were successful. No statistically significant difference in success rates was noted between these 2 groups. Of the 93 unsuccessful attempts, 7 were in patients who subsequently were successfully orally intubated in the field.

Forty-two patients (13.3%) experienced complications, but only 3 (0.9%) were serious. Epistaxis was the most common complication, accounting for 25 (58%) of the complications. However, none of the patients required nasal packing.

Of the 82 field paramedics, 49 attempted BNTI only 1–3 times during the 19-month study period. A significant increase in success was seen after a paramedic had attempted BNTI at least 4 times.

Because orotracheal intubation is often difficult to perform in cervically immobilized or noncooperative patients, BNTI appears to be a safe initial field airway approach in spontaneously breathing patients in whom no contraindications are evident. The procedure can be successfully and safely performed by properly trained paramedics.

▶ This study demonstrates that emergency medical systems should not be hesitant to implement the use of BNTI because of fear that the procedure cannot be adequately learned by paramedics. As with most other studies involving intubation, success rates increased and complication rates fell with more frequent utilization of the skill. Systems that do not have adequate patient contacts have to provide for ongoing training and monitoring of the skill, and the acceptable, minimal success rate should be established and adhered to. The Los Angeles emergency medical service system has used an 85% success rate as a training standard for oroendotracheal intubation and has demonstrated that it can be achieved with manikin-only training programs. Although the authors clearly elucidate the applications of this procedure in the field, those studies investigating the manipulation of the cervical spine and airway management have shown that BNTI does result in cervical spine movement. This procedure has been generally accepted as superior over other forms of intubation in patients with potential cervical spine injury, but the literature has not been generated to support that contention. This limitation should not detract from the reader noting that a majority of patients who benefited from this procedure were medical and not trauma.—W.J. Koenig, M.D.

---

### Endotracheal Intubation of Pediatric Patients by Paramedics

Aijian P, Tsai A, Knopp R, Kallsen GW (Valley Med Ctr, Fresno, Calif; Hennepin County Med Ctr, Minneapolis; Univ of California, San Francisco)
*Ann Emerg Med* 18:489–494, 1989                                         6–13

Children who arrive at the hospital in cardiopulmonary arrest have a very low survival rate. Endotracheal intubation, which can have a high success rate in adult patients in cardiopulmonary arrest, is used less often in pediatric patients.

The frequency, success rates, and complications of endotracheal intubation in children were retrospectively studied over a period of 38 months, during which 63 patients less than age 19 years had resuscitative efforts performed by prehospital personnel. Most of the children were less than 3 years of age. In 42 patients (68%), trained paramedic intubators were present. Endotracheal intubation was not attempted in 14 of these patients (group 1), was unsuccessful in 10 (group 2), and was successful in 18 (group 3).

Survival rates to hospitalization were 36% for group 1, 10% for group 2, and 50% for group 3. One child survived in group 1 and 1 child in group 3. Both survived drowning, and both had neurologic impairment. Most (67%) of the 42 intubated patients were less than 3 years old, but only 38% were infants. Endotracheal intubation achieved an overall success rate of 64%. In children more than 10 years of age, the rate was 75%. There were 28 complications, of which 2 were major.

These pediatric patients had rates of successful endotracheal intubation lower than those reported for adults. Children who underwent intubation fared no better on survival to hospital admission than those in whom intubation was not attempted or was unsuccessful. More specific training in performing endotracheal intubation may minimize complications and improve the rate of survival in pediatric patients.

▶ The findings in this study reiterate those of other studies that have looked at the resuscitation of children in cardiopulmonary arrest. Some facts are beginning to emerge in the literature: First, paramedics can be taught to perform intubation of children in the field, but the success rates are not so high as that of adult patients. Training standards and minimally acceptable success rates have not been generally agreed on. Second, success rates improve as the age of the patient increases, as demonstrated in this study. Finally, the etiology of cardiopulmonary arrest in children, unlike adults, is often respiratory, but successful intubation of children does not appear to alter the dismal outcome. Children less than age 18 months may be an exception, yet distressingly this is 1 of the age categories with the poorest success rates.

Further studies are necessary to assist medical directors in defining the appropriate place of this modaltity in emergency medical services. (See also Abstracts 4–65 and 4–56.)—W.J. Koenig, M.D.

---

**Models for Teaching Emergency Medicine Skills**
Nelson MS (Stanford Univ)
*Ann Emerg Med* 19:333–335, 1990                                    6–14

---

Learning to perform procedures is an important part of training in emergency medicine. The nature of the practice is such that it often is not practical to explain slowly and methodically how to do certain procedures. The use of animals is controversial today. Plastic models can be useful adjuncts, but even the best of them lack realism. Volunteers, paid or unpaid, are another alternative but are not practical as procedures become more painful and potentially dangerous.

Cadavers are excellent for teaching a variety of procedures, particularly those involved in airway management, chest procedures such as needle thoracostomy, wound care, and neurologic and neurosurgical procedures. Other procedures that are well taught with cadavers are nasogastric intubation, peritoneal lavage, Foley catheter placement, cutdowns, and arthrocentesis. Placement of central lines can be difficult to teach, and orthopedic procedures also can be a problem. Obtaining spinal fluid often is difficult. Very few procedures cannot be taught to some extent with cadavers.

Students may have concern over being disrespectful when using cadavers, but they do understand that it is for a good reason. Cadavers are a useful means of teaching procedures and should not be overlooked.

▶ I certainly agree with Dr. Nelson that the use of cadavers for teaching procedures to emergency medicine residents is an optimal experience. However, familiarity with the majority of the 26 procedures mentioned should be gained through repeated, firsthand experience with instruction. Chin lift, jaw thrust, suturing, local anesthesia, nerve blocks, nasogastric tubes, Foley catheters, arthrocentesis, and nail removal all are procedures performed on a frequent basis in any ED and to which residents should be exposed and have the opportunity to perform rather routinely. Most of the remaining procedures that may be encountered infrequently in clinical practice, such as cricothyrotomy, tube thoracostomy, thoracotomy, peritoneal lavage, and cutdown, are adequately taught on the dog or swine model. I do not believe that ethical concerns are valid with regard to the use of animals to teach physicians lifesaving procedures. The efficacy of cadaver use for teaching is unquestionable if the financial, laboratory, and support services needed can be mustered. If the use of cadavers is unfeasible, animal laboratories, coupled with bedside clinical teaching, are reasonable substitutes.—D.J. Cionni, M.D. (EMS Fellow), with S.J. Davison, M.D.

---

**Problem-Based ACLS Instruction: A Model Approach for Undergraduate Emergency Medical Education**
Polglase RF, Parish DC, Buckley RL, Smith RW, Joiner TA (Mercer Univ, Med Ctr of Central Georgia, Macon)
*Ann Emerg Med* 18:997–1000, 1989                                      6–15

---

The optimal approach to teaching advanced cardiac life support (ACLS) to medical students and other groups with little emergency experience has not been studied extensively. Most ACLS provider courses are taught over a 2-day period in a lecture-based format. In an ACLS provider course, emphasis was placed on interactive teaching and learning.

The self-directed problem-based learning model used a series of clinical problems that emphasized various aspects of the ACLS curriculum. The students then met with an ACLS instructor for weekly tutorial sessions. A specific set of learning objectives for the entire ACLS curriculum was developed into a study unit index and given to students at the beginning of the course. The students were offered enhanced practice time in the form of traditional teaching stations and skill laboratories.

Eleven sophomore medical students participated in the course. The students were tested using standard ACLS criteria, and none failed the course. These students achieved a higher pass rate on the written test and skill stations than senior medical students who underwent the standard 2-day course during the same period.

The problem-based ACLS instruction with enhanced practice time appears to be an effective alternative method in training groups having to acquire the basic skills needed in a resuscitation attempt but who have little previous experience in this area.

▶ Bravo! The importance of the material in the ACLS course is always overlooked, because the emphasis is consistently placed on passing the test. This problem-based interactive approach is an excellent format for conveying the needed information and skills to future physicians. Larger class size and a higher student/tutor ratio would probably be necessary if an entire medical school class were to take the course.—D.J. Cionni, M.D. (EMS Fellow), with S.J. Davidson, M.D.

## Triage, Planning, Emergency Department Operations

### Emergency Medicine: Winning the Revolution!
Anzinger RK (American College of Emergency Physicians, Dallas)
*Ann Emerg Med* 19:90–94, 1990                                    6–16

This presidential address was presented to the Council of the American College of Emergency Physicians (ACEP) in Washington, DC in September 1989. In addition to a discussion of policy changes within the ACEP itself, the revolution taking place in today's health care environment was reviewed.

Emergency medicine as a specialty began in the 1960s when the public demanded that expert care be available 24 hours/day, 365 days/year. The ACEP was founded to respond to that demand. Its original goal was to provide care to the patient from the time of onset of acute illness or injury up to and through disposition in the ED. These same goals are still valid today, but the specialty of emergency medicine has expanded to include a new system of ambulatory nonemergency care, most often provided in freestanding ambulatory care centers. In 1989 there were 3,900 freestanding ambulatory care centers seeing 50 million patients. It is projected that in 1991, there will be 5,000 freestanding ambulatory care centers seeing 85 million patients. To some extent, the ambulatory care centers may be viewed as the private practice of emergency medicine.

Today's revolution in health care involves issues of access, costs, and quality. Access to emergency care for the indigent has not been abandoned. However, hospitals and EDs are closing, EDs are functionally closed because of overcrowding, and ambulances are being diverted. This creates disruption within the prehospital system. The ACEP is working with Congress on the dilemmas surrounding indigent care because physicians cannot do it alone.

The need to lower costs has also affected the operations of EDs nationwide. In 1983, the ACEP cost-containment project defined a scientific method for cost reduction that should continue to be an effective mechanism for lowering costs. Outcomes research will provide answers to these cost-effective diagnostic and treatment efforts. Cost containment also involves promoting preventive strategies for reduction of illness and injury.

As for the quality of care, it is anticipated that emergency medicine will soon be awarded primary board status, which will allow the development of needed areas of subspecialty and improve the quality of the practice of emergency medicine. Personnel needs should also be addressed. There is an attrition study underway to measure the turnover of emergency physicians.

▶ The comments of a past president of the ACEP are worth reading in their entirety. As he points out, emergency medicine has now withstood the test of time and has been fully accepted into medicine's garden of specialties. We can now move forward to add substance to the structure.—D.K. Wagner, M.D.

---

## Use of Mildly Restrictive Administrative Protocol to Reduce Orders for Manual Blood Film Examination From the Emergency Department

Edelman BB, Groleau GA, Barish RA (Univ of Maryland, Baltimore)
*J Emerg Med* 8:1–13, 1990                                                                6–17

There is substantial evidence that manual blood film examination (BFE), which includes a 100-cell differential leukocyte count (DLC), evaluation of red blood cell morphology and platelet estimate, contributes little to clinical diagnosis or management. Given this, a mildly restrictive administrative protocol designed to reduce the number of BFEs performed in the laboratory was initiated. The protocol required a telephone request from emergency physicians or their designee to obtain a BFE. In lieu of a written request for a "differential count," 3-part electronic differentials (3PD) were performed.

With adoption of the protocol, the number of BFEs performed on ED patients decreased markedly from a previous level of 1 BFE for every complete blood cell (CBC) count. In addition, a retrospective review of the clinical course of 170 patients in whom no BFEs were requested showed no apparent adverse effect on patient care.

The number of manual BFEs performed for ED patients can be reduced to conserve laboratory resources, and the reduction does not adversely affect patient diagnosis and management. It is speculated that availability of the 3PD, which provides enumeration of lymphocytes and neutrophils with the CBC count partly facilitated the reduction in physician orders for manual BFEs.

▶ This is a most appropriate use of technology. The report strongly suggests that the automatic differential is as effective as the manual 100-cell differential for appropriate decision making. The details in the report itself discussing 50 physician-requested manual blood film examinations in which 24 examinations revealed 1 or more abnormalities of some apparent significance would not have influenced an emergency physician's practice, though they may well have an impact on the patient's inpatient management.—S.J. Davidson, M.D.

---

**Tetanus Immunity in Emergency Department Patients**
Stair TO, Lippe MA, Russell H, Feeley JC (Georgetown Univ Hosp, Washington, DC; Ctrs for Disease Control, Atlanta)
*Am J Emerg Med* 7:563–566, 1989                                    6–18

---

Despite the availability of an excellent vaccine, compliance with tetanus immunization is poor, especially among intravenous drug abusers, foreign-born young persons, and elderly persons. To ascertain the extent of tetanus immunity in ED patients, antitetanus toxoid antibody levels were measured in blood samples from 278 patients aged 8–91 years.

Mean antibody titer was 0.68 unit/mL. Of the 278 patients, 27 (10%) had inadequate antibody titers, defined as less than the 0.01 unit/mL considered protective by the Centers for Disease Control. Of the 27 with inadequate antibody levels, 14 were aged more than 70 years. Patients with inadequate immunization were more likely to be elderly (mean age 65 years) women, have fewer years of education, and be of non-U.S. origin than those with adequate immunization. Among the 84 patients who reported their immunization histories, 5 denied ever receiving the complete series of tetanus shots but had adequate antibody levels, whereas 3 who reported having completed the series had inadequate levels. Thirty patients had wounds, and 29 were correctly treated according to the recommended protocol: 5 required no additional immunization and 24 received tetanus toxoid. None of the 248 patients without wounds were immunized.

Patient recall of immunization history is not a reliable guide to tetanus immunity. It appears prudent for the ED physician to be liberal in prescribing tetanus toxoid and immune globulin for patients with incomplete or unknown immunization, particularly older women.

▶ This study serves to remind us all that tetanus is alive and well in this country and that a large percentage of ED patients are inadequately immunized. The antibody levels of the patients in this study who are most at risk for tetanus (i.e., those with wounds) are not reported. The fact remains, however, that it is our duty to identify those patients who are at risk for clarifying their immunization history and by treatment on "suspicion of need" if the history is unclear.— D.J. Cionni, M.D. (EMS Fellow), with S.J. Davidson, M.D.

---

**Emergency Room Use and Primary Care Case Management: Evidence From Four Medicaid Demonstration Programs**
Hurley RE, Freund DA, Taylor DE (Pennsylvania State Univ)
*Am J Public Health* 79:843–847, 1989                               6–19

Previous analyses have indicated that the majority of services rendered in the ED are for nonurgent care. Poor persons use hospital EDs more frequently for nonurgent care than do persons of more substantial means. Primary care case management programs might reduce reliance on the ED by the poor, possibly resulting in real savings for state Medicaid agencies. The results of 4 Medicaid demonstration programs aimed at replacing reliance on the ED with primary care case management are examined.

The 4 programs included 2 county-based demonstration programs in Monterey, California and Santa Barbara, California and 2 state-operated capitation programs in Kansas City, Missouri and New Jersey. All 4 programs used a gatekeeper or case manager model in which eligible persons were enrolled with a participating individual physician or primary care organization. The gatekeeper had to provide all primary care and had to approve all referral care, including all inpatient and nonurgent ED use. Information on age, sex, race (except in California), total months of eligibility, insurance coverage beyond Medicaid, and other variables were collected for each person in the 4 demonstration programs. For comparison, the same data from patients in traditional Medicaid programs were analyzed.

During the 1-year demonstration programs, large reductions occurred in the proportion of individuals with at least 1 ED visit, ranging from 27% to 37% for children and from 30% to 45% for adults, as compared with equally needy individuals who had not been entered in a demonstration program. Despite the reduced use of ED facilities, the number of primary care visits at most sites did not increase correspondingly. This finding suggests that formal enrollment with a responsible case manager provided improved continuity of care that reduced the need for such visits. These 4 capitated demonstration programs also appeared to provide a modest cost savings for the respective state Medicaid agencies as a result of reduced ED use.

▶ This is the kind of study that takes public health research of the current era into poor repute. Although the authors have successfully demonstrated the reduction in the number of ED visits without a concomitant increase in primary care visits, thus resulting in a modest cost savings, they have not, in fact, demonstrated cost effectiveness of the program. It is entirely possible that the health of those individuals in the program deteriorated. Without an effective means of determining health in the populations studied, and conducting both preassessments and postassessments of health in those populations, one cannot be certain that the reduction in the care provided did not also result in a reduction in overall health of 1 or more of these populations. Public health practitioners used to be more concerned with the health of populations than the cost of care.—S.J. Davidson, M.D.

---

**Community Hospital Transfers to a VA Medical Center**
Kerr HD, Byrd JC (Med College of Wisconsin, Milwaukee)
JAMA 262:70–73, 1989                                                    6–20

Cost-containment pressures have created the phenomenon of transferring medically indigent patients from community hospitals to public general and Veterans Administration (VA) hospitals. At the same time, funding for public and VA hospitals has been curtailed. Several reports have described the transfer of patients from community to public hospitals, but the transfer of patients from community hospitals to VA hospitals has not been examined. The volume of transfers from community hospitals to 1 VA hospital was determined, and the severity of illness, fitness for transfer, intended purpose of transfer, and health insurance status of the transferred patients were analyzed.

During a 7-month period, 352 consecutive patients aged 18–97 years were transferred from 61 different community hospitals to the VA hospital, 344 of whom were assessable. Most (98.3%) of the patients were men. Of the 344 patients, 199 (58%) were transferred directly from inpatient units; the remaining patients were transferred directly from EDs. Ninety percent of the patients were transported by ambulance; only 6% were accompanied by a nurse or physician. Of 344 transferred patients, 58% had no medical insurance.

Transfers from community hospitals totaled 4.7% of all VA hospital admissions for the period, but the transferees accounted for 19.1% of all hospital deaths. The mortality rate for transferred patients was 12.5% compared with 2.6% for all other acute admissions. The mean length of hospital stay for the transferred patients was 18.2 days compared with 10.1 days for all patients. At the time of transfer, 59 patients (19%) were considered unstable according to a modified APACHE II classification system, yet only 19 patients were cared for en route by a physician or nurse. The condition of at least 7 unstable patients deteriorated in transit; 1 experienced cardiac arrest and had to undergo intubation. Treatment such as cardiac monitoring, oxygen, intravenous fluids, and intravenous medications were discontinued before transfer in 76 of 200 patients for whom in-transit data were available. Five patients with gastrointestinal hemorrhage arrived at the VA hospital in shock. Seven others experienced cardiac arrest on the day of admission to the VA hospital; 3 died. A set of minimal requirements for interhospital transfer of critically ill patients should be developed.

▶ Unfortunately, this report confirms what we already know. Community hospitals dump patients whom they do not wish to care for, often on the basis of reimbursement. This study demonstrates an alarmingly high occurrence of transfer of unstable patients to a VA medical center with subsequent poor outcomes for many of these patients. The development of federal regulations of governing transfer of patients is an unfortunate, but probably necessary, response, which hopefully will result in the reduction of this behavior.

Emergency physicians must be particularly careful to document the reasons for a transfer and the patient's clinical condition at the time of transfer. Whenever there is any possibility that the patient is not sufficiently stabilized for transfer, transfer should be eschewed unless the receiving facility is aware of the situation and all agree that stabilization of the patient requires the care available at the receiving end of the transfer.— S.J. Davidson, M.D.

## Application of Clinical Indicators in the Emergency Department

O'Leary MR, Smith MS, O'Leary DS, Olmsted WW, Curtis DJ, Groleau G, Mabey B (George Washington Univ; Joint Commission on Accreditation of Healthcare Organizations, Chicago)

*JAMA* 262:3444–3447, 1989                                                         6–21

Clinical indicators, tools for measuring quantifiable aspects of patient care, are used increasingly for monitoring the quality and appropriateness of patient care. The overall discrepancy rate (ODR) is an indicator of discrepant interpretations between the ED and the radiology department (RD). Thus, the ODR measures the accuracy with which the ED interprets radiographs.

For all patients in whom discrepant radiologic findings are identified, the discrepancy is assigned to 1 of 5 discrepancy severity groups, with the group indicating the degree to which the patient was potentially exposed to the occurrence of a sentinel event. A sentinel event is an undesirable patient outcome characterized by preventable death or morbidity directly attributable to delayed accurate radiologic interpretation.

The study sample consisted of 23,500 radiographs from the ED during a 12-month period. A total of 776 ED-RD discrepancies were identified by the RD faculty, for an ODR of 3.3%. Three hundred fifty-two of the discrepancies were not related to the accuracy with which the ED faculty had interpreted the radiographs, nor were they associated with patient outcomes. The remaining 424 discrepancies resulted in a revised ODR of 1.8%. Of the 424 patients with confirmed discrepant radiographic interpretations, 412 were reassessed within 24 hours by the ED faculty, private physicians, or in-hospital staff physicians; 10 patients were asymptomatic and were not reevaluated, and 2 patients could not be traced. In none of the 422 cases for which follow-up information was obtained did the delay in accurate radiologic diagnosis lead to a sentinel event.

The use of clinical indicators enables health care professionals to manage the quality and appropriateness of care provided in their institution. The Joint Commission on Accreditation of Healthcare Organizations now requires the use of clinical indicators for accreditation.

▶ All of us practicing emergency medicine routinely conduct radiographic follow-up analysis to assure that our interpretations coincide with radiologist interpretations and result in appropriate diagnosis and patient care. This ongoing practice is generally considered a routine component of emergency medicine practice. This study takes this practice further by analyzing where and how discrepant interpretation occurred and what results transpired for the patient. I suspect that few emergency centers conduct that overall type of analysis, though proceeding with it and tracking it by physician would be a useful tool in improving overall quality. Again, this tool is most useful when the information about performance is regularly fed back to the involved providers so that they may alter or maintain behavior that is most important. In this case, of course, that behavior is optimal interpretation of radiographs.—S.J. Davidson, M.D.

**Emergency Room Visit Time: Changes Over a 16-Year Period**
Abramowitz S, Joy SA, Yurt RW (New York Univ Med Ctr; New York Hosp–
Cornell Med Ctr)
*NY State J Med* 89:446–449, 1989                                            6–22

In 1969, a prospective, 1-week time-and-motion study was conducted
at a large urban teaching hospital. In 1985, an identical 1-week time-and-
motion study was performed at the same hospital. Both studies surveyed
total visit time and time spent in the ED waiting to see a physician. In the
1969 study ED patients were seen first by the registrar and then by a
nurse who assigned priorities on the basis of need for immediate care. In
the 1985 study ED patients were seen first by a triage nurse who assessed
patient acuity and assigned the patient to medicine or surgery. The triage
nurse graded patient acuity as A (to be seen immediately), B (to be seen
within 10 minutes), or C (to be seen within 30 minutes).

Between 1969 and 1985, the number of ED patients increased by 36%.
The median total visit time in 1969 was 93 minutes, and in 1985, it was
115 minutes. However, in 1969, 32% of ED visits were completed in 1
hour or less, whereas in 1985, almost one half of the ED visits lasted for
at least 2 hours. In 1969, the median waiting time was 27 minutes; in
1985, it was 37 minutes.

Based on the data collected in these 2 prospective studies, specific steps
were taken to improve ED use and decrease patient waiting time. Because
many ED patients were categorized as C, an urgent care center was
opened adjacent to the main ED to handle selected C patients arriving
between 8:00 A.M. and 11:00 P.M. In addition, several physicians were
added to the ED staff to provide at least 1 full-time attending ED physician. These changes seem to have improved efficiency and shortened
waiting time.

▶ Of particular importance in this article is the fact that wait time to see a physician constituted only 33% of median visit time. The authors' suggestion of
implementing a tracking system to follow patient flow throughout their stay in
the ED is good. Particular emphasis would be placed on physician-related variables, such as wait times related to consultants and on-wait times related to
laboratory studies. This simple assessment would uncover the bottlenecks and
by its nature lead directly to solutions such as those implemented in this study.
In addition, study results will be a concrete piece of information to use in nego-
tiating changes with hospital administrators.—D.J. Cionni, M.D. with S.J. Davidson, M.D.

**Emergency Department Revisits**
Keith KD, Bocka JJ, Kobernick MS, Krome RL, Ross MA (William Beaumont
Hosp, Royal Oak, Mich; South Macomb Hosp, Warren, Mich)
*Ann Emerg Med* 18:964–968, 1989                                           6–23

Patients who return to the ED within 48–72 hours of an initial visit
are at high risk for errors in diagnosis or physician judgment in manage-

ment. The charts of patients returning within 72 hours to a single ED were reviewed to determine whether monitoring revisits is a useful quality assurance indicator.

Of 13,261 patient visits to the ED in 2 months, 455 (3.4%) were revisits within 72 hours; of these patients, the charts of 444 were available. The return visit and the initial visit were clearly related in 407 (91.7%) of these patients. Of 297 unscheduled related return visits, 96 (32.3%) were judged to be avoidable; of these, 39.6% involved management deficiencies, 14.6% had inappropriate prescribed follow-up, and 20.8% had not been properly instructed. Patient noncompliance was the cause of 35 (36.5%) visits. Of the unscheduled return visits, 146 (49.2%) of the patients returned within 24 hours; 89 (30%) returned at 24–48 hours; and 62 (20.8%) returned at 48–72 hours. Of the avoidable visits, 85% occurred within 48 hours, as did 92% of those involving medical management deficiencies.

Using a computer to monitor 48- rather than 72-hour unscheduled return visits in a suburban ED is an efficient quality assurance tool. This audit is useful to detect medical management deficiencies and other quality assurance problems.

▶ This report, a most appropriate process audit, is of interest to me for its potential application in training of emergency physicians. Although aggregate numbers are reported for only a 2-month period, this study, if conducted on a continuing basis, could be useful in tracking the progress of individual trainees over the course of their training program.

This type of process audit feedback to individuals, and monitored by them and program directors, can assist trainees in learning about many clinical and administrative problems in the emergency center. Patient care is bound to improve, and the process used is bound to gain the greatest cooperation because individual trainees will have an opportunity to change their own behavior in response to feedback about their performance. In industrial quality control circles, this is called a "quality improvement program." It is gaining adherents in medicine (1).—S.J. Davidson, M.D.

*Reference*

1. Berwick D: *N Engl J Med* 320:53, 1989.

---

**Health Care Needs of Homeless and Runaway Youths**
Council on Scientific Affairs (American Med Assoc, Chicago)
*JAMA* 262:1358–1361, 1989
6–24

Because little is known about the health care needs of homeless and runaway adolescents, the health care needs of homeless and runaway teenagers were reviewed.

Estimates of homeless adolescents range from 500,000 to 2 million. Some of these adolescents are runaways, others are homeless involuntarily, and some have been forced out of their homes. Most of these adolescents receive no help from social service agencies. Their lack of skills forces them to live marginally and makes them vulnerable to abuse. Health care problems include nutritional deficiencies, substance abuse, and high rates of psychiatric disturbances. General malaise and musculoskeletal, gastrointestinal tract, and genitourinary disorders are the most common ailments. Other problems include upper respiratory tract infections, minor skin diseases, and broken bones. Pregnancy and sexually transmitted diseases are included in genitourinary disorders; AIDS is of special concern. Health care is generally inadequate because of a lack of treatment facilities, the behavior of these adolescents, and the questionable legal status of homeless teenagers.

The health care needs of homeless adolescents are numerous, and health care provided is inadequate. The Council on Scientific Affairs has urged researchers to collect more reliable, up-to-date information on homeless adolescents to clarify the nature of their needs and to set guidelines for their medical care.

▶ Homeless and runaway youths appear with some regularity in the EDs of all hospitals. Though perhaps more common in the urban environment in which I practice, I suspect that many of us see these patients regardless of our practice environment and too commonly overlook the social aspect of the clinical circumstances around them. Since many EDs do not provide around-the-clock social service support, it is frequently difficult, at best, for the emergency physician to properly care for more than what may appear to be a trivial organic problem of the homeless or runaway youth.

In urban and near-urban EDs, where these problems are more common, perhaps we all should examine our approach to these children and access the resources we have available. As with many clinical diagnoses, including child abuse, an index of suspicion is important in recognizing a youth as homeless or runaway. These teens frequently avoid acknowledging that circumstance because they fear coming into contact with police authorities. Offering the youth a meal may be a means of retaining them in the ED while the physician and other staff pursue attempts to provide some meaningful social support. Once social support is provided, a resolution of longer-term health care problems becomes possible with more usual means of outpatient follow-up. In the absence of such social support, hospitalization, at a lower index of suspicion, may be a worthwhile practice to provide appropriate health care to a runaway or homeless youth.—S.J. Davidson, M.D.

---

**A Survey of Observation Units in the United States**
Yealy DM, De Hart DA, Ellis G, Wolfson AB (Univ of Pittsburgh, Ctr for Emergency Medicine of Western Pennsylvania, Western Pennsylvania Hosp, Pittsburgh)
*Am J Emerg Med* 7:576–580, 1989                    6–25

---

Observation units can help contain health costs and improve patient care. Previous studies of these units have been based on single facilities and have not been done on a national level. A survey of 250 hospitals and acute care medical facilities across the United States was undertaken to compile information on observation and holding units in the United States.

Of the 250 facilities surveyed, 27% had operational observation or holding units, and 16% planned to have them within 1 year. Nonteaching hospitals were significantly more likely to use observation and holding units than were teaching hospitals. There was a trend toward greater use of these units in suburban and urban centers than in rural facilities, but the difference was not significant. A majority of the observation and holding units (93%) were located within Eds, were staffed by emergency physicians, and were under the direction of ED administrators. Most were staffed by ED nurses and ancillary help. No hospital had both ED and non-ED units, and many units functioned as both holding and observation units. Administrators perceived these units to be advantageous for caring for patients and lowering health care costs.

Observation units are found in many hospitals in the United States, usually near or in EDs. These units may be beneficial for patient care, cost containment, and improvement of physician skills, but further prospective studies are warranted to objectively document these beliefs.

▶ It is important for emergency physicians to appropriately assess the ever-increasing emphasis placed on the use of the observation unit and its relation to emergency practice. The use of these units is economically driven, and it is incumbent on emergency physicians to ensure that the institution of these units does not compromise the care of their patients. Although the literature has demonstrated that many patients previously admitted to intensive care areas (especially to coronary care units) could safely be cared for in less labor-intensive and less expensive "step-down" units, we must ensure that quality of care is not compromised. Pressure to admit patients to areas with less-than-optimal staffing should be resisted. Emergency physicians must view these units as extensions of their practice and recognize the benefits that can accrue to our skills as a result of our involvement in the high percentage that were located administratively within the ED. The authors clearly identified that many of the beliefs that we have about these units need to be supported by additional prospective studies.—W.J. Koenig, M.D.

## Legal, Ethical Issues/Emergency Department Stress

### Litigation Against the Emergency Physician: Common Features in Cases of Missed Myocardial Infarction

Rusnak RA, Stair TO, Hansen K, Fastow JS (Hennepin County Med Ctr, Minneapolis; Georgetown Univ; Johns Hopkins Univ)
*Ann Emerg Med* 18:1029–1034, 1989                                   6–26

Missing myocardial infarction is the leading cause of malpractice losses in the ED setting. Adverse outcome data from 2 insurance companies were reviewed in an attempt to identify common factors in cases of missed acute infarction. Sixty-five cases of undiagnosed infarction seen in

EDs in 1982–1986 were included with an average insurance loss of $113,806. Fifty-three of the 65 patients died.

These 65 patients were significantly younger than concurrent controls and had more atypical signs and symptoms. They had fewer recorded ECGs, and fewer of these were diagnostic of acute infarction. The physicians who saw these patients had significantly less experience in the ED than others, they obtained less thorough histories, and they misinterpreted more ECGs.

Ten of the 65 physicians sued were board certified. One third of the group had 2 years or less of postgraduate training. Estimates of cardiac enzymes did not distinguish patients with missed infarction from control patients.

Physicians should obtain and document more detailed histories and consider atypical manifestations. They also should obtain more ECGs and should readily admit patients who have vague or suspicious symptoms. Emergency departments should be staffed by physicians who are board certified or who have had 3 or more years of ED experience.

▶ Research results reported here regarding malpractice losses secondary to the misdiagnosis of myocardial infarction are the kind of information that can contribute to the development of effective practice guidelines. The Massachusetts chapter of the American College of Emergency Physicians (MACEP) has similarly conducted a review of malpractice losses from 8 distinct entities, of which myocardial infarction was 1. The MACEP study (1) reported on the proposed use of practice guidelines, which, in their study, if applied, would have resulted in the avoidance of significant losses. The work by Rusnak et al. as well as the more recent MACEP report have fueled the development of practice standards for emergency physicians, the first 1 of which on chest pain was released in September 1990. The application of practice standards is likely to result in better patient care because of the effects their application has on the physician's organization of clinical information. Reduction in maloccurrences with concomitant reduction in malpractice losses is a subsidiary benefit (2).— S.J. Davidson, M.D.

*References*

1. Karcz A, et al: *Ann Emerg Med* 19:865, 1990.
2. Davidson SJ: *Ann Emerg Med* 19:934, 1990.

---

**Refusing Care to Patients Who Present to an Emergency Department**
Derlet RW, Nishio DA (Univ of California, Davis, Sacramento)
*Ann Emerg Med* 19:262–267, 1990                                    6–27

---

In mid-1988, a policy was adopted to refuse patients requesting admission to the ED who have no condition that is considered an emergency. Triage nurses evaluated patients, and those whose vital signs fell into specified categories and who had 1 of 50 minor chief complaints were refused care in the ED and referred to an off-site clinic.

A total of 4,186 patients were referred from the ED in the first 6 months of the new triage system, representing about 20% of all ambulatory patients seen in the triage area. Nearly 85% of them were referred to off-site nonuniversity clinics and the rest to a university-affiliated faculty-staffed clinic. Follow-up letters and calls to the clinics revealed no patient who required retriage to an ED. Fewer than 2% of patients complained about being referred out of the ED. Forty-two patients returned within 48 hours, but none had deteriorated to the point of requiring ED care.

A triage procedure will effectively decompress an ED through referring away many patients who do not require ED care. Further studies are needed to identify potential adverse outcomes even if these are rare.

▶ Derlet and Nishio have demonstrated that it is possible to refuse care to patients admitted to a university hospital ED without incurring legal sanction. Their procedure did include a rather unique intervention, the use of an assistance desk open 24 hours daily. They endeavor to assure that their patients did receive proper medical care, albeit in a somewhat less expedient fashion.

It is interesting to follow this tendency to refer patients away from the ED. Many EDs depend on a steady flow of nonemergent patients to support the overall economics of ED function. So I wonder whether patients directed away from the ED might turn out to have a different economic status then those seen in the ED. The study is silent on this point.—S.J. Davidson, M.D.

---

**Organ and Tissue Procurement in the Acute Care Setting: Principles and Practice: Part 1**
Rivers EP, Buse SM, Bivins BA, Horst HM (Henry Ford Hosp, Detroit)
*Ann Emerg Med* 19:78–85, 1990                                    6–28

---

With the tremendous progress in organ transplantation, the need for donor organs has increased dramatically. The ED provides an opportunity for improving organ-tissue procurement from the brain-dead patient. The financial, historic, organizational, legal, and psychosocial aspects of organ-tissue procurement in the ED were discussed.

The procurement process begins with the recognition of a potential donor, that is, a previously healthy person who has sustained an irreversible brain injury resulting in brain death. A uniform definition of brain death has evolved over the years in terms of clinical criteria and laboratory confirmation, as well as its legal implications. Four study groups have had a significant impact on brain-death certification in the United States, including the Committee of the Harvard Medical School, National Institute of Neurological and Communicative Disorders and Stroke Collaboration Study, Royal Colleges and Faculties of the United Kingdom, and the President's Commission for the Study of Ethical problems in Medicine and Biomedical and Behavioral Research.

The donation process involves the surviving relatives, and the process must be viewed as a continuum of care for both the patient and family. Factors that are related to family consent include certainty of brain-death declaration; appropriately timed request; informative and sensitive request; presence of other family members and friends for support; informal and private setting; knowledgeable, trained, and supportive personnel; and presence of a donor card signed by the deceased.

Several legal and organizational developments have been implemented to improve the procurement process, such as the Uniform Anatomical Gift Act, and various states have passed Required Request laws so that families may have the right to choose between voluntary donation and refusal. In addition to the decreased morbidity and mortality from end-stage organ disease, an improved procurement process will also be cost effective in terms of reduced expenditures, as in renal dialysis, and improved quality of life and ability to return to work.

▶ The state of Pennsylvania now requires the discussion of organ donation with all families of deceased patients. This includes corneal, skin, and bone donations in those patients who do not qualify as other organ donors. This is a most difficult process and I'm sure has been honored more in the breach than in performance in these early months that we have been subject to this law. Ross et al. (1) have recently concluded that "laws are ineffective in the absence of fundamental changes in the attitudes of the public and treating physicians."

Nonetheless, we have had occasional successes. My personal experience suggests that this is most likely to occur when the family has discussed the possibility of organ donation for whatever reason at some point in the past. It is often helpful to discuss the potential for organ donation with a family in the ED when the patient appears stable but the prognosis is grim. Planting the idea early on may well promote a favorable decision later on.—S.J. Davidson, M.D.

*Reference*

1. Ross SE, et al: *J Trauma* 30:820, 1990.

---

**Factors Associated With Stress Among Emergency Medicine Residents**
Whitley TW, Gallery ME, Allison EJ Jr, Revicki DA (East Carolina Univ, Greenville; American College of Emergency Physicians, Dallas; Battelle Human Affairs Research Ctrs, Washington, DC)
*Ann Emerg Med* 18:1157–1161, 1989                                     6–29

---

Levels of occupational stress and depression experienced by emergency medicine residents as a function of residency year, gender, and marital status were investigated using a survey of members of the Emergency Medicine Residents Association.

The 488 respondents provided demographic information and completed measures of stress and depression. Multivariate analysis of variance showed significant differences in stress and depression by year of training, gender, and marital status. Women had higher mean levels of stress and depression, and unmarried residents had more depressive symptomatology. There were no significant differences in stress or depression by year of training according to univariate analysis of variance.

These findings suggest that female emergency medicine residents experience more stress and depression than their male peers and that spouses can buffer some of the stress of residency training for both men and women. Residents apparently experience stress throughout the course of their training. Further research in this area is warranted.

▶ One of the paradoxes involved with medical education is that house staff are taught how to recognize and treat illness or injury in their patients, but caring for self is not emphasized. Job stress has been recognized as a concern for practicing emergency physicians for many years; however, little work has been done to identify strategies to deal with this issue. Unfortunately, at the resident level, it is often only when the resident profoundly compromises his or her position that the stress of training becomes apparent.—P.T. Pons, M.D.

---

**Substance Abuse Education in Residency Training Programs in Emergency Medicine**
Taliaferro EH, Rund DA, Brown CG, Goldfrank LR, Jorden RC, Ling LJ, Gallery ME (Am College of Emergency Physicians, Dallas)
*Ann Emerg Med* 18:1344–1347, 1989                                   6–30

Although emergency physicians encounter a high incidence of alcohol intoxication and alcohol abuse in the ED, they receive only minimal training in how to deal appropriately with these problems. How substance abuse education is taught in emergency medicine residency training programs was evaluated.

A task force composed of representatives of the American College of Emergency Physicians, the Society of Teachers of Emergency Medicine, and the University Association for Emergency Medicine drafted a set of objectives on substance abuse education in emergency medicine. The objectives were mailed to more than 200 persons representing academic emergency medicine and private practice. The respondents were asked to indicate whether they deemed the objectives appropriate to emergency medicine. On the basis of their recommendations, the objectives were modified and subsequently mailed to 65 directors of emergency medicine residency training programs who were asked to indicate to what extent the topics were covered in the training program at their institution.

Forty directors returned completed questionnaires. At least 50% of the respondents reported spending 1 hour or less on most topics, with many topics receiving less than 1 hour. The lecture method and bedside teaching were by far the most commonly used formats, followed closely by conference presentation.

Sixty percent of the responding directors were satisfied with the adequacy of the substance abuse training of the residents, but none was very satisfied. However, 74% of the directors were either dissatisfied or very dissatisfied with the adequacy of available substance abuse training materials. Finally, 58% of the directors were satisfied or very satisfied with the adequacy of the faculty's level of substance abuse training, 36% were dissatisfied, and 6% were very dissatisfied. Future studies should address not only what is taught in the area of substance abuse but also what the residents retain from their training.

▶ Substance abuse is prevalent in the practice of emergency medicine. Yet, Taliaferro et al. have demonstrated that in many emergency medicine residencies little formal teaching is devoted to this complex issue.

Emergency physicians often see the alcoholic or substance abuser as an unfortunate, or perhaps unpleasant, individual, best turfed to the detoxification center or social worker. Such resources do not always exist in the real world.

Taliaferro et al. point out that emergency medicine residents, though well trained both didactically and clinically in managing the acute overdose, probably lack expertise in other aspects of abuse problems (e.g., epidemiology, the ethical issues involved in reporting fellow physicians, and the ability to detect substance abuse problems in fellow health care workers). Such training needs support and development.—S. Jacubowitz, M.D. (EMS Fellow), with S.J. Davidson, M.D.

---

**Emergency Physicians' Responses to Families Following Patient Death**
Schmidt TA, Tolle SW (Oregon Health Sciences Univ, Portland)
*Ann Emerg Med* 19:125–128, 1990                                      6–31

---

Emergency physicians' responses to the death of a patient or their subsequent interactions with survivors have never been studied. However, because of the transitory nature of emergency physicians' interactions with their patients, they probably respond differently to a patient's death than do physicians in other specialties. One important difference is that deaths in an ED are much more likely to be unexpected by the family.

Emergency physicians' responses at the time of death of patients and their subsequent interactions with survivors were surveyed by means of a questionnaire, which was mailed to 138 Oregon ED physicians, 114 of whom (83%) responded after 2 mailings. Five physicians who had retired were excluded. Of the 109 participants, 86% were men with a mean age of 38.9 years.

The mean number of deaths encountered by ED physicians was 17 per year. Most (76%) usually notified the families in person, 20% used the telephone, and 1% sent the police to the home. The average time spent talking with families after a death was 15 minutes. Most physicians (70%) found notifying survivors of a death emotionally difficult at least one half of the time. Only 13% indicated that they usually or always requested autopsies. None of the ED physicians ever attended a patient's funeral, and very few had contact with survivors after a death. Only 32% of the respondents reported having residency training that dealt with the dying patient, and 48% reported some training during medical school related to those issues. However, 94% recognized the need for death education specifically related to responding to families immediately after a patient's death. Such educational programs for ED physicians should be implemented as part of the residency training, and outreach programs should be developed for survivors.

▶ The report by Schmidt and Tolle points to a significant failing in the education of emergency physicians. The intensity and stress of family reaction and grieving when informed of a death of a family member is a uniformly difficult experience, and regardless of how well prepared or experienced the practitioner is, this is a difficult, but necessary, component of practice. Sharing the news of a loved one's death, should be just that, sharing. Physicians should attempt, if even for a moment, to reach inside and find the empathy to acknowledge through even the briefest of human connections the tragedy that the individual or family is now facing. The aspects of training and outreach programs for survivors suggested by these authors are important components, but a human connection in this sharing of death at the bedside is basic to the physician's role. It has been said that physicians cure sometimes, relieve often, but comfort always.— S.J. Davidson, M.D.

---

### A Follow-Up Report of Occupational Stress in Urban EMT-Paramedics

Cydulka RK, Lyons J, Moy A, Shay K, Hammer J, Mathews J (Northwestern Univ; Cleveland Metropolitan Gen Hosp)
*Ann Emerg Med* 18:1151–1156, 1989                                6–32

---

Occupational stress among emergency medicine technician (EMT) paramedics has been the topic of a growing body of research. In addition to the variables causing stress in other health care workers, EMT paramedics are often forced to provide medical care in unfamiliar, inconvenient, and dangerous environments. To determine if EMT paramedics manifest stress differently depending on rank, job description, and area of the city served by the EMT paramedic's ambulance, 280 nonvolunteer, urban EMT paramedics completed a survey.

High levels of occupational stress were reported. A great deal of the variation in the manifestation of stress was explained by rank and job description, the district served, and the patient population served. Field EMT paramedics tended to manifest stress in more negative attitudes toward the patients. Administrative-level paramedics had more organizational stress. Age and length of employment correlated with level of occupational stress, as well as the recent occurrence of significant life events. Gender, marital status, and number of calls per shift were not significantly correlated with levels of occupational stress.

Occupational stress programs should be tailored to meet the needs of individual EMT paramedics; EMT paramedics who are undergoing stressful life events should be identified and counseled. Rotating EMT paramedics through various districts regularly may help alleviate the negative impact on patient care in particularly stressful areas.

▶ Stress in prehospital care providers has been well identified following high-intensity situations such as mass casualty incidents. Critical incident stress debriefing has been used to begin the process of recognizing and managing the anxieties created by such disasters. On a daily basis, however, the stressors that affect paramedics are often not dealth with. This is in contrast to departments such as law enforcement where programs for dealing with stress are commonly found. Similar programs designed to aid paramedics manage their stress will need to be created if paramedics are to have a lengthy career in EMS.—P.T. Pons, M.D.

---

**Violence in a Community Emergency Room**
Wasserberger J, Ordog GJ, Kolodny M, Allen K (Martin Luther King Jr Hosp, Los Angeles)
*Arch Emerg Med* 6:266–269, 1989                                          6–33

---

Violence is increasing in community and county hospitals in this country. Many ED employees suffer physically or emotionally from such violence. Because an agitated or assaultive patient provokes considerable anxiety in an ED, it is not unusual for inner-city EDs to confiscate weapons. Fatal episodes of ED violence have been described, and violence is not limited to inner-city hospitals.

Responses to violent episodes can be rehearsed. It is helpful to have a debriefing session after any major incident. Agitated patients should be seen immediately. Ways must be found for rapidly summoning the police, and removing a weapon should be left for the police. Overwhelming force by at least 5 persons should be used if restraining a patient is necessary. Straitjackets should be avoided. Patients should be sedated with intramuscular haloperidol or chlorpromazine or intravenous diazepam. All major episodes should be documented for medicolegal purposes.

▶ This case report reminds us all that violence strikes randomly. The measures suggested to deal with such an episode are good. I would place more emphasis, however, on the recognition and management of the potentially violent patient. As with everything in emergency medicine, prophylaxis is more efficacious than treatment. To wit, I would suggest the addition of a training session to improve the recognition of the potentially violent patient and detail the ways to possibly avert escalation to violence. The cardinal rule you should keep in mind at all times is that your own and your staff's safety is of primary importance. (See also Abstract 4–86.)—D.J. Cionni, M.D. (EMS Fellow), with S.J. Davidson, M.D.

# Subject Index

## A

Abdomen
  acute (*see* Pain, abdominal, acute)
  CT in children with neurologic
    impairment after blunt trauma, 66
  disease, acute, diagnostic peritoneal
    lavage in, 284
  pain (*see* Pain, abdominal)
  trauma
    blunt (*see below*)
    management, observation unit in, 30
    seat belt, 56, 67
  trauma, blunt
    amylase in, serum, 64
    CT in, for bowel and mesenteric
      injury, 60
    CT in, vs. peritoneal lavage, 63
    lipase in, serum, 64
    peritoneal lavage in, diagnostic, 60
    peritoneal lavage in, diagnostic, vs.
      CT, 63
    during pregnancy, 250
Abdominal
  aortic aneurysms, prognosis of, 133
Abrasion
  corneal, as cause of inconsolable crying,
    in infant, 248
Absorption
  aspirin, effect of activated charcoal on,
    177
  lidocaine and prolocaine, after EMLA,
    172
Abuse
  cocaine, and cerebral infarction, 179
  IV drug, and cotton fever, 157
  substance, education in residency
    training programs, 326
Acetaminophen
  overdose (*see* Overdose, acetaminophen)
  vs. sponging for fever reduction, 204
Acid
  -base status assessment in circulatory
    failure, 19
Acidosis
  metabolic, after naproxen ingestion,
    171
Adhesive
  cyanoacrylate tissue, for facial
    lacerations, in children, 207
Adolescent
  diabetic, insulin-dependent,
    hypoglycemic hemiplegia in, 223
  homeless, health care needs of, 320
  pregnant, with severe asthma, 256
  runaway, health care needs of, 320

  sickle cell disease mortality in, 230
  suicide attempt in, 237
  syncope in, 217
Adrenaline
  in topical TAC anesthesia for laceration
    repair, in children, 207
Advanced cardiac life support
  teaching to medical students, 312
Advanced trauma life support
  guidelines for C7-T1 fractures and
    subluxations, 42
  prehospital, for penetrating cardiac
    wounds, 304
Airway
  acute, cricothyroidotomy in, 265
  obstruction, upper, dystonia presenting
    as, 87
  pharyngeal tracheal lumen, training for,
    269
  pressure, nasal continuous positive, in
    sleep apnea syndrome, and
    pneumocephalus, 136
Alcohol
  intoxication, bedside diagnosis of, 289
  in saliva, colorimetric dipstick test for,
    290
Ambulance
  service, emergency, predicting demand
    for, 302
Aminophylline
  therapy, computer-assisted optimization
    of, 294
Amoxycillin
  /clavulanate after animal bites, 197
Amphetamine
  intoxication, haloperidol in (in rat), 182
Amylase
  serum, in blunt abdominal trauma, 64
Anaphylactic
  shock, outside hospital, 194
Anaphylaxis
  insect sting, 198
Anemia
  sickle cell (*see* Sickle cell, disease)
Anesthesia
  in "caine"-sensitive patients,
    diphenhydramine for, 161
  detection of knee injuries associated
    with tibial shaft fractures under,
    79
  for laceration repair, in children, 207
  topical
    absorption of lidocaine and prilocaine
      after, 172
    of eye, as diagnostic test, 246
Aneurysm
  abdominal aortic, prognosis of, 133

# Author Index